P. Doury Y. Dirheimer S. Pattin

Algodystrophy

Diagnosis and Therapy of a Frequent Disease of the Locomotor Apparatus

With a Foreword by J. Villiaumey

Translated by M.-Th. Wackenheim

With 46 Figures

Springer-Verlag Berlin Heidelberg New York 1981

Professeur PAUL DOURY
Service de Rhumatologie des Armées, Hôpital Bégin
F-94160 Saint-Mandé

Dr. YVES DIRHEIMER
Service de Neuroradiologie, Centre Hospitalier Universitaire
F-67091 Strasbourg Cédex

Dr. SERGE PATTIN
Service de Rhumatologie des Armées, Hôpital Bégin
F-94160 Saint-Mandé

Translator

MARIE-THÉRÈSE WACKENHEIM
Institut de Radiologie, Université de Strasbourg, 11, rue Humann
F-67085 Strasbourg Cédex

The cover design shows a classical algodystrophy of the wrist and of the hand

ISBN-13: 978-3-642-67991-9 e-ISBN-13: 978-3-642-67989-6
DOI: 10.1007/978-3-642-67989-6

Softcover reprint of the hardcover 1st edition 1981

Reproduction of the figures: Gustav Dreher GmbH, Stuttgart

2127/3130-543210

Foreword

It is with great pleasure and much interest that I accepted to write the foreword to this book by Paul Doury, Yves Dirheimer, and Serge Pattin on the subject of "algodystrophy." First, because I know the extent of their personal experience, from which they have selected the best for this book. Second, because it seemed to me that their detailed analysis of the numerous works on the subject, works which have been published all over the world and which provide diverse physiopathologic interpretations, would provide a comprehensive study meeting a real need.

Algodystrophy, to adopt the term used by the authors, merits rheumatologists' careful attention. It is indeed a frequent condition and, as is now well known, occurs in the most varied etiologic circumstances; it is not solely posttraumatic, a notion on which diagnosis had long been based. This variable etiology suggests the complexity of algodystrophy's pathogenic mechanism.

The condition usually shows a pseudoarthritic inflammatory pattern and/or localized and painful demineralization of the bones, which naturally leads the patient to consult a specialist. Recently much has been learned about algodystrophy, on the one hand as a result of modern investigation techniques such as bone scintigraphy, which make possible a more accurate diagnosis of the early stages or of the localized forms of the disease, and, on the other hand, with regard to the possibilities of a better adapted therapy, liable to modify markedly the evolution of the disease. The opening chapter of this book demonstrates the recent escalation of progress in this field.

This brief preface can unfortunately not provide an exhaustive account of the authors' personal contribution. I would, nevertheless, like to place special emphasis upon their essential conceptions. I feel that their governing thought has been to show the basic unity of the various types of algodystrophy, the clinical features and the mode of occurrence of which are so variable that one cannot wonder that so many authors have attempted to dismember this pathologic group and to individualize several related but nevertheless distinct entities. Doury, Dirheimer, and Pattin's approach is quite different and leads them to investigate uniting characteristics found in the fields of physiopathology and pathology and in the clinical picture of algodystrophy.

First of all, what is the genesis of this painful condition and of the trophic changes that characterize it? Many factors, from almost all fields of medicine and of surgery, seem to provoke or to favor algodystrophy. It seems, however that this condition never has one particular cause, but that it is nearly always the result of several pathogenic mechanisms occurring on receptive ground. This explains the absence of a strict or exclusive parallelism between the provoking or favoring factor and the resulting symptomatic and evolutive patterns. This is particularly so in cases following trauma, since the latter can be of vastly differing nature and severity, and it is far from true that the most severe always cause the most severe and most extended algodystrophic syndrome. The posttraumatic forms are considered to be the consequence of a pathologic reflex leading to direct lesion of the cutaneous, subcutaneous, muscular, tendinous, capsular, or bony tissues, or to the development of a large locoregional vascular disturbance with a complex evolution responsible for multiple alterations. – But it seems that such a reflex mechanism can also be the consequence of very diverse and nontraumatic affections of the locomotor apparatus or of visceral, coronary, mediastinal, and pleuropulmonary irritative stimuli. This mechanism can be determined or governed by central nervous system lesions or by neurosympathetic disturbances. Also involved are biochemic agents, such as serotonin, liable to be mobilized by metabolic disturbances or drug intoxications. Many unknowns still persist on the nature and evolution of the pathogenic process of algodystrophy, but it is very likely that there is a common response pattern to these very diverse stimuli.

A critical analysis allows the authors to describe a general symptomatology which is common to the different varieties of algodystrophy. They also underline the importance they attach to this unity by devoting a chapter to the general data on which the diagnosis of algodystrophy is based:

- A clinical syndrome comprising painful, mechanical, and inflammatory or mixed manifestations which affect more or less intensely the articular regions and are sometimes accompanied by synovial effusion of the mechanical type;
- Absence of any biologic changes of an inflammatory type;
- Radiologic changes not involving the interspaces and consisting predominantly of locoregional demineralization in differing degrees and times of occurrence;
- Almost constant and usually early occurring increased uptake of isotopes. This is, of course, not a specific but nevertheless a significant sign, especially when there is no radiologic evidence of the changes, in contrast to the clinical findings;
- A very peculiar cyclic development leading to spontaneous regression of the pseudoinflammatory clinical syndrome and of the scintigraphic and radiologic anomalies, occurring slowly with sometimes very marked tendinoaponeurotic sequels.

Quite naturally, this comprehensive study has led the authors to elaborate diagnostic criteria, the value and usefulness of which they have pertinently established. All this is the result of a detailed study of all clinical types of algodystrophy aimed at throwing light on the less well-known pecularities of the most classic forms as well as describing the hitherto undescribed features of the disease. The authors' personal experience makes this chapter a very original contribution. The description of the radiologic and scintigraphic anomalies is very carefully given, and abundant and accurate illustrations of remarkable quality are provided, for which the Editor must be congratulated.

In spite of their concern to demonstrate the unity of the disease, the authors also emphasize its polymorphism and describe in detail its many clinical forms, particularly their topography, evolution, symptomatology, and etiology. They thus draw attention to the localized variants of the algodystrophic syndrome, involving only the coxofemoral area and the knee. The latter forms, the diagnosis of which is difficult, have been made known thanks to the authors' personal studies. Equally fascinating is the description of the atypical evolutive forms, such as those which are immediately plurifocal, in a patent or latent manner, or secondarily plurifocal, in an extensive or recurrent way.

Finally, the authors rightly emphasize the incomplete or atypical forms, hyperinflammatory or pseudophlegmonous forms, and fibrous or pseudosclerodermal forms, demonstrating the extreme variability of the clinical features of the disease without casting doubt upon its fundamental unity. This polymorphism justifies the comprehensiveness of the chapter on differential diagnosis, which makes reference not only to the effusional type of rheumatic disease but also to the many conditions which may mimic, clinically or radiologically, some of the features of algodystrophy in their classic forms or in their unusual aspects.

Trauma remains by far the most frequent cause of algodystrophy, but several diseases as well as certain drugs can also be held responsible, as has already been shown. This has very important theoretical and practical implications. The authors have made a detailed review of such facts, providing an exhaustive summing up of all the available data.

The reader will also be interested by the other chapters of this book, for instance the pathologic study which includes an original description of a synovial involvement. The latter is all the more interesting as such documentations are very rare.

Finally, the treatment of algodystrophy has been dealt with in detail; the authors describe the drug and physical treatments which are applied simultaneously and the results which can be expected. Neither prevention nor medicolegal considerations are neglected, proof that Doury, Dirheimer, and Pattin wish to provide their readers with a complete handbook, combining theoretical data and the most useful practical indications. We can but congratulate them on their eclecticism and wish their book the success it deserves.

J. VILLIAUMEY

Acknowledgements

We are grateful to Prof. J. Villiaumey, president of the French Society of Rheumatology for having accepted to write the foreword for this book.

We wish to thank Prof. A. Wackenheim, Head and Chairman of Radiology, University of Strasbourg for his advices and constant support.

We thank also Mrs. M.-Th. Wackenheim for her English translation of our text and for her kindness and disponibility.

Many people in a variety of ways have made this volume possible and it gives us pleasure to identify them here: Prof. J. Arlet, rheumatology, Toulouse; Prof. R.P. Delahaye, radiology, Paris; Dr. R. Granier, nuclear medicine, Paris; Dr. L. Heraut, neurophysiology, Paris; Prof. R. Lagier, pathology, Geneva; Prof. P.J. Metges, radiology, Paris; Prof. P. Meunier, rheumatology, Lyon; Dr. B. Moyses nuclear medicine, Strasbourg; Dr. A. Norton, general practitioner, London; Dr. A. Ramsheyi, general practitioner, Teheran.

We thank also our technical assistants Mrs. C. Butterlin, L. Fischer, M. Reinheimer, R. Walter.

P. Doury
Y. Dirheimer
S. Pattin

Contents

Introduction

Chapter 1 Historical Review

In *Lessons on the Principles of Surgery*, published in France in 1766, J. Hunter [384] seems effectively to have been the first to draw attention to the distant effects of joint trauma, particularly effects on muscles. He said that it is worth noting that lesions of tendons, ligaments, aponeuroses, etc., especially those that take the form of a ligamentous strain, have a sympathetic effect on the muscles, which atrophy and lose their power.

Before the era of radiology, it was naturally impossible to give a complete description, but the clinical aspects and the natural history were remarkably well described during and since that period.

Also, in 1864, during the War of Secession, S.W. Mitchell et al. [575] gave an extremely precise and accurate account of the different aspects of the clinical syndrome of algodystrophy, which we recognize today in those patients who have sustained nerve trunk lesions. The "causalgia" which remains ascribed to the names of these authors, however, is only one of the aspects that they laid emphasis upon: "The skin affected in these cases was deep red or mottled, or red and pale in patches, ... the surface of all the affected part was glossy and shining as though it had been skilfully varnished..., in some form, pain has been an invariable attendant upon the diseased state of skin which we have tried to describe.... In the great mass of cases, it has been of that peculiar burning character of which we have spoken, ... in other instances, there was associated with this, acute or aching pain which extended beyond the diseased tissues."

These authors equally emphasize the articular manifestations of this condition: "It consists essentially of a painful swelling of the joints which may attack any or all of the articulations of a member. It is distinct from the early swelling due to inflammation about the wound itself, although it may be masked by it for a time."

Concerning the sometimes prolonged natural history of the condition, they note that "once fully established it keeps the joints stiff and sore for weeks and months, ... We have seen one instance in which the pain had lasted for twenty one months."

On the other hand, the vasomotor and trophic disturbances associated with central or peripheral nervous lesions of traumatic or non-traumatic origin were well known and described in the last century.

Just as J.M. Charcot [134] described "arthropathy that appears to be caused by a lesion of the brain or spinal cord," A. Vulpian [850] referred to associated trophic effects, and especially mentioned "the cyanotic or dark pink colour that the skin may exhibit, especially in the lower limb when the patient is standing,... the local cooling, the moisture of the hand or foot,... the edema." We may note that A. Vulpian also observed these effects after burns caused by flames.

In 1867, P.E. Chevallier [137] in his thesis "On the paralysis of vasomotor nerves" also drew attention to the trophic problems of nervous lesions. However it seems that these problems were less well known if not ignored in bone, joint, ligament, tendon, and muscular injuries.

Destot and Mouisset [201] in 1898 published the case of a 65-year-old lady who "after a fall on the right foot, had persistent severe pain in the region of the ankle joint. Radiography and autopsy subsequent to death from an intercurrent event, showed decalcification of the tarsal bones." The authors stressed the intensity of the pain and its traumatic etiology. In 1904, C. Destot [200] also wrote that "in certain bone conditions which develop after an insignificant trauma, there is skeletal resorption, without any subjective or objective evidence of a nervous lesion being found. Is one led to ascribe these lesions as well to a lesion of the sympathetic nervous system?" Moreover, R. Fontaine et al. [271] proposed to call these changes "Destot-Sudeck syndrome."

In 1900, at the 29th Congress of the German Society of Surgery, P. Sudeck [792] delivered a paper on "Acute inflammatory bone atrophy." It is useful to point out that this Hamburg surgeon, working under Kümmell, was already practising radiography which allowed him to interpret the clinically observed injuries. (In two articles published in 1901 [793] outlining his work, the author described an X-ray taken on

July 11th 1897, only 19 months after Roentgen's discovery. One can only be amazed by the swiftness of the widespread adoption of radiology, and the results which led to the characterization of a totally new form of pathology.)

In these two articles, if the clinical description of algodystrophy of the upper and lower limbs is very liberally treated, it is generally the radiological description that is very complete and thorough. Sudeck describes examples of osteoporosis occurring after acute inflammation of the digits, after fracture of the radius, fracture of the shoulder blade and of the scaphoid, after ligamentous tears, after infected soft tissue wounds, after nerve injury, and also after herpes zoster. It is therefore inaccurate to say that Sudeck only described painful posttraumatic osteoporosis. Besides, in 1901, Nonne [603] a neurologist working in the same Hamburg clinic as Sudeck, also published a series of case histories of radiologically demonstrable acute and chronic bone atrophies appearing on account of nervous conditions. (It is also interesting to note that from 1901, Nonne gave the name of "Sudeck's atrophy" to bone atrophy.)

But let us return to Sudeck and his radiological studies. He insisted on bilateral films to permit comparison with the healthy side for evidence of slight demineralization. He described the different aspects of his observations: "Irregular obliteration of the pattern of bony striation,... diffuse reduction in radiodensity of the bone image, with lacunae of spongiform bone,... the cortex is striated, especially in the digits, but does not show a reduction in thickness." In other cases there is almost complete disappearance of bone structure, much more visible in the extremities, however, than for example in the knee, where there is a much greater volume of soft tissue. Sudeck followed the evolution of demineralization by repeated X-rays. He said that this condition can disappear as fast as it appeared and result in *restitutio in integrum*. Yet, he observed that if the atrophy persisted for a long time, there is a chronic state. The bone structure is again visible, but the trabeculations are more slender and delicate. The bone seems less radiopaque. It is most often seen at this stage that the cortex has fine longitudinal striations. The outlines of the bone seem emphasized because the interior of the bone no longer has the same density, and in one case he notes that the image of the patella was no longer visible.

Here is what he said concerning the explication of this atrophy: "It is likely that, in sites distant from the site of the illness, it takes the form of an inflammatory irritation, which involves nutritional problems... and in consequence resorption of bone. Evidently, it is not by nature a physiological resorption of inactive bone, but if I may so put it, an active atrophy." Besides, it is not possible to say from radiographic studies that it is a lysis of calcium salts or accelerated resorption. But it is an atrophy of bone mediated by a local neurotrophic reflex, which is a different entity from trophic problems arising from central nervous system lesions.

To tell the truth, we must say that P. Sudeck [791], as well as R. Kienböck [407], recognized senile bone atrophy, disuse atrophy resulting from lack of functional stimulation (but always appearing late and sluggishly), and finally an acute inflammatory atrophy, which could be equally evident after septic arthritis or articular trauma.

In 1901, Secretan [735] observed tense posttraumatic edema always accompanied by rarefaction of bone. Likewise, further work by R. Kienböck [408], E. Delorme [190], and N. Allison and B. Brooks [5] did not attract the attention of surgeons, who despite the increased incidence of accidents, never looked at trauma from the point of view of tissue viability, but contented themselves with describing wounds and fractures, and knowing their infective, vascular, and nervous complications, but no more. Besides, a study of the trophic problems of bone after injury published by Cluzet in 1915 [141] separated different etiologies, but did not observe the cause and effect relation of early vasomotor responses and posttraumatic trophic problems.

In 1916, the First World War brought a new approach to algodystrophy. J. Babinski and J. Froment [25] and J. Babinski et al. [27] described "vasomotor and thermal problems of reflex origin" and incriminated these disorders in what they called "physiopathic problems or nervous problems of reflex origin."

These phenomena include: contractures, incomplete distal limited motor abnormalities, vasomotor and thermic problems (generally worse in winter), with associated cyanosis and hypothermia, hypotonia and mild or severe muscular atrophy, changes in cutaneous and tendon reflexes, corollaries of hypothermia, sensory problems associated with sudden pains and segmental hypothermia, exocrine gland disorder, trophic disorder (fibrotendinous and muscular contracture).

These descriptions bear the mark of J.M. Charcot, and his theory of hysteria [135].

In the same era, E. Delorme [189] reported "decalcification as a sequel of war wounds," and R. Leriche [488] by means of clinical observation and oscillometry, started a study of vasomotor disorders resulting from often minimal wounds where there appeared to be a lasting vasomotor derangement.

French work on posttraumatic osteoporosis are dominated by R. Leriche and his associates J. Policard [502], A. Jung [501], R. Fontaine [498] and their schools. They studied bone physiology, since alongside normal bone resorption and physiological osteolysis, there exist pathological bone rarefactions, one of the manifestations of which is painful osteoporosis. They were only interested in the sequels of trauma. From their work one came to speak of the "painful posttraumatic osteoporosis of Sudeck and Leriche."

This apart, the concept of algodystrophy was late in taking shape. In 1925, G. Maillard and G. Renard [529] described phenobarbitone-induced rheumatism, which was followed by the work of L. Beriel and J. Barbier [51] in 1934. However, it was not until 1966 that J.K. Van der Korst et al. [830] linked this phenomenon to the concept of algodystrophies.

In 1930, G. Kahlmeter [397] published a paper on "a form of omarthritis accompanied by vasomotor disturbances in corresponding hand and anxiety neurosis."

In 1931, E. May [548] described chronic vasomotor rheumatism and outlined the framework of the "ectosympathoses." The same year saw a publication by G. Maillard and P. Thomazi [530] describing 18 cases of painful syndromes observed in epileptics treated with barbiturates.

The work of the American school, especially between 1925 et 1945 produced many descriptions [107, 161, 339, 340, 360, 512, 570, 767]. In 1937, G. de Takats created the term "dystrophy of the extremities" to describe certain painful, motor, and trophic syndromes of the upper limb. The result of this was the magistral rediscovery of the shoulder-hand syndrome by O. Steinbrocker in 1947 [774, 775] in which he noted, like others [22, 84, 235, 374, 393, 459], the frequency of aortic and coronary artery disorders as a cause of this.

The Germans, ever faithful to P. Sudeck continued to describe the different traumatic forms, and limited themselves to certain aspects of the condition [62, 402, 443, 607, 663, 680, 795, 796, 797].

As regards the French, after the eclipse of the Second World War, there appeared a series of publications on the different clinical, topographic, and etiological aspects of algodystrophies.

In a thesis inspired by P.P. Ravault, M. Boucher [91] (1948) added the "painful decalcified foot" to the ranks of algodystrophy of the lower limb. P.P. Ravault [645] gave a clinical description of "neurotrophic rheumatism of the upper limb" and incriminated in its origin "trophic articular problems of nervous origin arising from organic shock or functional disturbance of the cerebro-spinal and sympathetic innervation of the upper limb." In 1951, S. de Sèze and A. Ryckewaert [759] proposed calling the effects on the upper limb previously reported by P.P. Ravault et al. "Sympathetic algodystrophy." Also, S. de Sèze et al. [758] in 1960 produced the first combined study of algodystrophy of the knee. Previously, only certain isolated cases had been reported by R. Leriche [494] (1939), J. Bernard [52] (1954), F. Coste and B. Piguet [154] (1956). In 1964, S. de Sèze et al. [760] unravelled scapulohumeral periarthritis and in so doing identified retractile capsulitis (frozen shoulder), the etiology which is identical to that of shoulder-hand syndrome. The majority of authors, and particularly M. Lequesne and L. Auquier [477] likened this capsulitis to a "shoulder-hand syndrome without the hand," but nobody would affirm that it was a reflex algodystrophy.

The same M. Lequesne [472] painted a complete picture of algodystrophy of the hip by virtue of ten cases published in 1968. It had, however, been previously identified by G. Vincent et al. [842] in 1962. P.H. Curtiss and W.E. Kincaid [168] described three cases of "transitory demineralization of the hip in pregnancy," but preferred to consider this an independent syndrome, without proposing any particular reason.

Although R. Leriche [494] suggested affliction of the spine, observations of vertebral algodystrophy are rare, almost as if the effects produced in the limbs cannot be produced in the spine.

Since 1895 and a communication entitled "*Ueber die traumatischen Erkrankungen der Wirbelsäule*" [424] H. Kümmell had treated "*rarefierende Osteitis des Wirbelkörpers.*" He returned to the same subject in 1921 [425]. After a generally mild trauma to the spine healing in a few days, intense pain appeared in the vertebral column after a period of several weeks or months. These attacks most frequently affect the thoracic spine, and the pain is accompanied by the appearance of a kyphosis or more or less localized gibbosity. The author thought that this was a process of rarefaction of vertebral bodies, leading to lysis, but could not prove it by autopsy. In 1892 Verneuil and Forestier [835] reported a similar phenomenon to that reported by H. Kümmell. A single examination, unavailable at this time, would have determined the nature of these lesions. That examination is radiography.

In his first work on posttraumatic bone atrophy P. Sudeck [793] noted in respect of one of his observations "*Der Ganze Verlauf des Falles... hat in der Tat... große Ähnlichkeit mit der Kümmellschen post-traumatischen Kyphose.*" With the introduction of radiology, the question took on a new interest. The cases reported multiplied until about 1935, but it is striking to note that after this time they became more and more rare. However, for R. Leriche and J. Policard [502], the affliction described by Kümmell was no more than a painful post-traumatic osteoporosis. The presence or absence of an initial vertebral fracture had little importance. The trauma created a new set of conditions in the static balance of the spine to which the vertebral column had to adapt. This adaptation was never satisfactory, resulting in "permanent trauma" involving hyperemia osteoporosis and compression.

Among the more recent observations, we must note those of J.A. Lièvre and A. Hubault [508], of J. Bacri and S. Mutin [29], and of H. Serre et al. [747], where the case took the form of an extensive involvement from the foot to the spine, and the two cases of A. Schiano et al. [727].

Even if the majority of cases concern a diffuse periarticular osteoporosis, localized forms have been described recently. M. Lequesne et al. [484] speak of "partial transient osteoporosis" and distinguish two different radiological forms: "the radial form, which involves only one or two rays of the hand or foot, and the zonal form in which the area of demineralisation is confined initially to such structures as one femoral condyle or one quadrant of a femoral head." P. Doury et al. [210] described an even more localized form, which they called "highly localized transient osteoporosis of the knee."

Besides these more and more localized forms, various multifocal types have been described: a bipolar form in the upper limb, giving rise to the classical shoulder-hand syndrome; a bipolar form in the lower limb; tripolar forms (shoulder-elbow-hand or foot-knee-hip); bilateral forms; and forms attacking the upper and lower limbs simultaneously.

Radiological signs of a clinically silent lesion, appearing in another site in the limb during the course of an algodystrophy are relatively frequent. However, the frequency of detection of subclinical lesions is now greater thanks to radioisotope investigations.

Finally, it is necessary to mention extensive forms which successively affect many articular areas, and multifocal relapsing types. Although some authors do not believe that properly defined relapsing algodystrophy exists, in this category we class the cases where different segments are successively affected, with free intervals of several months or years. P. Doury et al. [216] have also described this.

In this historical review we have spoken of a certain number of possible etiologies of algodystrophy in particular, nervous and posttraumatic origins – as well as the individual types of idiopathic forms. The last two decades have seen numerous publications on algodystrophy in numerous specialties: neurology, radiology, nuclear medicine, and cardiology, as well as rheumatology and orthopedics. We have already mentioned phenobarbitone-induced rheumatism. The introduction of isoniazid in the therapy of tuberculosis was accompanied by the appearance of a certain number of algodystrophies, which seem to be directly caused by it. In March 1961, G. Brouet et al. [104] published their first four observations of this, followed by the work of A.B. McKusick and J.M. Hsu [556] in the same year. Diabetes seems to be a factor, if not the determining one, favoring the appearance of an algodystrophy. M. Lequesne [476] recently emphasized the role of diabetes. The condition can occur in a known treated diabetic, or a diabetic diagnosed on that occasion, after systematic examination which excludes the culpability of oral hypoglycemic agents.

The association between locomotor dysfunction and thyroid dysfunction has long been recognized: thyrotoxic rheumatism during the course of hyperthyroidism; postmenopausal myxedema; hyperthyroid osteoporosis; thyroid-related peripheral circulatory disorder. Besides, in 1928, W.S. Duncan [230] noted the relative frequency of scapulohumeral periarthritis in thyrotoxicosis. But it seems that treatment with methylthiouracil, as reported by S. Sitaj et al. [770], and especially with radioactive iodine are more directly to blame than G. Methlin et al. [563] reported.

Among diseases of the heart and great vessels, coronary artery disease is the most frequent. Since the first description by W. Osler [612], innumerable reports of algodystrophy of coronary etiology have appeared.

Although numerous meetings have been devoted to algodystrophy, amongst which we must mention those of the Belgian Association of Surgery and the Belgian Societies of Surgery and Orthopedics in 1956 (10th Belgian Congress of Surgery) and that of the German Orthopedic Society of the same year, it is essentially since the 5th International Conference on Rheumatic Diseases (Aix les Bains, June 1972) that a number of afflictions given different names by their authors, who insisted on various aspects of localization, etiology, or mechanism, can be considered parts of the same entity. History must also remind us of the different pathogenic theories and treatments that were successively proposed. We will consider these in the respective subsequent chapters.

The variety of names ascribed to this syndrome over the years calls for a list of synonyms. However, the list is inevitably incomplete.

In the English literature:
- Acute bone atrophy
- Algoneurodystrophy
- Migratory osteolysis or regional migratory osteolysis
- Posttraumatic painful osteoporosis
- Posttraumatic sympathetic atrophy
- Reflex dystrophy
- Reflex sympathetic dystrophy syndrome
- Shoulder-hand syndrome
- Sudeck's atrophy
- Sympathetic reflex dystrophy
- Transient or transitory osteoporosis

In the French literature:
- *Algodystrophie* or *algodystrophie décalcifiante*
- *Algodystrophie réflexe* or *algodystrophie sympathique*
- *Algoneurodystrophie réflexe*
- *Ostéoporose algique post-traumatique*
- *Ostéoporose algique essentielle du pied*
- *Ostéoporose-ostéoarthrite dystrophique*
- *Pied décalcifié douloureux idiopathique*
- *Pseudo-rhumatisme* or *rhumatisme neurotrophique*
- *Syndrôme de Sudeck-Leriche*

And in the German literature:
- *Algodystrophien*
- *Akute Knochenatrophie*
- *Pseudoarthritiden*
- *Reflexdystrophische Pseudoarthritis*
- *Sudeck'sche Dystrophie, Sudeck'sche Erkrankung, Sudeck'sches Syndrom,* or simply "*Sudeck*"

The term algodystrophy which we have used seems the most satisfactory, because it does not imply involvement of any particular tissue. The term reflex dystrophy, sometimes used in publications in English is a reasonable approximation. Nevertheless, only the painful forms are seen in the clinical situation, and therefore the definitive term we propose should be adopted is ALGODYSTROPHY.

Chapter 2 Why Study this Condition?

Where there exist a large number of clinical descriptions and different titles of what we think may only be particular aspects or different varieties of the same condition, a work of synthesis and condensation is worthwhile. This is possible in the light of our experience and the results of modern investigation.

The attentive reader of the early authors on this subject will have noticed how these authors observed facts that were later forgotten. From 1901, Sudeck described many circumstances in which one might observe the syndrome of painful osteoporosis.

The large number of works appearing under various titles, which have been published every year for the last eighty, demonstrate the frequent occurrence of algodystrophy.

Despite this literary abundance, the actual number of cases is inevitably underestimated, mainly because of its great clinical polymorphism, its incomplete, atypical, and misleading forms, which may pass unrecognized or only be recognized very late.

Besides painful posttraumatic and postoperative osteoporosis, largely seen and recognized by surgeons (at least in its more violent forms), more recent work, generally by rheumatologists, has emphasized the numerous etiologies of algodystrophy, which cover almost every branch of medicine and surgery. These works have particularly shown the large incidence of primary algodystrophy.

On our part, algodystrophy seen in a rheumatology practice represents 1%–2% of our clientele, amounting to 250 new cases over a period of 10 years. Our work is based on this experience.

Systematic employment of radiological examination and especially scintigraphic exploration of the skeleton have shown the frequency of initial multifocal forms, or alternatively have shown that specific localizations are only manifestations of the same disease.

Knowledge of these multifocal forms has allowed confirmation that some very atypical forms exist, manifest in a clinical syndrome, a radiological syndrome, or a scintigraphic syndrome.

Finally, as regards therapeutics, calcitonin and the beta-blockers have now been added to classical medical and occasionally surgical treatment. In certain cases, remarkable results have been obtained, the usual slow and sometimes heart-breaking evolution of the condition being dramatically cut short.

Part 1 Symptomatology

Chapter 1 General Data in Algodystrophy

The fully developed form of algodystrophy consists of five fundamental features:

1) A pseudoinflammatory clinical syndrome
2) A biochemical syndrome characterized by the absence of inflammatory signs
3) A radiological syndrome with more or less extended homo- or heterogeneous locoregional demineralization
4) A scintigraphic syndrome with marked and almost constant increased uptake
5) More or less rapid regression of the condition with or without sequelae

A. Clinical Syndrome

Following a discernible initiating factor in the recent or distant past (which will be considered in Part 6), or without apparent cause, *pain* develops suddenly or progressively in an articular area. This pain may be provoked by mobilization of the joint or weight-bearing, or it may occur spontaneously, even overnight. It has either a mechanical, or an inflammatory, or a mixed character; its intensity varies from one case to another. *Swelling* appears more or less rapidly in the articular area. It may be localized to or extend beyond the tender area. Its degree is very variable: a pseudophlegmonous condition can occasionally lead to inopportune surgery. The local temperature may be increased. The teguments are pink, red, or even purplish. Clinical examination shows unaffected joints, with slightly diminished amplitude of passive movement and pain occurring only at the limits of movement. However, the intensity of the periarticular pseudoinflammatory features can be such as to cause functional disability mimicking articular involvement. In some instances when the knee is affected, one can note intraarticular effusion, usually of the mechanical type. More or less marked muscle wasting is noted more or less early. There is never any adenopathy. The range of intensity varies from barely perceptible forms, clinically within normal limits, to the most dramatic clinical conditions. There exists a large degree of clinical polymorphism depending on the intensity of each of the above-described signs. There is no repercussion on the general state, no fever, weight loss, anorexia, or systemic involvement.

B. Biochemical Syndrome

There are no biochemical inflammatory signs. The erythrocyte sedimentation rate is normal, as is the serum fibrin and serum protein electrophoresis. Nevertheless, a preexisting or associated pathologic condition may affect the laboratory findings and raise difficult problems of differential diagnosis. Classically, it is assumed that the metabolism of calcium and phosphorus is normal. However, since Leriche's studies [494], hypercalciuria has been reported. In the last 10 years or so, stress has been laid on the frequently elevated hydroxyprolinuria.

C. Radiological Syndrome

Demineralization is the common factor. It may be homogeneous or inhomogeneous and of very variable intensity, ranging from radiologically silent forms to complete radiologic disappearance of the bone structure. The extent of bone involvement varies from one case to another: demineralization may involve a very confined part of a bone, or affect the epiphysis, metaphysis, and diaphysis on each side of a joint, or even an entire limb.

Demineralization may be a very early radiological feature or appear only after a few weeks' or months' evolution; it may involve only the clinically affected area or extend to one or several other areas. The integrity of the articular interspace is a fundamental and constant negative feature.

D. Scintigraphic Syndrome

Bone scans with technetium-99m marker on pyrophosphate molecules show almost always, and usually very early, increased uptake. The increased activity is particularly marked and may be confined to a region of a bone part or involve the entire articular area, or even several other clinically and/or radiologically affected or unaffected parts.

E. Clinical Course

Spontaneous regression is the rule. The pseudoinflammatory clinical syndrome regresses within a variable period, as does demineralization and increased radionuclide uptake. There may exist clinical and/or radiological sequels. Clinical sequels are especially marked in the upper extremities, especially on the hands.

The very polymorphous appearance of algodystrophies has for a long time been responsible for extremely different descriptions.

Chapter 2 Clinical Description

Whatever the etiology and the affected site, algodystrophy will cause general pathologic changes of both soft parts and bone, so that a common symptomatology can be described.

The onset is very variable, characterized by sudden or progressive occurrence of pain in the articular area, either following a known initiating factor or without apparent cause.

After a few days the clinical picture is evocative, characterized by the association of pain, swelling, vasomotor disturbances, and articular stiffness: this is the "hyperemic" or "warm" stage of algodystrophy.

The pain is of variable type: mechanical pain provoked by mobilization or weight-bearing on the joint, pseudoinflammatory pain, spontaneous and even nocturnal pain, and sometimes a mixture of these. The patient very often describes them as nagging or tearing pains. In about 10% of cases they are of the more characteristic causalgic type (burning pain). The intensity of the pain varies from a moderate and tolerable one, well relieved by rest, to intense, lancinating and terebrating pain with paroxysms at the least attempt at mobilization, exacerbated by mere contact with the bedclothes, persistent at night and thus interfering with sleep. Finally, these pains are not adequately relieved by immobilization and trivial antalgic drugs, but respond somewhat better to anti-inflammatory therapy.

Edema and vasomotor disturbances are particularly significant in the forms affecting the distal segments of the extremities, where they are responsible for a pseudoinflammatory condition, particularly evocative at the level of the hand or foot. These signs are never seen in the hip or shoulder. Edema causes diffuse, succulent and pitting swelling, with pudgy fingers or toes, effacing the cutaneous folds and the relief of the tendons. It may be localized to or more or less overlap the painful area. Its degree varies from person to person; extreme forms may take on a pseudophlegmonous appearance. *Vasomotor disturbances* occur frequently but with variable intensity: the skin is tight, pink or frankly erythrotic, even erythrocyanotic. The area is warmer than usual with an increased sweating that is responsible for a peculiar smell (sui generis).

The clinical examination reveals moreover a more or less painful *limitation of the articular mobility*. Passive movements are relatively preserved, pain being felt only at the limits of movements. The periarticular pseudoinflammatory symptoms may sometimes be responsible for almost complete functional disability.

When the knee is affected there may be hydrarthrosis; the removed joint fluid proves to be of the mechanical type.

There is more or less marked *amyotrophy*, depending on the duration of the disease.

In the great majority of cases the *systemic signs* are lacking and apyrexia is the rule. There is never any locoregional adenopathy, the distal pulses are always well perceived. The neurological examination may be normal; in some cases osteotendinous hyperreflexivity may be present, as reported by Babinski and Froment [25] and also by Ravault [645]: the reflexes are strong and may even be exaggerated. In one of our cases of involvement of the foot inexhaustible epileptoid trepidation of the foot was seen without any other pyramidal sign; it finally regressed in parallel with the regression of the algodystrophic episode.

The presence of a peculiar psychological *background* is often reported, associating emotivity, anxiety, and a depressive tendency. We have found this condition in about half of our cases.

We would also like to point out the very great clinical polymorphism of the condition, depending on the intensity of the above-described signs: minor forms occur as well as the most striking ones. It should also be pointed out that the hyperemic stage may be very short, so that the patient may be examined for the first time at the ischemic or "cold" stage.

The clinical course varies with the site of the algodystrophic process. In the distal forms affecting the hand or the foot, pain is attenuated within a few weeks or months, swelling regresses, and the vasomotor disturbances progressively disappear and are replaced by changes in the skin, nails, and hair, and in the tendons and muscles. The skin becomes pale, glistening, and atrophic; the local heat diminishes but profuse sweating persists for a long time. This corresponds to the second, ischemic or cold stage of algodystrophy.

Articular stiffness secondary to capsuloligamentous and tendinous retraction is particularly evident at the level of the hands and may even be responsible in severe forms for the classical neurotrophic clawhand. At this stage spontaneous pain has disappeared or become minimal and only forceful movements of the various joints may provoke it. As concerns the shoulder, the prominent clinical feature is always the capsular retraction, which is responsible for the so-called frozen shoulder.

The ulterior course is most often favorable since the great majority of patients affected with algodystrophy recover without sequels. Complete recovery occurs usually within a few months or several years; the delay has been considerably diminished by modern therapeutics. Nevertheless, sequels may persist, particularly on the hands. Besides this usually favorable course, there are other evolution modes which are dealt with in more detail Part 3, Chap. 2. They comprise:

1) Early or delayed bilateralization of the process, in particular in the upper limbs
2) Extensive involvement, particularly of the lower limbs
3) Polytopic forms characterized by the simultaneous or slightly retarded involvement of two or several articular areas
4) Plurifocal forms, in which the different episodes are separated by free intervals of a few months to several years
5) Exceptional recurrent forms.

Chapter 3 Topographic Forms

In the previous chapter we described the general symptomatology of the algodystrophic syndrome.

In practice the clinical picture depends on the localization of the pathologic process. Thus, we shall distinguish schematically four topographic forms: algodystrophy of the upper limb; algodystrophy of the lower limb; algodystrophy of the spine; and algodystrophy in other sites.

A. Algodystrophy of the Upper Limb

In 1946 Ravault et al. [650] provided the first clinical description of "neurotrophic rheumatism of the upper limb." One year later Steinbrocker [775] reported his observation of a symptom he picturesquely called the shoulder-hand syndrome. This terminology is now widely accepted.

Because of its very evocative clinical features, we shall take the posttraumatic form as the typical form of algodystrophy, although this etiology is not the most frequent one: 10% according to Steinbrocker [775], 25% according to Ravault and Durant [648], 30% in the series of Schiano's et al. [727].

I. Onset

The first signs appear after a free interval of variable duration ranging from a few days to a few weeks (average of 5 months according to the statistics of May et al. [549], 2 months in the report of Schiano et al. [727]).

Pain of variable character and intensity is usually the first symptom. The shoulder is first affected in most cases; but the hand may be the first affected part, and the clinical picture is an acute one with painful and inflammatory edema.

II. First Stage

(Stage I according to Ravault and to Steinbrocker)

After a few days this stage is characterized by the association of pain, swelling, articular stiffness, and vasomotor disturbances.

1. Involvement of Hand and Wrist

Pain is of variable type: mechanical, i.e., provoked by mobilization of the joints, pseudoinflammatory (spontaneous or even noctural), or the association of these two types constituting a mixed-type pain. The intensity varies from one subject to another. This pain is aggravated by passive or active movements, and by palpation of and pressure on the affected segment. In some instances, the pain has a neurologic origin due to entrapment at the level of the osteofibrous tunnels (carpal tunnel syndrome).

Swelling and vasomotor disturbances produce an evocative pseudoinflammatory pattern: soft, succulent, pitting edema, infiltrating the palm of the hands, giving the fingers a pudgy appearance, effacing the cutaneous folds and the relief of the tendons. The skin is stretched, has a pink, red, or sometimes purplish color. The local temperature is usually increased and sweating is frequent, predominantly on the palm (9 cases out of 20 in May's series [549]). This edema masks a more or less marked muscle wasting.

Stiffening of the wrist and of the fingers occurs concomitantly with the painful edema. As concerns the wrist, there is limitation in the flexion-extension movements with antalgic attitude in semiflexion. At the level of the hands, flexion and especially complete extension of the fingers cannot be performed; the fingers adopt a slightly flexed position. The thumb is usually spared or only slightly affected.

2. Involvement of the Shoulder

This presents as the clinical picture of the so-called fibrotic scapulohumeral periarthritis. Painful stiffening is the prominent feature of the clinical symptomatology, but the signs are less marked than on the distal part of the limbs. The pain is of variable type and intensity; it may radiate to the arm, the armpit, and exceptionally to the cervical spine. Movement restriction is always rather global, affecting the internal and external rotation as well as abduction and retropulsion. Palpation of the joint triggers diffuse painful spots. Edema and vasomotor signs are always lacking, whereas amyotrophy is not present at the onset of the disease.

III. Second Stage

(Ravault's stage II, Steinbrocker's stages II and III)

This stage is dominated by the onset of trophic disturbances. It progressively follows on the previous stage within a period of a few weeks to several months. While pain is decreasing, swelling regressing, and vasomotor disturbances are becoming less prominent, changes occur in the periarticular structures. The main aim of treatment is to prevent these changes.

1. Hand and Wrist

The skin becomes pale, glossy, atrophic, and thin; in some cases, however, it becomes thicker or takes on a sclerodactylic appearance. Schiano et al. [727] have seen in one of their patients a vitiligo-type depigmentation at the level of the metacarpophalangeal and interphalangeal joints. The hair comes out or becomes thicker; the subcutaneous tissue is atrophied;

the nails are friable, but hippocratic fingers are never seen [645]. The local temperature is lowered and the algodystrophic hand becomes colder than a normal hand [253]. Hypersudation of the palm, already present in the first stage, may however persist for a long time.

Stiffening of the metacarpophalangeal and interphalangeal joints is secondary to capsuloligamentary and tendinous retraction fixing the fingers in the semiflexed position producing the classical "neurotrophic claw." The palmar fascia may be the site of longitudinal nodular indurations also producing retraction, responsible for the clinical picture of Dupuytren disease. The wrist is more rarely affected by the stiffening which would tend to fix it in a slight dorsal flexion.

Spontaneous pain is at this stage either absent or minimal; pain is only produced by forced movements.

Amyotrophy affects especially the thenar and hypothenar eminences as well as the interosseous muscles; the forearm is spared.

General signs are always lacking at this stage. The distal pulses are normal; the neurologic examination is most often negative but occasionally shows osteotendinous hyperreflexivity.

2. Shoulder

Spontaneous pain also diminishes and disappears. However, palpation may provoke it, particularly at the level of the anterior part of the articular interspace and at the insertion of the supraspinous muscle [253].

Limitation of movement persists and may even be aggravated by capsuloligamentous retraction, becoming responsible in the most severe forms for what Anglo-Saxon authors call "frozen shoulder." Diminished mobility in the glenohumeral joint is always more marked than the patient was aware of, on account of the possible scapulothoracic compensation: by immobilizing the inferior angle of the scapula while performing passive movements one may notice extremely reduced abduction – less than 45° – as well as adduction; there is also almost complete absence of external and internal rotation. The limitation of all shoulder motions is characteristic of capsular retraction.

Amyotrophy is of variable degree; it involves especially the deltoid muscle.

3. Elbow

The elbow is usually not affected, at least not clinically; it is not uncommon for the roentgenogram to show a certain degree of demineralization, witnessing latent algodystrophy.

IV. Evolution

The evolution is usually favorable and complete recovery occurs within several months to two years. Modern therapeutics aim at decreasing this delay.

There may however be sequels; they consist of mild cutaneous trophic disturbances, limited extension of the fingers, restriction in the amplitude of the movements of the shoulder, and declivity erythrosis [670]. Palmar nodules may persist, as well as retraction of the palmar fascia.

V. Topographic Forms

The bipolar form we have described as the shoulder-hand syndrome is the most evocative but perhaps the least frequent form; a certain number of algodystrophies of the upper limb remain confined, at least clinically, to a single joint: hand or shoulder.

1. Isolated Involvement of the Hand

This condition, which according to Faulong [253] is very exceptional, is responsible for what Ravault and Bouvier [646] have called the "isolated neurotrophic hand." It is mainly encountered in traumas to the hand, as pointed out in May's statistics [549]. In their series of 53 algodystrophies of the upper limb, Schiano et al. [727] report 14 cases involving exclusively the hand and the wrist, of which 9 were of traumatic origin.

2. Isolated Involvement of the Shoulder

This condition has been individualized and termed retractile capsulitis; it is much more frequent than the previous one. For most authors as for ourselves it is merely a peculiar form of algodystrophy.

Its diagnosis may be difficult because there are no superficial, that is, distal signs. Such signs should be carefully searched for: they can be very discreet, and for instance consist only of slight diminution of the finger movements. Algodystrophy should be suspected in case of painless or almost painless blocked shoulder, in which the X-ray showed normal features or a slight demineralization. Two additional examinations might be useful but not indispensable for the diagnosis: bone scan, which shows obvious increased uptake, and contrasted arthrography which gives evidence of the capsular retraction.

3. Associated Involvement of the Elbow

The tripolar form in the upper limb exists according to Ravault [645] in one-third of the cases, and more rarely according to Steinbrocker [775]. May et al. [549] found it clinically 3 times out of 20, and radiologically 6 times out of 20. Schiano et al. [727] report associated involvement of the elbow 6 times in 34 cases of shoulder-hand syndrome, of which 4 had clinical symptoms and 2 had only radiological signs. The symptomatology usually consists only of pain, either spontaneous or provoked by palpation; complete extension cannot be achieved and prosupination movements are painful. This usually transient involvement of the elbow regresses without sequels.

4. Associated Involvement of the Sternoclavicular Articulation

This is exceptional (a single case published by Ravault [645]), producing painful swelling of the articulation which regresses before the end of the first stage.

5. Algodystrophy Localized to Two or Three Fingers of One Hand

Three such cases were reported in 1972 by Damman [170]. More recently, Lequesne et al. [484] have also reported a very confined form involving one or two metacarpophalangeal rays for which they proposed the term "radial form of partial transient osteoporosis"; this form remains partial throughout its evolution, without showing secondary extension.

6. Bilateral and Extensive Forms

Algodystrophy of the upper limb may however take on an *extensive pattern and bilateralize*. These bilateral forms would be seen in more than a third of the cases (19 times out of 52, according to Ravault and Bouvier [646]).

The condition starts usually on one side, the other side being only secondarily affected, often to a lesser degree, and the shoulder more often than the hand. But there exist also some peculiar cases with simultaneous involvement of both shoulders and both hands. These bilateral forms seem to have a more severe prognosis.

In some exceptional cases the already bilateral shoulder-hand syndrome is accompanied by *extension to the lower limbs*, in particular hip or knee. Three cases of this type have been reported by Schiano et al. [727]. Such an extensive involvement is nevertheless very rare and should not raise doubt as to the mainly regional character of the disease.

Finally, we would like to underline that no multiple episodes of algodystrophy affecting the upper extremities have been reported, such as are known in the lower limbs.

B. Algodystrophy of the Lower Limbs

Algodystrophies involve the lower limbs more frequently than the upper limbs, but this is not entirely accounted for by the larger number of traumas and orthopedic operations.

Algodystrophies of the lower limb have a less evocative clinical picture, since they are usually confined to a segment of the limb (foot, knee, more rarely the hip) and do not produce the so suggestive bipolar involvement of the shoulder-hand syndrome.

On the other hand, the vasomotor disturbances of the lower extremity are of variable intensity and display different clinical features from one patient to another. This accounts for a very wide symptomatic polymorphism, comprising slightly painful, minimally invalidating forms as well as hyperalgic conditions responsible for complete incompetence.

The clinical picture depends mainly on the site affected.

I. Algodystrophy of the Foot

This condition was described for the first time in 1900 by Sudeck [793] under the term "acute inflammatory bone atrophy" and then by Leriche and Fontaine [498] in 1930, who termed it "posttraumatic painful osteoporosis."

It constitutes the most frequent localization in the lower limb and has an often prolonged evolution which may cause difficult diagnostic problems.

In a recent series, Serre et al. [754] counted 122 involvements of the foot in 188 localizations in the lower limb.

Schiano et al. [727] report 48 algodystrophies of the lower limb, among which the foot is affected 41 times: 30 times in isolation and 11 times concomitantly with another joint of the lower limb.

In our series of 250 cases we found 92 involvements of the foot among 168 algodystrophies of the lower limb: 49 isolated localizations and 43 cases with another clinical, radiological, and/ or scintigraphic localization.

In the traumatic, i.e., the most frequent etiology (56% in Serre's series [754], 44% in Harif's [351], and 65% in ours), the first signs appear after a free interval ranging from a few days to several months, the average delay being 1 month. Most often the *onset of the disease* involves a single foot, but it may also involve both feet, or concern the foot and the knee. According to Serre et al. [749] the onset is characterized by pain alone in 60% of cases, pain associated with swelling in 35.5%, and swelling alone in 4.5%.

The onset is seen to be *progressive* in the majority of cases (86% in Serre's series, 66% in our series). It is a matter of painful incompetence of the lower limb, which may or may not be associated with segmental changes in the foot: swelling, vasomotor disturbances. The patient avoids weight-bearing on the foot and walks with a crutch.

Sudden onset is more rare: the patient experiences sudden pain in the forefoot or in the toes, more rarely in the posterior bony tarsus or in the tibiotarsal joint.

At the full development stage, painful disability is a constant sign dominating the clinical picture. It becomes worse and renders walking impossible, so that two crutches are necessary. It may be the only sign, the clinical examination remaining entirely normal. As has been pointed out by Serre et al. [749], the contrast between the absence of objective signs in the clinical examination and painful disability in walking, which could even lead one to suspect the patient's good faith, is highly evocative of algodystrophy of the foot. Most often this disability is associated with swelling, cutaneous changes and articular and muscular stiffness.

Swelling is frequent (78% of cases, according to Serre et al. [754]): it is usually diffuse over the whole foot and extends sometimes as far as the lower third of the leg; in about one-fourth of cases it may also remain confined to the ankle or to a part of the foot. It is a pitting edema, increased by tiredness and prolonged standing.

Cutaneous changes are seen in only half to the cases. They consist of erythema with increased local temperature and sweating producing a pseudoinflammatory appearance, or of objective cooling down of the foot often associated with a cyanotic appearance of the teguments provoked or aggravated by a sloping position.

Stiffness in the various articulations of the foot is difficult to elicit since examination is painful. Marked stiffness of ankle and foot seems to be relatively rare (20% of the cases according to Serre).

We would like to point out that all these signs may occur on their own or associated in variable proportions, but that the major symptoms are always pain and swelling. It is noteworthy finally that there is no locoregional adenopathy, and no general signs or fever.

At a later stage, after several weeks' or months' spontaneous evolution the clinical picture has changed: pain decreases and disappears, swelling also regresses, but trophic disturbances appear which affect all tissues. The skin becomes thinner and colder, but abnormally profuse sweating persists. The plantar fascia may retract and produce the appearance of Ledderhose disease.

Retraction of tendons and of joint capsules witnesses the articular stiffening. Moderate atrophy of the calf (1–2 cm) is present in about 20% of cases; more rarely it concerns the quadriceps muscle.

Evolution is usually favorable, but, on the whole, algodystrophy of the foot has a slower evolution than algodystrophy of the knee or hip. Healing occurs after 12 months on the average (delays ranging from 4 to 28 months). In our series of 53 cases the duration of evolution is as follows: less than 1 month in 8 cases, from 1 to 3 months in 20 cases, 3 to 6 months in 8 cases, 6 months to 1 year in 13 cases, more than 1 year in 4 cases.

The mean duration of interruption of professional life is 11 months in Serre's statistics [749]. The only sequels – which are rare – consist of pain occurring with tiredness or with weather changes, associated with slight limping. Early and adequate treatment would seem to diminish the duration of evolution.

Some clinical varieties deserve individual mention on account of the association of the different signs. Among the symptomatologic forms, the following can be individualized:

The isolated painful foot or "demineralized foot." Walking has become impossible but the clinical examination is normal. The X-rays show characteristic demineralization and the bone scan reveals indisputably increased uptake.

The atrophic form, a delayed or inadequately treated form, exhibits a predominance of trophic disturbances.

The painless form has been described by Coste and Piguet [154] under the term "painless reflex dystrophy." This is a very uncommon variety with a characteristic clinical and radiological picture of algodystrophy of the foot, but with absolutely painless evolution from beginning to end.

The rightaway bipolar forms are characterized by the simultaneous involvement of two articular levels. Serre et al. [754] has observed 19 cases, including 14 with bilateral involvement of the feet and 5 with involvement of foot and knee. In our series, involvement of both feet was noted in 7 cases and involvement of foot and knee in 10 cases.

In the extensive forms the algodystrophy extends to other articulations of the homolateral lower limb (28 cases in Serre's series, 6 in ours). Bilateral or contralateral recurrent forms are more rare. In some exceptional instances, the extension concerns the spine, causing the problem of vertebral algodystrophy, which will be dealt with later on. The evolution of these extensive forms is longer but still favorable.

Finally we should mention the forms where successive episodes occur: a new algodystrophic affection occurs one or several years after the initial episode and involves a different joint (3 cases in Serre's material, 3 cases in our series).

II. Algodystrophy of the Knee

The first exhaustive study of algodystrophies of the knee was performed in 1960 by de Sèze et al. [758]. Other studies are due to Rénier [669], and to Blauth [76].

Before that, some isolated cases had been described by Leriche, 1939 [494], Bernard, 1954 [52], Coste and Piguet, 1956 [154].

Though in this localization it is classically considered a rare condition, algodystrophy of the knee is in fact very often not recognized as such. Schematically, algodystrophy of the knee occurs in two types of circumstances, of unequal interest. It may be a secondary localization of an algodystrophy which started in another segment of the limb, in particular the foot; in this case there is no diagnostic problem. Alternatively, it may be the main site of a process which starts in the knee, and may remain unique or isolated or extend secondarily to other segments of the lower limb. In this second instance, the diagnosis is more difficult.

The relative frequence of these two possibilities varies from author to author. In their first study, of 12 cases, de Sèze et al. [758] reported 9 cases of isolated or primary involvement of the knee and 3 cases of secondary localization following involvement of the foot. In the study of Schiano et al. [727] on 15 cases of clinical involvement of the knee, the authors note 4 cases with isolated involvement of the knee, 8 cases with involvement of the knee associated with localization in the foot, 2 cases with simultaneous involvement of the knee and the hip, and 1 case of triple involvement of the knee, the foot, and the hip. In our series of 168 algodystrophies of the lower limb, we noted 49 isolated involvements of the knee.

Most often, subsequent to a traumatic factor or without apparent cause, the onset is either progressive (31 cases out of Serre's 35 cases) over several days, and characterized by the appearance of pain and swelling of the knee, or sudden (17 times out of 49 in our series).

At the fully developed stage, *three schematic clinical pictures* may be described:

1. The Classical Form

Pain is permanent and deep, increased by active and passive movements and by weight-bearing on the lower limb. There may exist misleading nocturnal recrudescence. Swelling is seen in about one-third of cases (12 of 35 in Serre's series): it is diffuse and responsible for the globulous appearance of the knee, where the temperature is increased relative to the unaffected side. Coloration of the skin is usually normal.

The mobility of the knee is restricted both in extension and in flexion. Pressure on the articular interspace and bone extremities is painful. A discreet layer of hydrarthrosis is frequently present (14 cases out of Serre's 35). Amyotrophy of the thigh is noted two times in three, and of the calf one time in three.

One can even observe limitation of the extension movement with an irreducible antalgic flexed attitude. In one of our cases the onset had been characterized by sudden pain caused by forceful flexion of the knee, with irreducible flexion. A diagnosis of lesion of the meniscus and retractile capsulitis was considered, but the arthrography was normal. Subsequent roentgenograms and bone scanning were typical of algodystrophy. The patient recovered rapidly with calcitonin treatment. In this case it was very certainly a matter of a predominantly tendinous involvement. In another of our cases the onset was also sudden and characterized by marked swelling of the quadricipital tendon and of the patellar tendon, with antalgic attitude in the extended position, flexion being almost impossible. The clinical course of this very peculiar and very longstanding tendinitis was characterized by radiologic and scintigraphic signs typical of algodystrophy; the very slow evolution of this condition ended up with recovery within one year.

The clinical evolution of this complete form is usually recovery without sequels within a few months (according to Serre, an average of 7 months) the extreme durations being a few days and 12 months.

2. Partial Algodystrophy

Partial algodystrophy has been recently described by Lequesne et al. [484] in 7 cases, in 4 of which the knee was affected. The clinical picture is almost the same as in the classical form but pain is selectively confined to the lateral femoral condyle in two cases, and to the medial femoral condyle in the two other cases. The main interest of this new form of algodystrophy lies in the difficulty of its diagnosis during the 2 or 3 months when radiological demineralization remains partial. This appearance raises suspicion of a possible infectious, acute inflammatory or even tumoral process.

3. Highly Localized Algodystrophy

Highly localized or parcellar algodystrophy has been very recently reported by two of us with reference to seven cases, in six of which the condition was confined to the knee [211].

It is characterized clinically by the classical symptoms of algodystrophy: pain with progressive or sudden onset, of mechanical or mixed type (in 5 cases out of 6 it shows the pattern of a femoropatellar syndrome); usually moderate and inconstantly present pseudoinflammatory local signs; and mainly, very severe localized pain on extremely limited palpation of a femoral condyle or of a tibial plate (medial femoral condyle in 4 cases, lateral femoral condyle in 1 case, medial tibial plate in 1 case). Differential diagnosis is even more difficult than in partial forms and concerns mainly osteoid osteoma and necrosis of a femoral condyle.

The evolution is regressive, either spontaneously within a few months, or more rapidly (sometimes in a few days) in response to the treatment which consists mainly of calcitonin, without development of significant locoregional demineralization. This particular evolution clearly differentiates this clinical form from partial dystrophy as described previously. Like all other forms of algodystrophy, parcellar algodystrophy may present with a monofocal or plurifocal pattern, either right at the onset or somewhat delayed with regard to the initial episode; these facts lead one to consider this new radioclinical form as a mere modality of algodystrophy of the limbs, intermediate between the forms without any radiological anomalies (Harif) and the complete and extensive forms with major radiological signs.

III. Algodystrophy of the Hip

This is a relatively rare site for algodystrophy, since we could find only 160 cases in the literature, In fact, it is very likely more frequent, but the diagnosis of algodystrophy is not always considered.

The condition has been known for quite a long time; as early as 1916 Babinski and Froment [26] reported 9 cases concerning patients with injuries to the lower limbs: following a slight trauma these patients showed a very marked claudication of the lower limb with significant functional incompetence, with faulty attitude of the lower limb, i.e., external rotation and abduction, slight pain at mobilization of the hip, and above all, limitation in the passive movements of internal rotation and flexion, with moderate atrophy of the thigh. Examination performed under chloroform anesthesia allowed a hysterical origin for these manifestations to be ruled out.

In 1956 Ravault and Durant [647] report involvement of the hip in "neurotrophic rheumatism of the lower limb" which had however already been related by Leriche [494] in 1939.

Isolated involvement of the hip was described for the first time by Curtiss and Kincaid [168] in 3 cases occurring in women at the end of their pregnancy, and termed by these authors "transient demineralisation of the hip."

In 1962, Vincent et al. [842] reported a case of neurotrophic rheumatism of the hip.

In 1966, de Marchi et al. [191] published 6 new cases of "peculiar rarefying arthropathy of the hip."

Lequesne [472] was the first to speak about "transient osteoporosis of the hip," with reference to 10 cases reported in 1968.

The same year, Hunder and Kelly [382] reported 9 cases, with a histological study of the synovial membrane.

Since then, there have been more publications referring to this localization of algodystrophy [24, 35, 42, 56, 149, 171, 205, 331, 354, 419, 514, 542, 687, 717, 725, 788, 790, 806, 818, 827, 841]. In our series of 250 cases of algodystrophy, 21 concern isolated involvement of the hip.

1. General Data

Algodystrophy of the hip is seen predominantly in males, in the ratio of three males to one female. In our series this ratio is even higher: 17 males to 4 females.

The average age of occurrence is 41, i.e., 10 years earlier than for other localizations.

The left hip is more frequently affected than the right (57% to 43%). Bilateral involvement, either simultaneous or successive, was seen in 21% of the cases. Our findings corroborate those in the literature: left hip 11 times, right hip 9 times, simultaneous bilateral involvement 1 case.

All authors agree that algodystrophy of the hip seems to be more often *idiopathic* and primary than algodystrophies affecting other sites. Such was the case in 6 of the 10 cases in Lequesne's first series [472] and in 16 of our series of 21. On the other hand Serre et al. [754] found only 37% of primary forms in their 30 cases.

As concerns the *secondary forms*, the most frequent cause is a traumatism, but unlike what happens with other localizations, this plays a less important role; it appears always to be minimal (effort, muscle strain) and ill-defined. In their series, Serre et al. [754] elicited a history of a traumatism in 26% of the cases, but this rate is lower in our statistics (3 of 21 cases). In females, algodystrophy of the hip may occur during pregnancy. Among the 16 cases, including 3 personal cases, reported by Vinceneux et al. [841], the age ranges from 28 to 43 years (average: 32 years); the disease commences after the 4th month, in three cases it seemed even to have been provoked by the term of pregnancy (3 deliveries and 1 cesarean section). Our series of 21 cases includes a case which developed during the 7th month of pregnancy.

2. Clinical Signs

Pain is the cardinal symptom, but its mode of occurrence, site, and character vary greatly.

The onset is often sudden (in 6 of Lequesne's 10 cases [473] and in 6 of Hunder's 9 cases [382]). The onset is sometimes so well-defined that the patient is able to indicate the precise moment of its occurrence and thus to correlate it to a slight injury or to muscle strain. According to Grosclaude [331] pain more often develops progressively. Whatever the mode of onset, the pain becomes worse and reaches maximum intensity after several days to 1 month, sometimes 2–3 months.

The site of the pain is also variable: in half of the cases its inguinocrural topography draws attention to the hip; more rarely gonalgia is the revealing sign.

The character of the pain also varies from one patient to another: it is most often of the mechanical type, appears on weight-bearing or on walking, or during motion, and is entirely relieved at rest; in some cases it may persist during the night, either at a minor level and transiently, or severe enough to cause the patient to search for an antalgic position (sitting, for instance). But on the whole, the pain is of moderate intensity.

Functional disability is quite surprising, since most of the time there is a striking discrepancy between the degree of disability and the moderateness of the pain. All authors report a discrepancy between often total functional disability and the pain described by the patients as very mild. Disability on weight-bearing may cause a limp. The patient describes a feeling of feebleness and unsteadiness on weight-bearing, which rapidly necessitates the use of one or two crutches.

The clinical examination discloses a certain number of signs.

The skin has a normal color and the local warmth is not increased. There is no palpable adenopathy, nor any swelling. Limitation in the hip motion is often moderate and dissociated: flexion is relatively less restricted than abduction or rotation, as has been pointed out by Lequesne [485], Dini and Faussone [205], and Hasche and Meyer [354]. Other authors, however, such as Ayrolles et al. [24] report limitation of motion affecting all movements. Grosclaude [331] found this to be the case in 25% of his material. Limitation in the hip motion may be so severe as to cause certain authors even to consider it a entity in its own right, which they termed "capsular retraction of the hip" [478]. In one of our cases and in one of Curtiss and Kincaid's the hip movements were not limited, but painful at the end of range.

Pain provoked by pressure on the ischiopubic ramus and the greater trochanter has been reported [35]; according to these authors it is evidence of diffusion of the process to a larger part of the pelvic skeleton.

Atrophy develops rapidly during the second or third week; it is mainly located in the buttock and in the quadriceps muscle, as was noted by Serre et al. in 21 of 31 cases, but sometimes in the calf, in 5 of the 31 cases [754]. In our series of 21 cases the atrophy varies from 1 to 4.5 cm.

The rest of the clinical examination of the affected lower limb is normal, both from the articular and from the neurologic point of view.

3. Clinical Course

Algodystrophy of the hip evolves spontaneously in three phases, as Lequesne [474] accurately demonstrated.

The first phase consists of a progressive aggravation lasting 1 month or less.

The second phase concerns the full development, when all clinical signs have reached their utmost degree and remain stationary for 1 or 2 months.

The third phase, finally, commences at the end of the second or the beginning of the third month; it corresponds to regression of the clinical signs.

There is general agreement that algodystrophy of the hip is characterized by a shorter evolution than other loclaizations. Thus, in their study of 188 cases of algodystrophy of the lower limbs Serre et al. [754] report an average duration of 12 months in involvements of the foot (from 4 to 28 months), of 7 months in involvement of the knee (from 3 to 12 months), and of 5 months for the hip (from 2 to 11 months).

Modern treatment with calcitonin has markedly reduced this duration. In our 21 cases, recovery was obtained within 3 days to 6 months; in 6 the duration was less than 21 days.

Recovery occurs most often without sequels. Very exceptionally there may persist slight pain on weight-bearing, moderate restriction in the movement, and amyotrophy of the quadriceps. Moderate and persistent osteoporosis may be shown on X-ray examination. Longer evolutions with significant sequels have however been noted: it is then a matter of true capsular retraction, either idiopathic or secondary to the various usual causes of algodystrophy.

Algodystrophy of the hip does not in principle recur. Nevertheless, two cases of homolateral recurrence have been reported [354, 806], in patients who had had alternating forms.

These *alternating forms* occur in 21.5% of cases, this percentage attaining 36.5 in pregnant women. In our series of 21 cases, 4 occurred within 1–3 years after the initial episode. Finally, algodystrophy of the hip can be followed by involvements of the lower limbs and, more rarely, of the upper limbs, whence the extensive forms described by David-Chaussé et al. [177] and Serre et al. [747].

When the successive episodes are separated by free intervals of several months or years, two of us have proposed calling the condition the *"plurifocal recurrent form."*

C. Algodystrophy of the Spine

The notion that algodystrophy might affect the spine is relatively recent, but some cases already reported in the literature make it reasonable to consider this possibility.

The first case was published by Lièvre and Hubault [508] in 1951; it concerns a patient who, after a fall due to electrization, presented compression fractures of vertebrae T4 to T6. After the patient had spent 3 months in a plaster cast he returned to work. Two months later, a slight trauma brought about severe lumbalgiae; X-rays performed 8 days later showed marked demineralization of the whole spine, extending to the sacrum and iliac wings with squeezing of the body of L1. The authors attribute this evolution to phenomena "analogous to traumatic osteoporosis of the limbs" and discuss the causal factor, i.e., electrization or traumatism.

The same year, Bacri and Mutin [29] reported a case of marked demineralization of C6 occurring in a shoulder-hand syndrome of herpes zoster origin. The patient recovered within a few months, and by the 8th month the C6 vertebra had regained a normal X-ray appearance.

In 1966 Gougeon and Moreau-Huttin [320], discussing recurrent forms of reflex algodystrophy, reported a case with spinal localization, but they hesitated to include it in the group of algodystrophies. Their case concerns a 64-year-old man who had had gastrectomy performed, and who had experienced, between his second and third episode of algodystrophy of the lower limbs, pain in the spine with appearance of a kyphosis and radiological signs of rarefying osteosis in the thoracolumbar spine. Stabilization was obtained after a few months.

In 1968 Serre et al. [747] reported a conclusive case concerning a 55-year-old woman who presented an initial episode of post traumatic extensive algodystrophy of the left lower limb, followed 6 months later by a severe syndrome of rarefying osteopathy with multiple flattened vertebrae.

In 1974 the same authors [753] reported two other cases of secondary involvement of the spine from a series of 54 patients with extensive algodystrophy of the lower limbs.

In 1975, Simon [765] reported a privileged case; it concerns a 31-year-old man in whom an accident on November 12, 1975, had produced a fracture with flattening of T5 and T12, giving rise to thoracic kyphosis. After $2^1/_2$ months' treatment the patient resumed his professional activity in spite of the persistence of pain. Control X-rays performed 6 months later gave evidence of rather diffuse bone rarefaction. Two years after the initial trauma, the thoracic pain became worse, and there was now marked thoracolumbar kyphosis. Medical treatment and kinesitherapy resulted in partial reduction of the kyphosis.

In 1969 a second road accident caused a fracture of the pelvis and a significant flattening of T12 and L1, on a preexistent marked bone rarefaction. In February 1970, there was some stabilization from the radioclinical viewpoint, but the patient's height had diminished by 10 cm. From this date on the patient improved clinically, his pain gradually disappeared and the X-rays showed signs of bone repair, confirmed by follow-up films carried out in 1973.

Schiano et al. [727] reported in 1978 two cases of demineralization of the lumbar spine occurring during extensive algodystrophy of the lower limbs in elderly women.

Finally, Delbart et al. [187], in 1978, published a case of a 66-year-old male with retractile capsulitis of the right shoulder and a clinical picture of cervical myelopathy of arthrotic origin, treated by C1-C5 laminectomy. Six months after surgery severe cervicalgiae appeared and the X-rays revealed besides the very marked cervicarthrosis, diffuse demineralization of the cervical spine. Bone scans showed increased activity in the right shoulder, and in the cervical area. Treatment with calcitonin relieved the cervicalgiae within a few weeks; a bone scan performed 10 months after the first showed no increased uptake. According to these authors, this case could be considered as an algodystrophy of the cervical spine.

An analysis of the different cases reported in the literature provides a certain number of criteria, viz., algodystrophy affects predominantly the lumbar or the thoracolumbar spine; it causes incapacitating pain and sometimes leads to kyphosis; radiologically, it is characterized by regional demineralization with one or several flatted vertebrae. In the few published cases, the spinal involvement is said to occur often at the same time as algodystrophy of the lower limbs or to follow it after a short interval;

sometimes it is part of an algodystrophic condition with successive episodes. The evolution seems to be cyclic and to end up with clinical recovery and radiological stabilization.

The existence of algodystrophy of the spine could allow some of the clinical descriptions made by Kümmell [424] in 1895 and by Verneuil and Forestier [835] in 1892 to be reconsidered.

Let us recall that this Kümmell-Verneuil syndrome is characterized by an evolution comprising three stages: a direct or indirect benign trauma to the spine causes thoracic pain confined to one or two vertebrae, without significant functional disability. There then ensues a free interval from several weeks to 6 months during which patients resume their normal activity. During the third stage, pain reappears progressively or following an effort, accompanied by a deformation of the spine (kyphosis or kyphoscoliosis) and radiologic evidence of flattened vertebrae and increased bone translucency (rarefying osteitis of Kümmell). However, though the clinical data were the same, the physiopathologic mechanism differed from one author to the other.

At the beginning, Kümmell thought that the painful kyphosis was due to a nutritional disturbance caused by tearing of vessels; later, in 1928, he incriminated a vertebral fissure into which the disk protrude and cause flattening of the vertebral body.

According to Verneuil and Forestier the trauma produced multiple fractures of the trabecula, whereas the corticalis remained intact. The body weight exerts pressure on these fractures, and because of its spongy nature, the vertebra becomes flattened.

Leriche and Policard [502] thought that Kümmell's syndrome was only a peculiar localization of "post-traumatic painful osteoporosis."

Later on the Kümmell-Verneuil syndrome gave rise to numerous publications, including the study of Froelich and Mouchet [285].

Recent studies (Thomas [810], Demilly [192]) have been aimed at showing that no valid demonstration allows the anatomic basis of such a syndrome to be established. In 1958, Decoulx and Rienau [182], in their contribution to the French orthopedic congress, stated: "The Kümmell-Verneuil syndrome does not exist." According to these authors posttraumatic pain in the spine has only a discal or muscular origin.

In 1968, and also in 1974, Serre and Simon [747, 753] proposed the hypothesis of an algodystrophic factor playing a part in the aggravation of an up to then quiescent rarefying osteopathy. They thereby rehabilitated the Kümmell-Verneuil syndrome insofar as they reconsidered Verneuil's hypothesis concerning the existence of microfractures aggravated by bodyweight. These microfractures release a veritable storm of sympathetic activity which accentuates, through vascular and trophic mechanisms, the bone rarefaction and produces squeezing of the vertebrae.

According to these authors, the Kümmell-Verneuil syndrome is a manifestation of what they term "spinal neurotrophic rheumatism" in which algodystrophy is added to the preexisting osteoporosis; this would account for the failure of already osteoporotic vertebrae to return to normal appearance.

In 1977, Simon [766] reported an interesting observation of a 71-year-old woman who, after a benign fall on the buttocks, had shown an indisputable Kümmell-Verneuil syndrome. For him, one could say the posttraumatic secondary flattening of a vertebral body does exist. The subsequent kyphosis seems in this case to have been the first stage of spinal algodystrophy, of which the radiological evolution is continuing, although there is a regression of the functional signs.

The problem of the Kümmell-Verneuil syndrome remains unsolved, but one may ask oneself whether it were not in fact an algodystrophy of the spine.

One fact nevertheless remains disturbing and not properly explained: despite often marked demineralization, no fractures are reported in algodystrophy of the limbs. One may wonder why only algodystrophy of the spine should cause flattening of the vertebrae, unless it occurs on an already osteoporotic spine.

Systematic bone scans with technetium-99m would be of interest to give evidence of possible algodystrophy of the spine, since in this case the increased activity would be diffuse and not solely confined to the flattened vertebra, if any; it would also persist for a long time, whereas there is no increased uptake with vertebrae that are only osteoporotic and not flattened.

In the present state of our knowledge it is difficult to have a definite view. By analogy with algodystrophy of the limbs, the application of our criteria (Part 5) will perhaps allow a better diagnostic approach for further studies.

Major forms of algodystrophy of the spine are certainly rare, but we believe that many patients complaining of posttraumatic spinal pain actually suffer from a minor form of algodystrophy.

D. Other Localizations

We did not find in the literature any facts convincing enough to prove that the algodystrophic process could also affect other parts of the organism. Nevertheless, such an eventuality is theoretically possible; it is hardly believable that skeletal parts other than spine and limbs should not be involved.

However, some conditions presenting with clinical or etiopathologic relationships deserve to be reported and discussed.

In 1934 Costen [157] and, later Hennebert [359] noted an algodystrophic syndrome in patients who had lost some or all of their teeth, and who had no prostheses or poorly fitting ones. Some have though this condition to be an algodystrophy affecting the *mandibular joints*. But, considering the description these authors made of their cases, we cannot agree that it is algodystrophy.

The syndrome of the *anterior thoracic wall* described by Dulap and Ivins [225] in 1952 and by Prinzmetal and Massuni [640] in 1955 seems very similar to algodystrophy in its symptomatology and mode of occurrence. This syndrome is usually seen following a myocardial infarct; it is characterized by pain confined to the sternochondral joints. In spite of its possible association with a shoulder-hand syndrome, its cause remains unknown and there is no valid argument to connect it with an algodystrophic process.

In 1956 Griesmann et al. [327] reported 4 cases of involvement of the *pubic symphisis* among 100 prostatectomies performed with the Millin technique. This condition is characterized by osteoporosis of both pubic rims and could, according to the authors, be considered a postsurgical algodystrophy.

Finally, it should be mentioned that no case of algodystrophy affecting the *skull* has ever been reported.

Part 2 Complementary Investigations

Chapter 1 Biochemistry

For a very long time it was assumed that algodystrophy was not accompanied by significant biochemical modifications. Only recently has evidence been provided of variations of certain biochemical constants.

A. Nonspecific Indicators of Inflammation

No biochemical signs of inflammation are usually seen in algodystrophy: the erythrocyte sedimentation rate as well as protein electrophoresis and fibremia are normal. Serre et al. [749] found a normal sedimentation rate in 41 of 45 algodystrophies of the foot, in the 4 remaining cases its elevation was related to intercurrent diseases. In forms with acute and "pseudophlegmonous" onset, Ravault [645] observed transient elevation of the sedimentation rate. The findings deserve some critical remarks. Indeed, Schiano et al. [727] studied the sedimentation rate in 78 patients allocated to three groups according to the stage of their illness, both from the clinical and from the radiological viewpoint: the sedimentation rate had a mean value of 28 mm after 1 h in stage I conditions, 30 mm in stage II, and 20 mm in stage III. After ruling out an intercurrent disease which would have accounted for the increased sedimentation rate, these authors found a moderate increase of the sedimentation rate in a nonnegligible number of cases, whatever the stage of algodystrophy. In our series of 250 cases, moderate and isolated elevation was found in 29 cases. From these data we may conclude that the sedimentation rate in algodystrophy is normal and its moderate increase very rare.

B. Calcium and Phosphorus Levels in Blood and Urine

Most authors agree that the values for blood calcium, phosphorus and alkaline phosphatase are usually normal in algodystrophy. On the whole our data corroborate these findings. Note however that Belenger [44] found some cases with significant hypercalcemia and clearly increased ionized calcium levels. In 5 of their patients with a stage I disease, Schiano et al. [727] found increased alkaline phosphatase levels; they consider these findings as proof of osteoblastic hyperactivity in the early stages of algodystrophy, subsequently confirmed by the histologic studies.

Tests with calcium 45 or 47 have been carried out exceptionally. In a patient with a shoulder-hand syndrome of 4 months' duration, Huaux and Nagant de Deuxchaines [376] found an increased calcium pool and increased speed of uptake and resorption of calcium in the bone. In a patient with a stage III algodystrophy Schiano et al. [727] note a normal pool (5,850 mg/day) and a slightly diminished turnover (490 mg/day).

The average value of calcium in urine usually remains within normal limits. Obviously increased values – above 250 mg/day – have been found by several authors [44, 271, 494, 727]. Among 17 cases Belenger [44] found 4 with an average 24-h urine calcium of 275 mg. According to him, elevated urine calcium values correspond to recent or still evolving algodystrophies. Schiano et al. [727] report 12 of 57 patients as having a urine calcium level above 250 mg (7 of 31 patients had a stage I disease, 3 of 16 a stage II, and 2 of 10 a stage III disease). In our series of 250, a 24-h urine calcium level of more than 6,250 mmol was found in 8 cases, one of which consisted paradoxically of parcellar algodystrophy of the knee. There does not seem to be a parallelism between the existence or the degree of hypercalciuria and the apparent extension of the algodystrophic process.

The phosphate level in the urine, which is known to depend on diet, is usually within normal limits in algodystrophy.

C. Calcitonin Test

Injection of a single dose of calcitonin induces hypocalcemia, the degree and duration of which depend of the dose and on the mode of administration of the drug. This test is also called "calcitonin-induced acute hypocalcemia"; it induces in fact several other side effects [72, 90, 277, 769, 828, 839], such as lowered serum phosphorus level and hydroxyprolinuria, increased calciuria, and increased levels of parathormone in the blood and of cyclic AMP in the urine; there are no changes in the alkaline phosphatase level. According to Bordier et al. [90] and to Singer et al. [769], the immediate response to calcitonin is proof of changes in bone resorption function.

It should thus be interesting to study the response to this test in algodystrophies, since the number of osteoclasts is often increased in this condition.

Blanc [71] carried out this test in 13 cases of algodystrophy at the warm stage and in 15 controls. His protocol was the following: Intramuscular injection of 100 units MRC salmon calcitonin was given. The calcium level in the serum was determined 3 h prior to the injection, and 3, 6, 9, and 24 h after the injection. In the controls the calcemia was lowered on the average by 2.3 mg/l (in 11 of the 15 cases the lowest level was recorded 6 h after the injection). In the algodystrophies the average reduction was 3.5 mg/l, recorded in 8 of 13 cases 6 h after the injection. According to the author, there was no statistical difference between hypocalcemia in algodystrophy and in the control group. Fournié et al. [277] performed this test in 22 cases with algodystrophy at different stages and in 15 controls, by injection of 160 units of pork calcitonin. The average decrease in serum calcium is 4.44 mg/l in algodystrophies and 2.83 mg/l in the control group. The difference between the two groups is not statistically significant.

In 1979 Fournié et al. [276] presented the results of a simplified induced hypocalcemia test in 16 cases of algodystrophy: in one-third of the cases the hypocalcemic response suggested increased osteoclastosis. Ten of these 16 patients were treated with calcitonin: 5 did not show induced hypocalcemia and did not improve as a result of the treatment; in the other 5 there was a clearly positive response, i.e., induced hypocalcemia equal to or above 6 mg/l, and the treatment was successful.

For our part, we have performed this test with an injection of 100 units of salmon calcitonin in 44 patients presenting various stages of algodystrophic processes. The results were very discordant and paradoxical. The decrease in the serum calcium level was equal to or above 0.1 mmol/l in 14 cases and below 0.1 mmol/l in 15 cases; but in 15 other cases an increased serum calcium level, reaching a maximum 6 h after the injection, was noted; however, the result of the calcitonin treatment was good in about half of these 15 cases.

From these different findings we must conclude that it is not possible to anticipate the efficiency of calcitonin therapy from the acute test; moreover, satisfactory results seem to be related to the vascular effect of the hormone rather than to its effect on the bones.

D. Hydroxyproline in the Urine

Since it reflects bone metabolism, the urinary excretion of hydroxyproline proves the most interesting biochemical parameter to study in algodystrophy.

Eisinger [240] was the first to report significant increases of hydroxyprolinuria in 8 cases of algodystrophy. Eisinger et al. [243] confirmed these results in 1972, with reference to 33 patients, and observed that hydroxyprolinuria is markedly more elevated during the first clinical manifestations of the condition. Subsequent studies [242, 513] bearing on a larger number of patients afford additional details.

Determined by the method of Prockop in a patient on a gelatin-poor diet, the average hydroxyprolinuria in the adult is 25 ± 15 mg/24 h according to Dreux [223], which corresponds to a rate ranging from 75 to 300 μmol/24 h.

A certain number of physiologic variables may influence the rate of urinary excretion of hydroxyproline. Among these, age is the most important, which is quite understandable given the origin of hydroxyproline. Leroy, quoted by Dreux [223] provides the following particulars concerning the period from 0 to 25 years: from 0 to 1 year the average value is 33 mg/24 h; from 1 to 10 years, it is 67 mg/24 h; from 11 to 16 years, one observes the highest excretion rate (143 mg/24 h), probably due to the rapid growth characterizing this period; from 17 to 24 years the average is 50 mg/24 h; above the age of 24 years the normal rates are about 25 mg/24 h. The diet must also be taken into account to explain the wide dispersion of the normal values. The daily excretion rate is more constant when the diet does not include meat, jelly, ice-cream, and certain jams which are rich in gelatin and collagen. Finally, Eisinger [240] estimate the variation from day to day in the same patient to be 25%. This variation is reduced when the average hydroxyprolinuria over three consecutive days is taken and when the ratio urinary hydroxyprolinuria over urinary creatinine is used.

Eisinger et al. [242] studied hydroxyprolinuria in 67 algodystrophies, comprising 37 women and 30 men of an average age of 56 years; in 31 cases the algodystrophic process affected the upper limb and in 36 the lower limbs. The average hydroxyprolinuria was 42 mg/24 h, i.e., twice the normal level, estimated by the authors to be 21 mg ± 12/24 h in 15 controls aged 50–60 years. The results with regard to the stage of the condition are the following: 41 stage I conditions had an elevated hydroxyprolinuria of 51 ± 29 mg/24 h; in 17 patients at a stage intermediate between the warm phase and the cold phase the hydroxyprolinuria was moderately increased (36 ± 15 mg/24 h); finally, 9 patients with tendon retraction had a normal rate (22 ± 12 mg/24 h). There is a statistically significant difference between stage I and stage II ($p<0.01$) and between stage I and stage III ($p<0.05$) but not between stage II and stage III ($p<0.1$). The same authors demonstrated that hydroxyprolinuria diminishes progressively over the first 4 months of the spontaneous course of the disease: 1st month: 75 mg/24 h, 2nd month: 56 mg/24 h, 3rd month: 41 mg/24 h, 4th month: 30 mg/24 h. Later the level stabilizes at about 30 mg/24 h until the 10th month. The authors did not note significant differences between hydroxyprolinuria in algodystrophies of the upper limbs (42 mg/24 h) and of the lower limbs (43 mg/24 h). They also found no difference between patients with a single articulation affected and those with several. Moreover hydroxyprolinuria follows the course of the disease: it diminishes following classical therapy and may increase again when there is a clinical recurrence.

In our series the hydroxyprolinuria was determined in 78 patients with algodystrophy at various stages. Our results differ considerably from those of Eisinger et al. [242]. We found a normal rate of hydroxyprolinuria in 44 patients and an increased rate in 34. The highest rate (1,230 μmol/24 h) was observed during the cold phase of an algodystrophy of the foot in which a bone scan had shown hypofixation. We were astonished to find a clearly increased hydroxyprolinuria (518.5 μmol/24 h) in one case of parcellar algodystrophy of the knee.

To sum up, increased hydroxyprolinuria remains a useful but inconstant clue in the diagnosis of algodystrophy.

E. Parathormone

Leriche and Jung [501] have considered the possible existence of a parathyroid factor in the long course of certain posttraumatic algodystrophies. With regard to 2 cases presenting a marked aggravation of the local state and extension of the disturbances to the contralateral side, these authors recorded a marked hypercalciuria of 300–400 mg/24 h, without any other anomaly in the phosphocalcic metabolism. After failure of usually efficient treatments, parathyroidectomy was performed, when the parathyroid glands were found to have an increased volume. Surgery was followed by rapid regression of the clinical changes and of the hypercalciuria. These facts led the authors to believe that a parathyroid factor had appeared subsequently in the course of a primarily localized condition.

To our knowledge no study has since been published about the possible role of the parathyroids and the changes in the level of parathormone in algodystrophies.

F. HL-A Antigen

We have not found in the literature any studies concerning the distribution of HL-A antigen in algodystrophy.

We summarize below the results of our first 24 studies bearing on locus A and B.

HL-A A2	13	52%
HL-A A9	8	38%
HL-A B12	7	28%
HL-A BW15	6	24%
HL-A B27	3	12%

Dausset [172] recorded the frequency of HL-A alleles in the French population as follows: A2, 44.8%; B12, 32.5%; BW15, 12%. There is no marked difference between these results and our own short series.

No conclusion can however be drawn from such fragmentary results, which need to be confirmed by subsequent studies.

G. Synovial Fluid

Not uncommonly there is an intraarticular effusion, for instance in the knee, usually of the mechanical type, i.e., containing less than 500 cells/mm^3. In our series of 250 cases the synovial fluid was examined in 12 cases and shown to contain few cells.

H. Muscular Enzymes

To our knowledge no studies have reported changes in the muscular enzymes in algodystrophy.

Predisposition to Algodystrophy in Certain Preexisting Metabolic Disturbances

Stress has been laid recently on certain metabolic factors predisposing to algodystrophy; these factors are dealt with in greater detail in Part 6.

1. Diabetes Mellitus

In 1970 Lequesne [476] already pointed out the role played by diabetes mellitus; this role is now recognized by most authors. The series of 103 algodystrophies reported by Schiano et al. [727], however, includes only 2 diabetics. In a series of 108 of our algodystrophy patients we found 8 patent or latent cases of diabetes. But since the oral glucose tolerance test was not performed in all these patients, the frequency of diabetes in our series might have been underestimated.

2. Hyperlipidemia

Pinals and Jabbs [628] reported in 1972 the existence of type IV hyperlipoproteinemia in 3 patients affected with algodystrophy.

Very recently Amor et al. [7] reported the results of a study of lipid metabolism in 34 patients with algodystrophy (of the hip and other sites) and in a group of 11 controls. By means of the hypertriglyceridemia test induced by alcohol ingestion these authors demonstrated that the increase of the rate of triglycerides is significantly more elevated ($p<0.02$) in the diseased group (+64%) than in the control group (+16%). Moreover, simultaneous determination of glycemia and uricemia disclosed 5 patients with diabetes and 5 with hyperuricemia in this group of 34 patients, and gave evidence of a triple metabolic syndrome, gout – diabetes – hyperlipidemia, existing in certain algodystrophies.

These findings suggest a peculiar metabolic background which should be systematically searched for in posttraumatic as well as apparently idiopathic algodystrophies.

The metabolic disturbances are the same as those found in aseptic osteonecrosis.

Chapter 2 Radiology

Although for 80 years all studies have stressed the usefulness of radiography for establishing the diagnosis of algodystrophy, and all workers from Sudeck on have devoted a great part of their publications to radiology, only a few papers deal specifically with the radiological appearance of cases of algodystrophy. We would like to quote here Hermann et al. [360], Ecoiffier and Geerts [233], and Genant et al. [305].

Up to the last few years, the roentgenographic investigation was the main examination, necessary although not absolutely indispensable for the diagnosis. Even when the clinical data pointed to algodystrophy, nobody dared affirm this diagnosis in the absence of typical radiologic signs, though some, in particular Reichle [660], had repeatedly stated that the diagnosis was mainly based on clinical features and that radiography was only useful to confirm it.

Since the clinical signs most often precede the radiologic evidence by several weeks (on average by 4–6 weeks), the classical authors recommend repeated X-raying for assessing the diagnosis. This is no longer the case. As we shall see further on (Part 2, Chap. 3), bone scanning provides much earlier and more convincing data. The precedence of scintigraphy over radiography is accounted for by the fact that increased activity shown on the bone scan is correlated to the development of immature bone collagen [815], whereas radiologic evidence of demineralization depends mainly on the loss of calcium. To say that the boundary between the normal and the pathologic image in radiology is difficult to define and often quite subjective is a frequently repeated truism. It is classically believed that demineralization can be identified on an X-ray picture as soon as the proportion of bone calcium is diminished by 15%–30%. From 50% on – a very high level – it becomes significant. This shows how approximate is the appreciation of calcium loss on the basis of radiographic translucency. (Moreover, it should be kept in mind that these figures relate to experimental conditions, i.e., radiographs of dried bones, particularly vertebrae, which have the greatest homogeneity of bone structure).

Already in 1902, Exner [251] had studied the ratio of bone weight per cubic centimeter in three cases of acute bone atrophy. In all three cases he found the values were diminished, by 30%, 7%, and 67%, respectively. This does not, however, mean that the reduction in bone weight corresponds only to loss of mineral salts. Besides, the method he used was very imperfect and approximate and thus bound to be criticized. Finally, it should be mentioned that even the case with a 7% weight loss showed marked radiological osteoporosis. Pursuing his work Exner established the ratio of organic substance to inorganic substance by means of biochemical studies. In a single case, the third one, he noticed a reduced proportion of calcium, which he believed to be due to the presence of noncalcified bone substance, this being either demineralized or not yet mineralized.

Under these conditions, it is important that the roentgenographic technique be as perfect as possible and that new advances in radiology be exploited to the utmost.

A. Techniques

Standard roentgenographs with conventional projections are very often quite sufficient, although some special projections may sometimes be useful. Ravault et al. [652] pointed out that demineralization is visible earliest and best in the sesamoid bones. There is no special projection for the hand; for the forefoot it is advisable to use the tangential Müller's projection (Fig. 14). Finally, for the patella, the axial projection of the femoropatellar interspace provides the most data (Fig. 18). X-raying the knee in the false lateral projection may be useful for displaying successively the anterior and the posterior part of each condyle (Fig. 6). In practice, it is advisable in each case to use the projection best suited to the clinical findings.

I. Magnification Radiology

The magnification obtained by the geometry of positioning (i.e., placing the hand at a distance from the film) produces a larger image, but when a screen is not used the result is usually of poorer quality than that obtained by the conventional technique. Direct magnification makes it possible to obtain at once an image two to three times enlarged. A very fine focus and slow screens with high definition should be used. Genant et al. [305] employ "fine grain industrial film (Kodak type M) with exposure conditions of 50 kVp 500 mA and 0.8 s at a 48 in. focus-film distance. A contact exposure is made with a 1.2 mm focal spot tube. The radiographs are processed in a Kodak Industrial B processor and viewed by optical magnification using either the Schneider-Kreutznach lupe (4×) or the Leitz Macro Promar projector (5–10×). We use a similar technique (Figs. 8, 11).

II. Tomography

Tomography is useful in obliterating overlapping shadows that interfere with visualization of the area in question. Tomography is not very often used for the phalanges, since they can usually be demonstrated by simple radiographic techniques.

Tomography with simple or, better, complex linear movement must allow a clear image of the selected section to be obtained and above all as complete as possible an effacement of images in other planes. But the tomographic image shows little contrast, the more so when the section is precise and the over- and underlying cuts well effaced. When there is bone demineralization of a structure with a specific opacity close to that of the neighboring tissues, the structure will be poorly visible in tomography and quite invisible on thin cuts. However, a thin and well-contrasted structure in dense surroundings may sometimes be well visualized thanks to a complex tomographic movement (Fig. 12).

III. Xeroradiography

In xerography the image is first formed on a photosensitive plate and then transferred to a sheet of paper. Xeroradiography records X-ray images by means of alterations in charge on semiconductors. X-radiation causes local alterations in the charge on a selenium plate. A charged powder distributes itself, depending on the intensity of the charge on the selenium plate, producing an image. Because of its ability to display on a single film two anatomic structures with different densities (contrast compression), xeroradiography is indicated each time it is necessary to demonstrate the relations between bone and soft tissues. This method can thus be useful for studying articular and periarticular edema in algodystrophy (Fig. 1).

Another advantage of xeroradiography is its relatively large latitude, and the fact that a high kilovoltage can be used while maintaining an adequate image. Optimal hand xeroradiographs can be obtained with a kilovoltage of 12 kVp.

IV. Electron Radiography

As quoted by Poznanski [636], electron radiography is a newly described method in which an image is formed of a charged distribution on a dielectric plate. This is converted into an image by exposure to a toner in a development chamber, and finally the image is fixed. The resultant image somewhat resembles that seen in xeroradiography with enhanced edge effect.

V. Logetronography

By means of a photographic process this method improves the image quality. The film to be processed is placed in contact with an unexposed film. Very narrow bands of these two films are successively exposed to a light ray the intensity of which is regulated by means of a photoelectric cell. The ray of light is intensified or weakened according to whether it concerns a dark or a bright part of the radiograph: the result is a harmonized reproduction. The image thus obtained gives an impression of relief, but causes certain details to disappear.

Once more we would like to point out the necessity of X-raying the unaffected side as well, for comparison.

As concerns the description, we distinguish involvement of the soft parts, involvement of the bone, and involvement of the joints.

B. Involvement of Soft Tissues

Swelling of the soft parts may be either diffuse or only periarticular, but most often the two types are associated. Genant et al. [305] have provided a detailed description of this type of lesion, which we have also seen in our cases (Fig. 1). Their criteria for "*diffuse swelling* included generalized prominence or thickening of the soft tissue, obliteration or narrowing of interdigital skin folds and a reticulated appearance of the soft tissue which was thought to be related to edema of the subcutaneous fat." In their series they found 91% of involvements of this type, but this percentage depends of course on the stage at which the X-rays were performed. "*Periarticular* accentuation of the *soft tissue swelling* or capsular distension is identified by a prominence of the soft tissue around joints, associated with obliteration of the normal periarticular fat planes."

Appreciation of the thickness of the soft tissue has been mainly used in acromegalia, but could be used in algodystrophy as well. Lin and Lee [509] have described a soft tissue index at the level of the second phalanx. They define this index as the ratio between the thickness of the phalanx in its median part and the thickness of the soft tissues at the same level. The index in normals was 0.45 with one S.D. = 0.05.

C. Involvement of Bone

I. Elementary Radiographic Signs

The most obvious bone lesion is the radiologic hypertranslucency of the bone skeleton or osteopenia, but other changes can be studied.

1. Osteopenia

As with soft tissues, two types of change are to be distinguished: diffuse, and juxta- or periarticular changes.

Diffuse osteopenia is ultimately only a subjective evaluation, and we have already mentioned the difficulty of evaluating bone loss. We shall study in more detail the different methods for measuring bone density in Part 2, Chap. 4.

Peri or juxta-articular osteopenia is explained by the accentuation of the demineralization process of the trabecular bone in the epiphyseal area which is seen, radiologically, as a periarticular hypertranslucency. This is due to thinness or even complete disappearance of the epiphyseal bone trabeculae, a particularly evocative sign of algodystrophy (Fig. 2).

Lacroix and Ponlot [436] believe that the subchondral area is not the only area to be demineralized and that the metaphysis is also be affected. They report cases in which this has become abnormally translucent. "At this stage it does not affect the transverse area which in the adult marks the spot where, at the end of growth, metaphysis and epiphysis join; it corresponds precisely to the metaphyseal trabeculae which lead to the transverse area... : the metaphyseal borderline area tends to disappear, whereas the epiphyseal borderline area persists." This demineralization is transient, but according to the authors it is at least as characteristic for posttraumatic osteoporosis as is subchondral demineralization (Fig. 3). Stern [782] who speaks about "acute transverse bone atrophy" has also reported a similar image. Stern's cases, with but one exception, were confined to the long bones of the lower extremity, usually to the lower end of the tibia. A certain number of surgeons – it is indeed most often a matter of posttraumatic findings – consider these data as a precursor of algodystrophy. In the book he published in 1960, Wagner [851] presents a certain number of radiographs with such features but does not comment on them.

According to Lacroix and Ponlot [436] this metaphyseal demineralization is better visible in young adults; it becomes less obvious in patients above 50, and is almost invisible in older people. There are two bone extremities which are usually spared since they are affected by more diffuse demineralization, namely the upper extremies of the humerus and the femur.

2. Subchondral Lysis

Subchondral lysis, or, rather, subchondral bone resorption, is one of the earliest signs. Leriche [494] stresses this: "Often the cartilaginous border appears more distinctly than normally. It looks as if the bone had been stylised, as if a black line had been drawn to underline its limits." He called this sign the "gouache-sign." But in fact it is not a cartilaginous line (Figs. 4, 10), but the subchondral bone lamina. This lamina may disappear more or less completely over a greater or lesser distance. Such features are seen particularly on the femoral head, where they cause unsharp contours (Fig. 5).

As concerns the subchondral bone proper, resorption may be homogeneous (Fig. 2) or lacunar. It is often at this level that the lesions are the most significant; the lacunae are of very variable size (Fig. 7).

3. Resorption of Cortical Bone (Figs. 8–10)

Thinning of the diaphyseal cortical layers on the hand and the foot is a characteristic sign. There is usually *subperiosteal resorption* responsible for irregular lysis of the external limits of the cortical bone, producing an undulated appearance of the edges of the shaft. This appearance is similar to that encountered in mild forms of fibrous osteitis in primary hyperparathyroidism.

Endosteal resorption is characterized by a scalloped internal borderline communicating with the medullary space, producing an extremely irregular and rough endosteal surface with marked variations in the thickness of the cortical layer.

When algodystrophy passes from the acute to the chronic phase, the irregular resorption of the endosteal surface causes remodeling of the endosteum and thus produces a large medullary canal and a thin cortex. At this stage, the lesions can no longer be distinguished from those of chronic osteopenia, i.e., postmenopausal or senile osteoporosis.

The use of the *thickness of the cortical layer* of the second metacarpals as a measure of mineralization has been suggested by various workers including Virtama and Mähönen [844], and Barnett and Nordin [33]. Use of the second metacarpals correlates well with other methods of bone measurement. According to Genant et al. [305], "a reduction in cortical thickness for the involved hand of all patients was evident when compared to either the uninvolved hand or to expected normal values. Serial examination in 3 patients revealed progressive bone mineral loss in the affected hand, while the contralateral hand remained essentially unchanged... The mean cortical thickness of the diseased extremities was 3.5 mm compared to 4.59 mm for uninvolved hands and 5.17 mm for controls. This represents approximately a one third loss in cortex, primarily from the endosteal surface, since the outer cortical dimensions of the three groups (involved, uninvolved, and controls) were nearly identical" (Fig. 11).

Finally, there also occurs *intracortical resorption,* especially clearly visible in the phalangeal diaphyses, and less obvious in the metacarpals and metatarsals. The cortical layer has a striated appearance and is more visible on frontal than on lateral films. Criteria have been established for grading cortical striation or tunneling in the metacarpals or metatarsals, as described by Meema and Schatz [558]: grade 0 for uniformly compact cortical bone, to grade 3 for marked striation extending throughout the cortex.

4. Juxta-articular Erosions

Genant et al. [305] report about three degrees of juxta-articular and subchondral erosive changes (the grading criteria are: 0 = none; 1 = borderline; 2 = surface erosion; 3 = pocket erosion). Grade 2 erosions were of two types: "the first consisted of surface erosions producing a 'saw-tooth,' 'dot-dash' or 'bare trabeculae' appearance of the subchondral cortical bone. The second and more common pattern of grade 2 erosion was an unusual ragged appearance resulting from irregular resorption and fragmentation of juxta-articular cortical surfaces accompanied by reactive bone formation." The author illustrates his paper with some radiographs which are far from convincing. The subchondral erosion, called in France subchondral lysis, would be more adequately termed subchondral resorption, but it certainly exists. On the other hand, we think that the juxta-articular erosion "appearance" is correlated to so advanced a thinning of the cortical layer that it becomes optically invisible, though it is still present (Fig. 12). Another mechanism would be the presence of microfractures in the bone trabeculae. Reactive bone formation could subsequently occur, which would also account for the *"proliferative erosions"* described by Genant. But this hypothesis has not been proven histologically.

Classically, *one of the criteria of the diagnosis is the absolute integrity of the articular interspaces.* Referring to Rutishauser's et al. [708] pathologic investigations, it appears that this worker's case 1 showed macroscopically "irregular erosions of the articular surfaces of the wrist bones with a finely gnarled appearance of the border of the cartilage." None of our 250 cases of algodystrophy showed evidence of narrowing of the articular interspace.

II. Association of Primary Lesions Producing Different Types of Image

Osteopenia with generalized involvement of the bone trabeculae is the most significant feature in algodystrophy, but the association, at various degrees, of the elementary radiological signs already described produces different radiological types of algodystrophy. These types depend however on the stage at which the roentgen examination is performed and on the site and intensity of the algodystrophy.

The most characteristic image is produced by *mottling or vacuolar osteoporosis.* In his first case report Sudeck [793] noted it, with the following description: "...Irregular spotty hypertranslucency of the bone shadows, producing a striking peculiar dappled image. On the hand this dappled appearance is seen first in the spongious bone." Later these features were seen by all workers; they consist usually of individualized rounded or oval images without precise limits, present in large amounts. Not uncommonly there are also more diffuse demineralization areas, giving the impression that the bone architecture has been irregularly rubbed out, or on the contrary there may be smaller, punctiform images (Fig. 13).

The anomalies of the bone architecture sometimes have other appearances, which may exist alone or be associated to produce the background for vacuolar osteoporosis.

There may be a mere *rarefaction* of the bone trabeculae, producing a homogeneously increased translucency of the bones, the evaluation of which requires excellent films and comparison with the unaffected side. The other trabeculae can appear thickened exaggeratedly underlining the force lines of the bone to which they give a roughly combed appearance.

These *hypertrophic, rarefied trabeculae* give rise to an irregular and anarchic trabeculation when some of them have lost their normal orientation.

The trabeculation can even disappear almost completely, so that the bone seems washed, devoid of any apparent structure, with a blurred bone architecture. This anomaly has been termed "glassy" or "vitrified bone," or "*glass bone.*" In extreme cases one could also speak of "*phantom bone.*"

III. Evolution Features

1. Early Demineralization

We have already mentioned that osteopenia is quite delayed with regard to the clinical signs; this latency varies from 15 days to 12 weeks, with an average of 4 weeks. Belenger [44] retains the average of 3 weeks. Therefore it should be said that, in cases where algodystrophy is suspected, the radiologic investigation should be repeated when the first is negative. Depending on the intensity of algodystrophy, osteopenia occurs more or less early, but its intensity is not proportional to the intensity of the provoking factor or to the degree of clinical changes in the soft tissues. We could not give evidence of a correlation between the degree of osteopenia and hyperthermia measured by thermography. According to Wagner [851] the latency is longer in winter than in summer, owing to vitamin deficiency. As we have already said, the early signs should be searched for in the thin bones, i.e., the distal epiphyses of the forearm or leg bones, the small bones of hand and foot, the sesamoid bones, and the patella.

2. Evaluation of the Radiologic Intensity of Algodystrophy

The degree of osteopenia certainly varies from one case to the other; in some instances it may even be disputable whereas in others it is quite definite. Moreover, during evolution of algodystrophy it may be difficult to appreciate changes occuring between two radiologic investigations. As concerns the hand, Hackethal [343] has proposed a classification into 8 stages based on three data: 1) osteoporosis extends from the proximal to the distal extremity; 2) osteoporosis affects first the spongious tissue and later the cortical bone; 3) osteoporosis of the cortical bone becomes evident earlier on the small than on the larger bones.

This classification seems interesting but its value has not been demonstrated. Besides it has not been tested on larger series, nor by different workers. As for ourselves, we could not decide to undertake this somewhat fastidious task.

3. Classification into Stages

The intensity of the radiologic changes depends partly on the stage at which X-raying is performed. From the clinical point of view (Part I, Chap. 2) two or three stages are usually distinguished; also in pathology, it is possible to distinguish different stages (Part II, Chap. 8); and in radiology, finally, a certain chronology does seem to exist. Nevertheless, clinically, radiologically, and pathologically, the passage from one stage to the next is not always quite clear. Around 1940 to 1950 a great debate among German traumatologists concerned the determination of the radiological stage I. According to them, stage I was a physiological stage of repair from which evolution could lead to recovery or to true algodystrophy. Later, some of them reconsidered this view when they noticed that there were no undisputable signs characterizing the different stages, but multiple transitional forms, so that classification was only approximate.

What is certain, however, is that the vacuolar, dappled microlacunar appearance corresponds to the acute phase, whereas subcortical atrophy with thickened trabeculae corresponds to a later phase. Besides, this latter can persist indefinitely, so that after 5 or even 10 years it is possible to recognize this form as a sequel of cured algodystrophy. According to Hackethal [343], only stage I recovers entirely; all other stages lead to recovery with sequels responsible for what Sudeck [793] described as "hypertrophic atrophy."

According to Belenger [44] the radiologic regression depends mainly on the appearance, thus on the evolution stage. Thus mere osteoporosis would as a rule be followed by restitutio ad integrum; the vacuolar appearance might regress completely or partly; the glassy appearance would persist even after clinical recovery, or in any case, regress incompletely.

We believe that three radiological stages can be schematically distinguished. The first stage is characterized by the absence of radiological anomaly or by the presence of simple diffuse demineralization. The second stage consists in marked local or locoregional demineralization, with a homo- or heterogeneous pattern and blurred appearance of the bone trabeculae and/or lacunar images with ill-defined margins. The third stage comprises regression of the radiologic anomalies or, more often, rarefied bone trabeculae, which appear denser and thickened, and thinning of the cortical bone. There may also be lacunar images but these are well delimited, with clear-cut margins: stage 3 represents a sequellar appearance (Fig. 15). The three radiological stages have variable durations, stage 2 and stage 3 may even be lacking.

4. Forms Without Bone Demineralization

There certainly exist algodystrophies without radiological manifestations, as there are algodystrophies without pain. Harif [351] reported 3 cases out of 85 who showed no radiologic signs during the entire course of the disease. Among our 250 cases we found 8 cases without radiological changes throughout the course of the disease, including one case of involvement of the foot with hyperactivity at bone scanning in the course of a Lobstein disease. The absence of radiologic evidence may be due to the fact that the pathologic changes produce a demineralization of less than 15%–30%, below which the mineral loss is not visible even on good quality films. Therefore the diagnosis of algodystrophy without radiological signs becomes difficult and requires the concordance of all other data, i.e., etiologic, biochemical, clinical, evolutive and, above all, scintigraphic. We shall consider this problem again when dealing with the diagnostic criteria of algodystrophies (Part 5). One could even consider the hypothesis of algodystrophies which do not affect the bone tissues.

D. Topographic Forms

The above description could be applied to all localizations of algodystrophy, but there indisputably exist regional variations. Before studying these particular forms we would like to discuss the localized forms, described recently.

I. Partial Algodystrophy [484]

Two different radiological manifestations of "partial transient osteoporosis" have been observed: the radial form, which involves only one or two rays of the hand or foot, and the zonal form in which the area of demineralization is confined initially to such structures as one femoral condyle or one quadrant of the femoral head.

The radial type of algodystrophy tends to affect one or two rays of hand or foot. These changes may extend from the carpus through the metacarpals to the phalanges of the hand or, equally, from the tarsus to the metatarsals and phalanges of the foot. The condition is extremely rare, but is easy to recognize radiologically. The radial form of partial algodystrophy has remained partial throughout its whole course, as occurred in Lequesne's case 1, where the thumb and index finger alone were affected. On the other hand, it may extend, as in Lequesne's case 2, in which the osteoporosis spread from initial involvement of the third ray to affect all the bones of the foot.

Only Dammann [170], as early as 1972, published a report of similar forms. With reference to three cases of Sudeck syndrome, affecting only two or three fingers of one hand, he confirmed that the Sudeck syndrome is a matter not of a general disease but of locally restricted neurodystrophic disturbance of the tissue vascularization.

In *the zonal type*, the localized area of demineralization, particularly in relation to the hip or the knee, was observed to involve either the medial or lateral condyle of the femur or a single quadrant of the femoral head. The resultant radiographic pattern is unusual and is open to serious diagnostic error. The zonal form appears to be the first manifestation of the more generalized disorder. This zonal form of algodystrophy appears to be somewhat rare and so far unappreciated. This partial form was not mentioned by Schiano et al. [727] who collected 479 references on this subject and presented 103 personal cases of algodystrophy in 1976. Serre et al. [754] described a few rare instances of monostotic involvement, involving the patella alone. Corbett et al. [146] published four cases of pain in the knee associated with osteoporosis of the patella. In three a neurologic lesion at the appropriate spinal segment was present, and the fourth patient, who was hysterical, had an anatomic disturbance. The authors believe that these four patients had a "neurovascular dystrophy similar to that described by Sudeck." Bacri and Mutin [29] observed a local osteoporosis of the sixth cervical vertebra after herpes zoster.

We have observed two cases of partial algodystrophy involving only the head of a metatarsal (Fig. 18), of which one showed a secondary extension to the second and third rays of the foot.

II. Highly Localized or Parcellar Algodystrophy (Fig. 19)

Two of us [210] have described a form of algodystrophy which may, like all other forms of algodystrophy, present in a mono- or plurifocal form, either from the onset, or delayed with regard to the initial episode; this leads one to consider this new radioclinical form as a simple modality of algodystrophy of the limbs, intermediate between the forms which show no radiologic anomaly during the entire course, and the complete and extensive forms with major radiographic signs. With reference to 7 cases, the authors described a peculiar form of algodystrophy characterized by an almost punctual pain. The roentgenograms show an extremely confined area of demineralization with unsharp limits, the contours of the cortical bone remaining unaffected. This demineralization is only visible on axial projections of the knee flexed at 90°, in 4 cases, whereas all other projections showed no anomaly. In two cases it was the lateral projection of the knee which displayed the small demineralized area. In one case, it was located on the cuboid bone.

In 6 of the 7 cases the affection remained strictly confined and parcellar. In the seventh case, it later showed the classical locoregional extension as in Lequesne's cases of partial algodystrophy.

III. Algodystrophy of the Upper Limb

In their most complete forms, algodystrophies of the upper limb affect both the shoulder and the hand together, producing what is generally called the shoulder-hand syndrome, in spite of the criticisms to which this term is open. Radiographs demonstrate the increased radiotranslucency of the bones of the hand; demineralization extends more or less far to the bones of the forearm and arm. Besides the strictly bipolar changes, demineralization spreading to the skeleton of the upper limb, including the diaphyses, may be seen, but this is rare. In 53 algodystrophies of the upper limb, Schiano et al. [727] only twice noted *diaphyseal demineralization.* Less rarely one sees radiologic *involvement of the elbow* with or without clinical and/or scintigraphic involvement. May et al. [549] report 6 such cases among 30 patients. Schiano et al. [727] found it two times in 30 shoulder-hand syndromes without clinical involvement of the elbow.

Involvement of the hand alone is exceptional, according to Faulong [253]. According to Ravault and Bouvier [646] it constitutes the "isolated neurotrophic hand." It is mainly seen in traumatisms to the hand proper, as shown by May et al.'s statistics [549]. Finally, in their series of 53 algodystrophies of the upper limb, Schiano et al. [727] counted 14 involvements confined to the hand and/or the wrist, of which 9 had a traumatic origin.

Exceptionally, the *sternoclavicular articulation* may also be affected in the shoulder-hand syndrome, as was seen in a case published by Ravault [645], but in that case there were only clinical manifestations, without a radiologic lesion of the sternoclavicular articulation.

Involvement of the shoulder alone (Fig. 22). In our opinion, all cases of retractile capsulitis of the shoulder should be classified as algodystrophies. Some other cases of isolated periarthritis of the shoulder, which are apparently trivial from the clinical point of view, could also be placed in this group. This is certainly so for cases of isolated scapulohumeral periarthritis secondary to angor, infarction of the myocardium, hyperthyroidism, etc. The same considerations hold for cases of periarthritis observed in different nervous diseases (hemiplegia, herpes zoster, and perhaps cervicobrachial neuralgia), but also in iatrogenic periarthritis (isoniazid, barbiturates, radioactive iodine). In comparison to the distal extremity of the upper limb, the radiologic involvement of the proximal extremity is less frequent and less marked. Bone demineralization may not be present but it is sometimes possible to observe dappled osteoporosis of the humeral head, on the great tuberosity, extending sometimes to the glenoid cavity and the acromion.

IV. Algodystrophy of the Foot
(Figs. 2, 3, 9, 13, 15)

The foot is indisputably the most frequent site for algodystrophy. Serre et al. [754] report 117 cases of involvement of the foot out of 188 involvements of the lower limb. In their series, Schiano et al. [727] report 48 algodystrophies of the lower limb in which the foot was affected 41 times, in 30 of which the foot alone was affected, and in the other 11 with another articulation of the lower limb (knee and/or hip).

The delay between the occurrence of the clinical and of the radiological signs seems to be less marked than with the upper limb, the first changes being noticeable after 2 weeks' clinical course, but on the average, according to Belenger [44], after 3 weeks.

The radiological signs are quite similar to those seen in the upper limb, but the diffuse and glassy appearance of algodystrophy is a more frequent feature in the lower than the upper limb. In our experience, algodystrophy of the foot presents radiologically in most cases as a heterogeneous demineralization, ending up with a fibrillar appearance.

Demineralization of the sesamoid bones is a particularly early sign, and should be looked for on the specific radiologic projections (Fig. 14).

Extension of the demineralization to the diaphyses of the bones of the leg is frequent (Fig. 13). Finally, although clinically only the foot seems to be affected, a radiologic investigation of another segment of the same limb or of the contralateral limb may reveal distant signs of algodystrophy. Therefore it is necessary, in algodystrophy of the foot, to carry out roentgenograms of the other foot, of both knees, and of the pelvis.

V. Algodystrophy of the Knee
(Figs. 4, 6, 12, 20, 23)

According to de Sèze et al. [758], to whom we owe the first description, algodystrophy of the knee is rather uncommon. In fact it is quite frequent in rheumatologic practice but often not recognized as such. Sometimes it is a matter of a secondary involvement in an algodystrophy which has already affected another segment of the limb, sometimes it is the only site affected.

The radiological signs appear relatively early; the delay between occurrence of the clinical signs and the appearance of radiologic anomalies is often only 2 weeks. We have already pointed out the usefulness of the axial projection of the femoropatellar interspace for the study of the femoral condyles (Fig. 17) or the patella. For studying the intercondylar area, which is also often demineralized, it will be advisable to performs X-rays on curved films.

Demineralization may be confined to the anterior part of one or both femoral condyles, or to the anterosuperior part of the tibia, or even to the patella. We have seen that in "highly localized algodystrophies" described by Doury et al. [210] the affected area is even more restricted (Fig. 19). Conversely, the extension may occur toward the femoral or tibial diaphyses or to another segment of the limb, or even to the contralateral limb (Fig. 20).

VI. Algodystrophy of the Hip

This is a relatively rare localization in its isolated form; we have found only 160 cases in the literature, but it seems that this condition is also often misdiagnosed. We have seen that association with algodystrophy of the foot and/or of the knee is frequent, in particular in the asymptomatic clinical or radiological form. The radiologic signs usually come 3–6 weeks after the clinical onset, but the delay of appearance of demineralization can be 3 months or even more. Thus, a normal early roentgenographic investigation does not rule out a diagnosis of algodystrophy.

A small number of algodystrophies of the hip are characterized by the absence of a significant image of demineralization, or merely by a moderate perifoveal demineralization. In the classical form, the film conveys the impression, on the affected side, of being blurred or out of focus.

Diffuse rarefaction of the bone architecture produces three sorts of sign: bone hypertranslucency, effacement of the contours of the femoral head, and accentuation of the force lines.

Bone hypertranslucency is especially marked in the femoral head, where it predominates in the superoexternal and inferointernal area, and on the cotyle, where it is most marked in the upper part.

Effacement of the contours of the femoral head is a frequent sign reported in numerous observations (Fig. 24). Effacement of the border of the epiphysis produces a blurred appearance and may be so alarming as to lead one to perform tomography and even synovial or bone biopsy. The modifications in the femoral head may be associated with those of the neck and, to a lesser degreee, of the cotyle. Finally, *accentuation of the force lines* may be seen in some cases (Fig. 20).

Demineralization of a heterogeneous, multilacunar type is only seen in one-third of the cases and, above all, is an almost pathognomonic feature. It is responsible for spotty, dappled, speckled, and flecked images. While Lequesne [473] found this image 7 times out of 10, Serre [754] saw it only 7 times out of 30 (Figs. 26 and 28).

One can see both bilateral forms (1 case in our series of 21 algodystrophies of the hip) and alternative forms (4 cases in the same series of 21). Contralateral involvement of the hip may occur after a variable delay (1 to 3 years in our 4 cases) (Fig. 24b).

Finally, there may be *total disappearance of the bone architecture,* making the bone look rubbed out, washed out, and optically empty, either delimited or not by a finely traced line. This glass bone appearance corresponds to complete disappearance of the bone trabeculae. When the rubbed out appearance corresponds also to the cortical bone, the hypothesis of an infectious disease or malignant osteolysis is sometimes considered (687, 727).

Whether it is diffuse or heterogeneous, demineralization may overlap onto the femoral neck and the cotyloid area, the iliac wing, the ischiopubic ramus, and even the femoral diaphysis (Fig. 26).

VII. Algodystrophy of the Spine

The problem of spinal involvement was treated in Part 1, Chap. 3. To be able to make such a diagnosis on radiological evidence, it is necessary for the demineralization, which exactly resembles that of osteoporosis, to overlap considerably the possible perifractual area and for there to be no doubt as to the radiologic integrity before or at the time of the traumatism. In conclusion, there exists no pathognomonic image for the vertebral spine.

E. Articular Involvement

All authors without exception agree that algodystrophy *never affects the joint space.* French authors in particular, consider this negative sign an important element for the differential diagnosis. We have included this sign among the criteria of algodystrophy (Part 5). Throughout the evolution of algodystrophy, there is never any evidence of narrowing of the articular interspace, proof of involvement of the cartilage, nor any erosion or subchondral destruction. We have already said what should be thought of Genant et al.'s "juxta-articular erosions" [305].

Only the Geneva school of pathology, with Rutishauser et al. [708], Rohner [691], and very

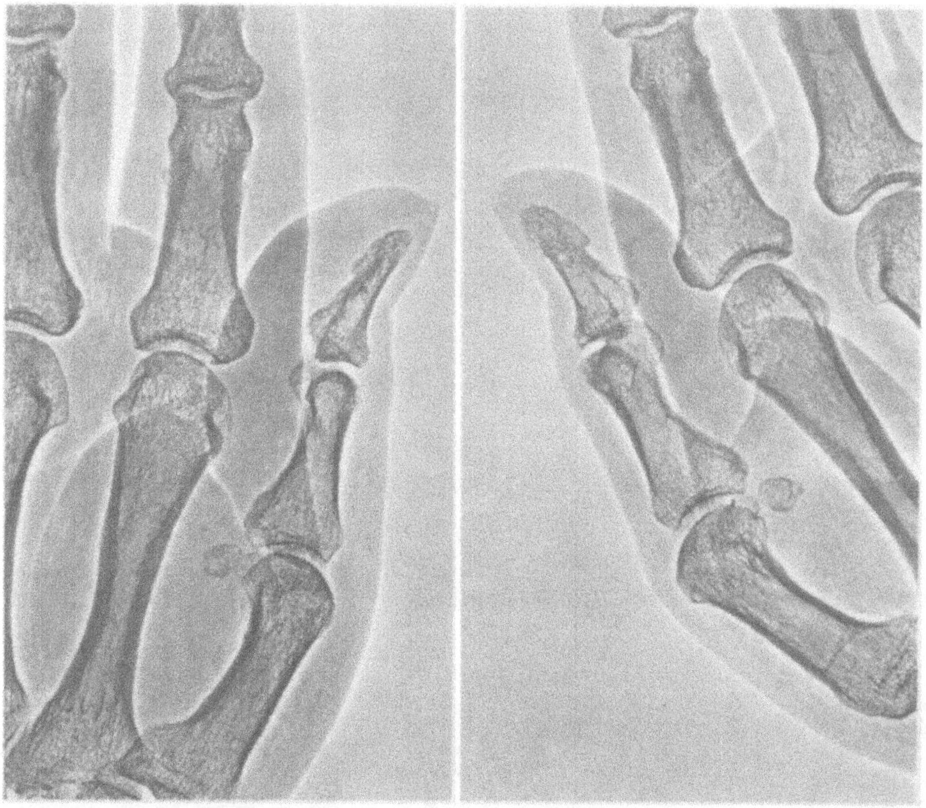

Fig. 1. Xerography performed during the first stage of algodystrophy of the hand, after treatment with phenobarbital. Note on the left the edema of the soft tissues, mainly visible on the thumb. The diameter of the thenar eminence is increased by 5 mm. Changes in the bone structure are better visible on the radiographs than on the xerograph

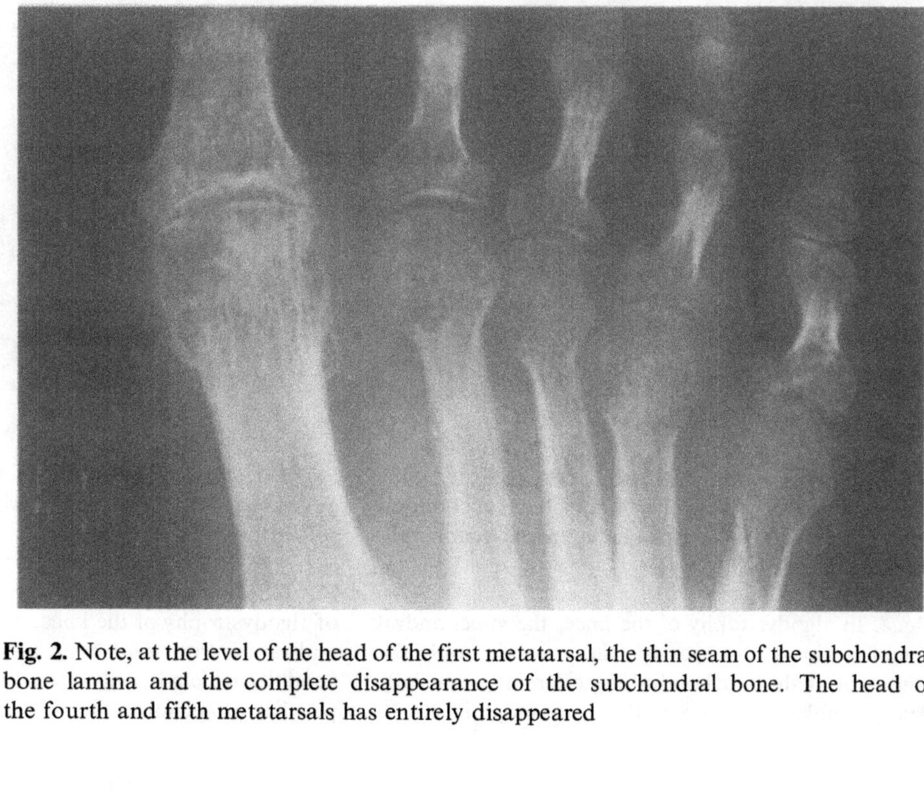

Fig. 2. Note, at the level of the head of the first metatarsal, the thin seam of the subchondral bone lamina and the complete disappearance of the subchondral bone. The head of the fourth and fifth metatarsals has entirely disappeared

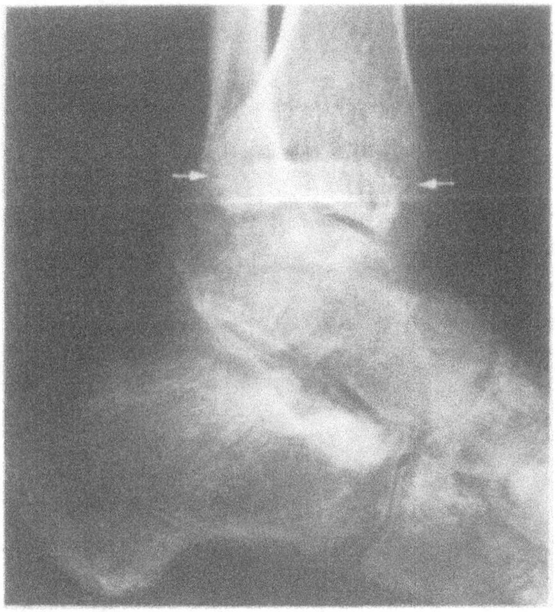

Fig. 3

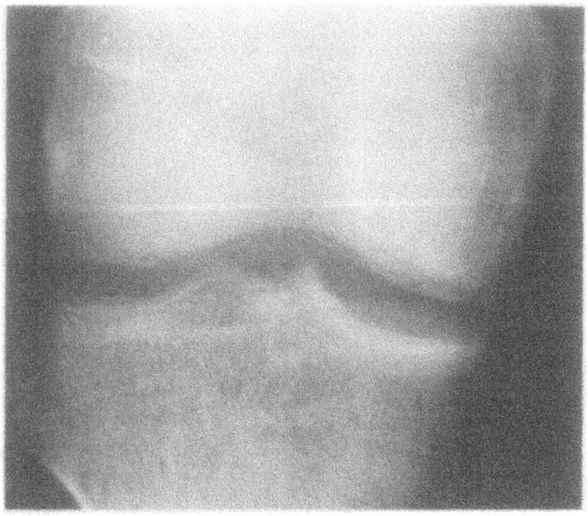

Fig. 4

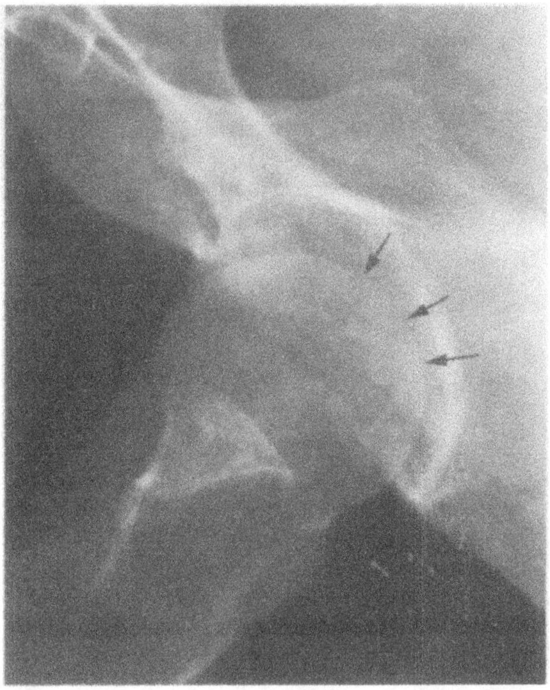

Fig. 5

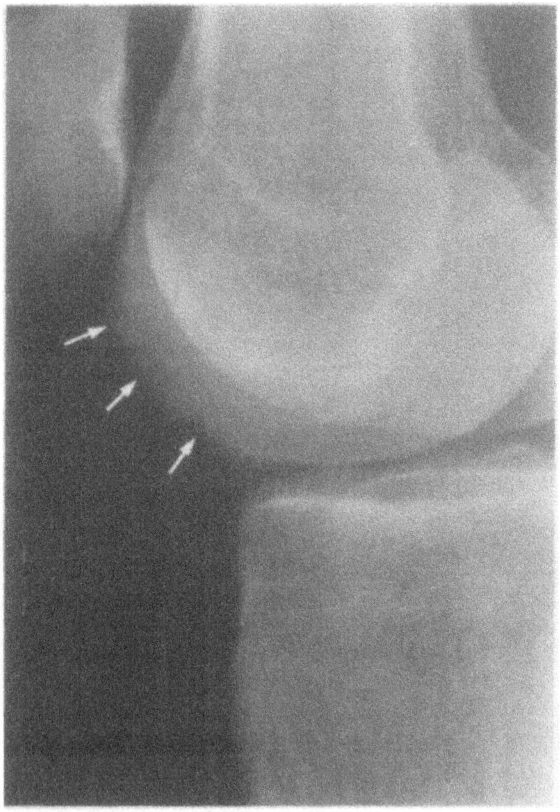

Fig. 6

Fig. 3. Heterogeneous demineralization of the ankle and tarsus. Abnormally clearly visible subchondral bone lamina. Note the strip of metaphyseal demineralization (→)

Fig. 4. In algodystrophy of the knee, the subchondral bone has almost disappeared; there remains only the thin seam of the subchondral bone lamina, especially clearly visible in the area of the intercondyloid notch

Fig. 5. Unsharp appearance of the contour of the femoral head, the axial part of which has almost disappeared (→)

Fig. 6. False lateral projection of the knee, in a case of algodystrophy of the knee. Note the marked demineralization with total bone loss involving the medial condyle, which is only visualized by means of this peculiar projection (→)

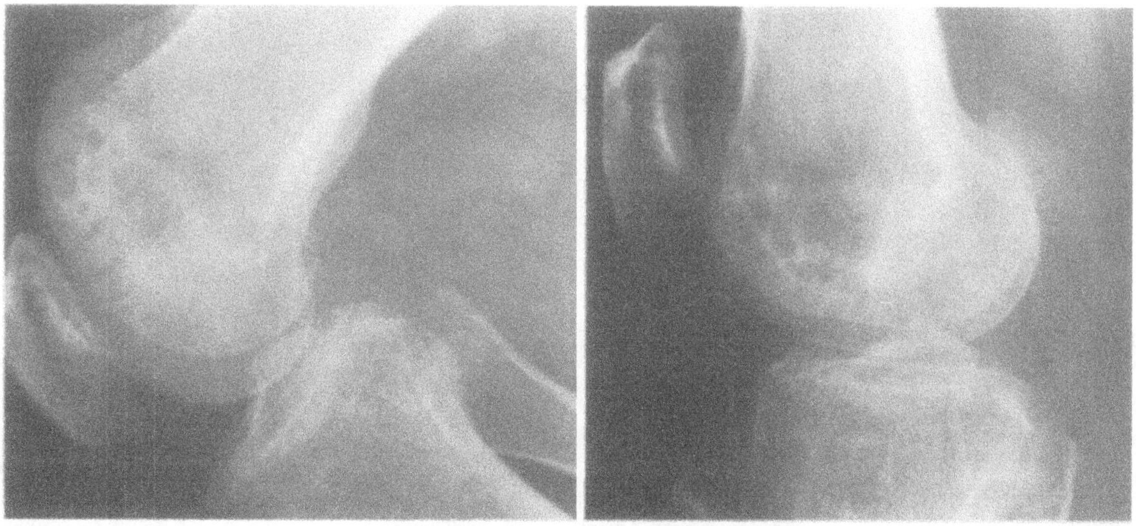

Fig. 7

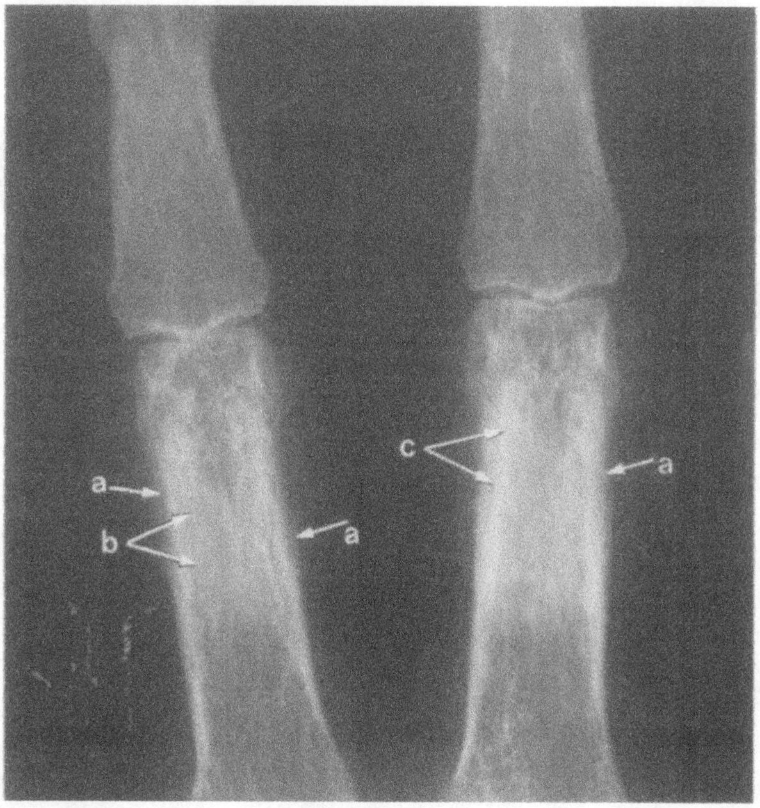

Fig. 8

Fig. 7. Lacunar demineralization of the subchondral bone in two cases of algodystrophy of the knee. The size of the lacunae is variable

Fig. 8. Resorption of cortical bone. *a* (→) subperiosteal resorption providing an irregular appearance of the external aspect of the cortex; *b* (→) endosteal resorption with irregularities of the inner surface; *c* (→) Intracortical resorption with the image of elongated cavities within the cortical bone (direct magnification)

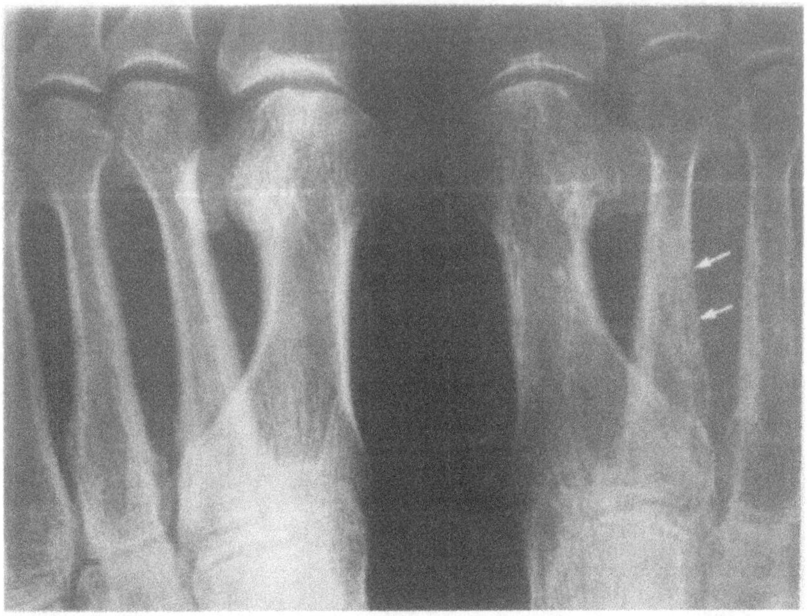

Fig. 9

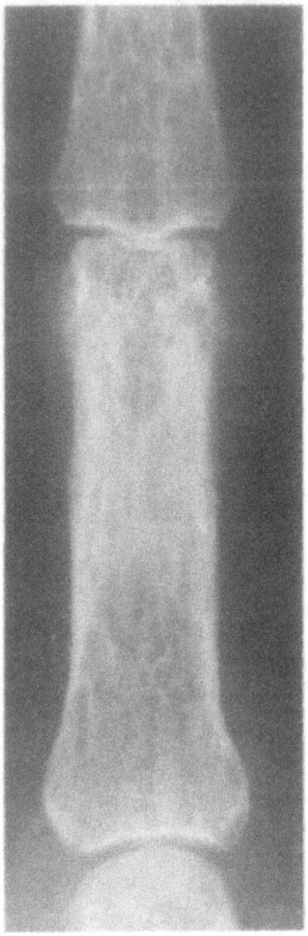

Fig. 11

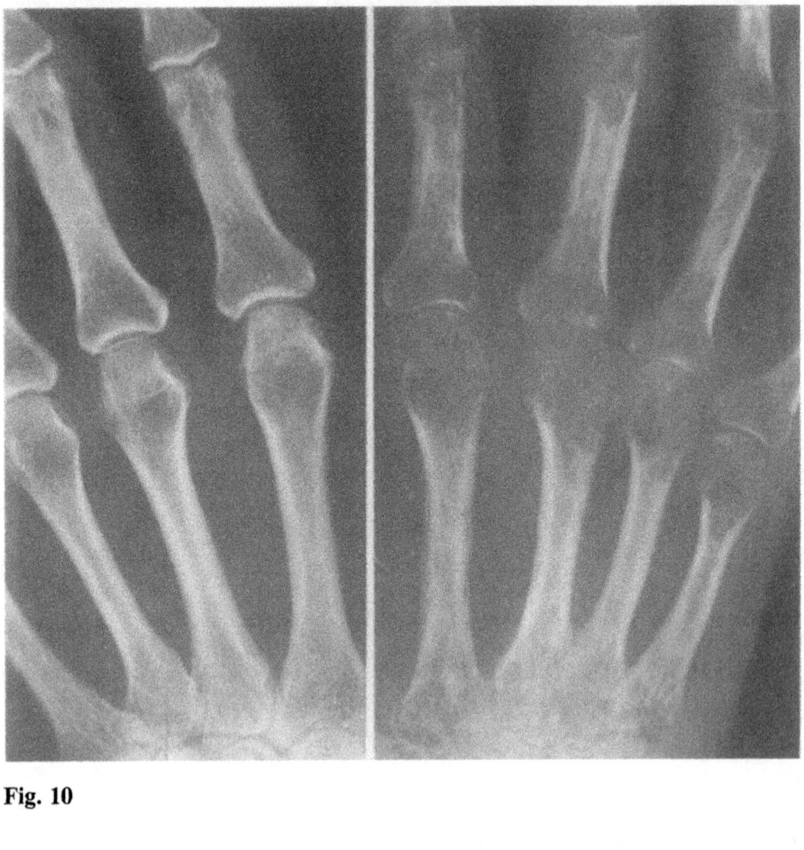

Fig. 10

Fig. 11. Thinned cortices and irregular appearance of the internal surfaces. The cortical bone has a lamellar and striated appearance (direct magnification)

Fig. 9. Note on the right the thinning of the cortical bone of the second metatarsal. In some places it has almost disappeared (→). The opposite side is reproduced for comparison

Fig. 10. On the right, irregular margins; thinning and intracortical resorption of the metacarpals and first phalanges. The opposite side is shown for comparison

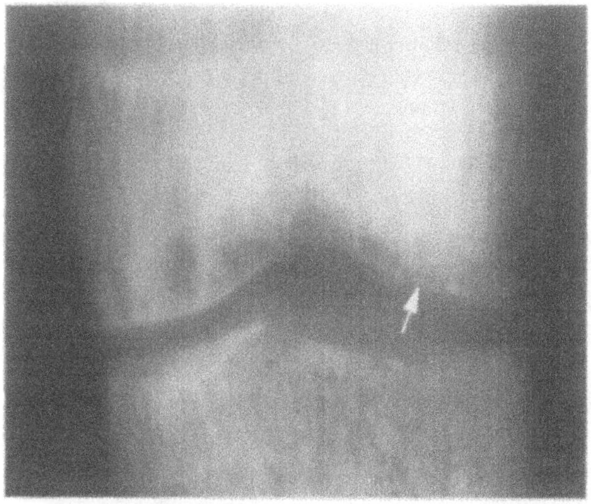

Fig. 12. Frontal tomogram of an algodystrophic knee. Juxta-articular erosion by resorption of subchondral bone (→) on the lateral femoral condyle

Fig. 13. Patchy osteoporosis of the ankle and of the foot. Note disseminated lacunae of variable size in the epiphyses of both bones of the leg up to the diaphyses. This image is also seen in the bones of the tarsus, in particular on the lateral view of the calcaneum. On frontal and lateral views of the talus, note areas of homogeneous demineralization caused by the confluence of the lacunae (→)
▼

recently Lagier and Van Linthoudt [439, 440], reports macroscopic, histologic, and radiologic articular lesions.

The question arises whether it is a matter of algodystrophy appearing in articulations previously affected by arthrosis or arthritis, which is not exceptional. Indeed, in our series of 250 cases, algodystrophy occurred three times in rheumatoid arthritis, one time in a Reiter syndrome and one time in ankylosing spondylarthritis.

Review of the various published cases seems to show that articular involvement occurs in long-standing and severe algodystrophies, although Rohner [691] has published cases with this type of lesion in evolutions of less than 1 year. Lagier and Van Linthoudt [439] recall the pathologic signs: dissection in depth with duplication of the subchondral bone plate; superficial dedifferentiation with fibrous or even bony ankylosis. There can be additional capsuloligamentary ossification and corticoperiosteal remodeling. According to these authors, there could exist a dystrophic factor affecting the soft tissues of the articulation. They think it more realistic, however, to attribute the condition to immobilization. Going even farther, these authors believe that such cases are reason to reconsider the possible participation of immobilization in the genesis of some rheumatic changes

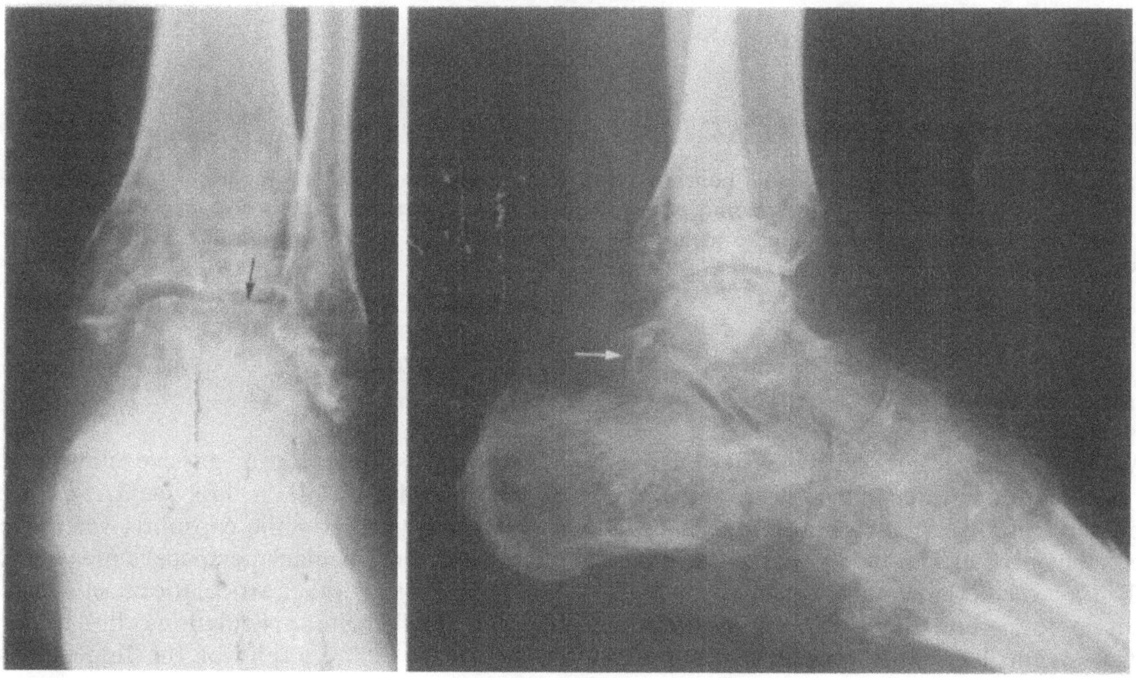

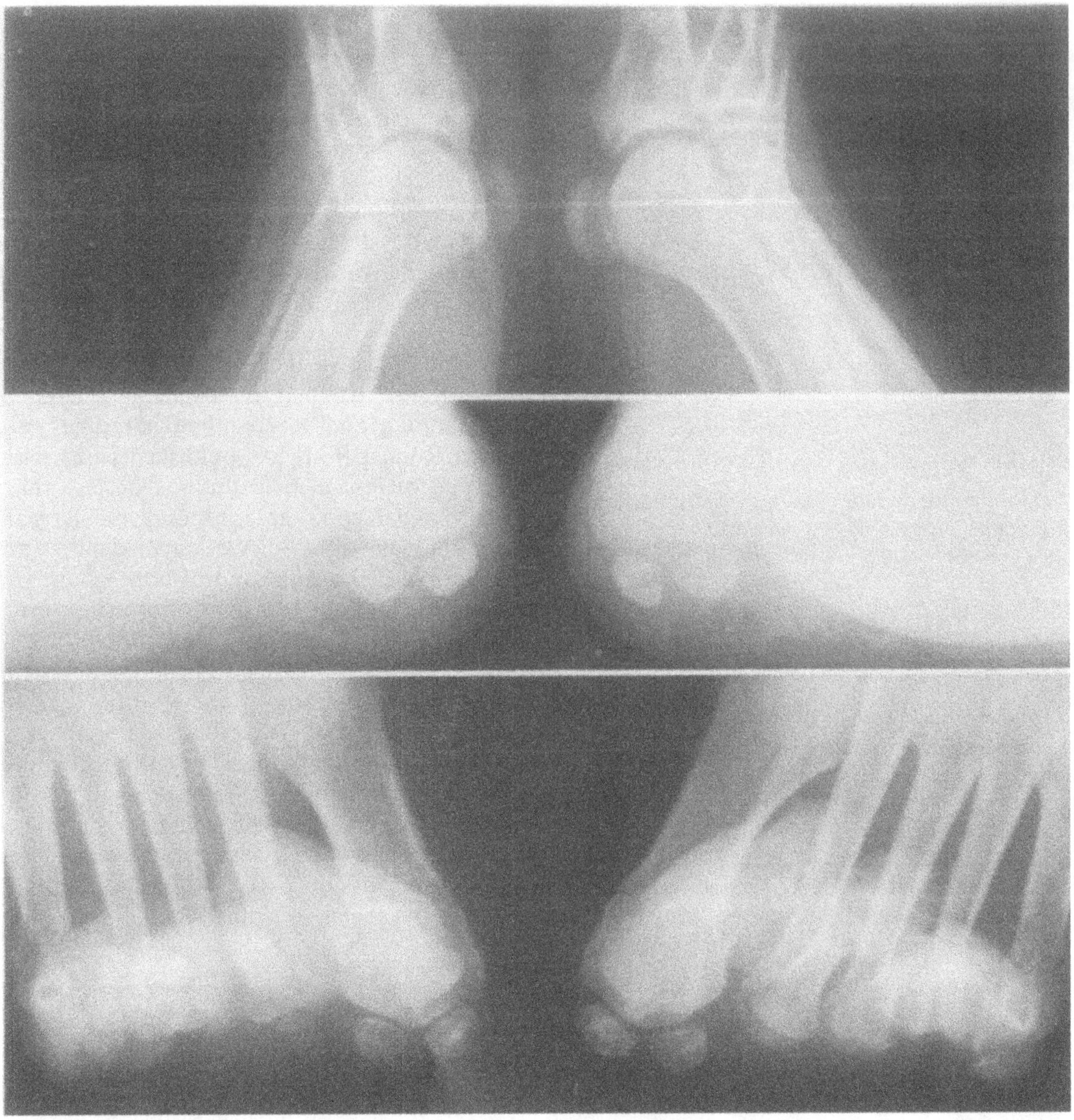

a

b

c

Fig. 14a–c. Involvement of the sesamoid bones: **a** on the left, in lateral projection of the sesamoid; **b** on the right, involvement of the sesamoid evidenced by a Walter-Muller projection; **c** on the right, sequellar form of algodystrophy; on the left, alternative evolutive form. Note the smooth and well-delineated appearance of the microlacunae in the sequellar form

classically attributed to inflammation of the synovial membrane, such as cartilaginous pannus and ankyloses.

We have observed a case of synovial or capsular calcification in isolated algodystrophy of the shoulder (Fig. 16). In our series of 250 cases this is the only articular involvement. One might well ask whether including articular involvement in the group of algodystrophies would not mean too large an extension of the limits of algodystrophy.

F. Arthrography

When there is limitation of passive movement of the shoulder or of the hip, we know that it is a matter of retractile capsulitis when the integrity of the articular interspace is preserved. The same goes for other articulations, in particular the small digital articulations, but as far as we know, arthrography of the fingers has never been performed in algodystrophy.

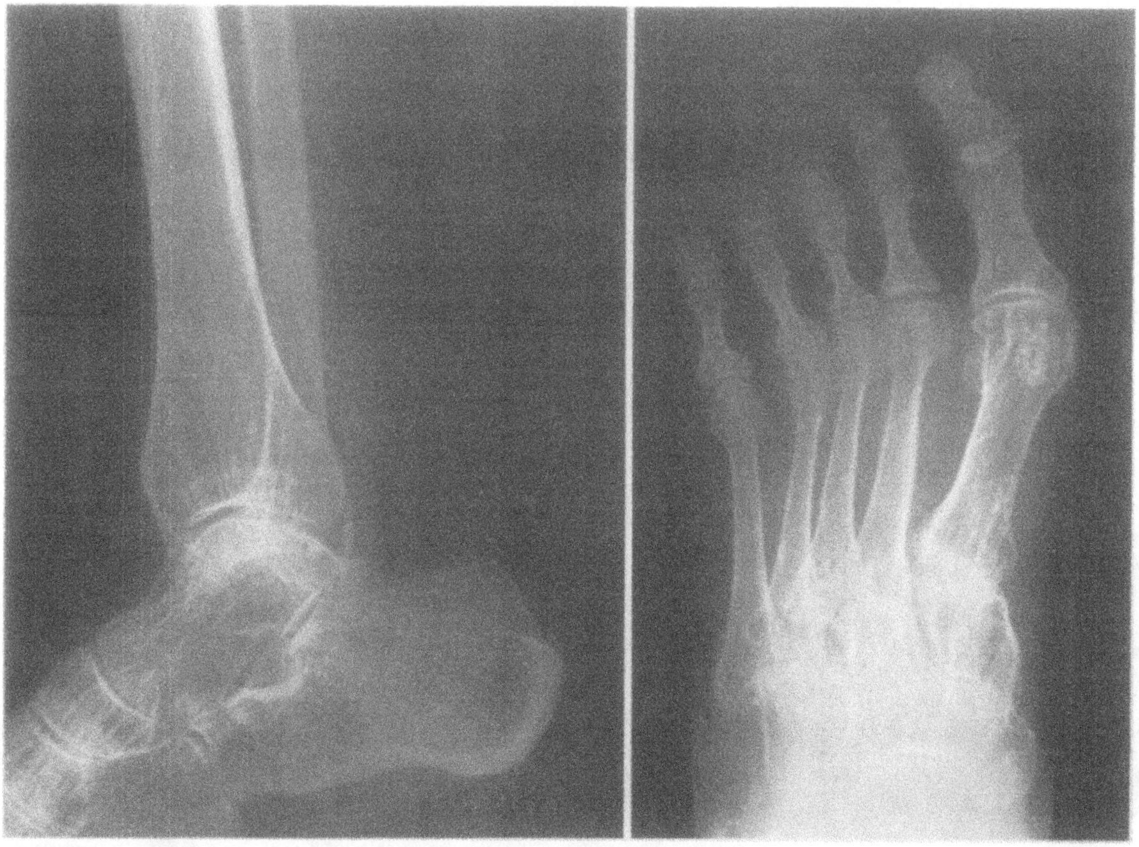

Fig. 15

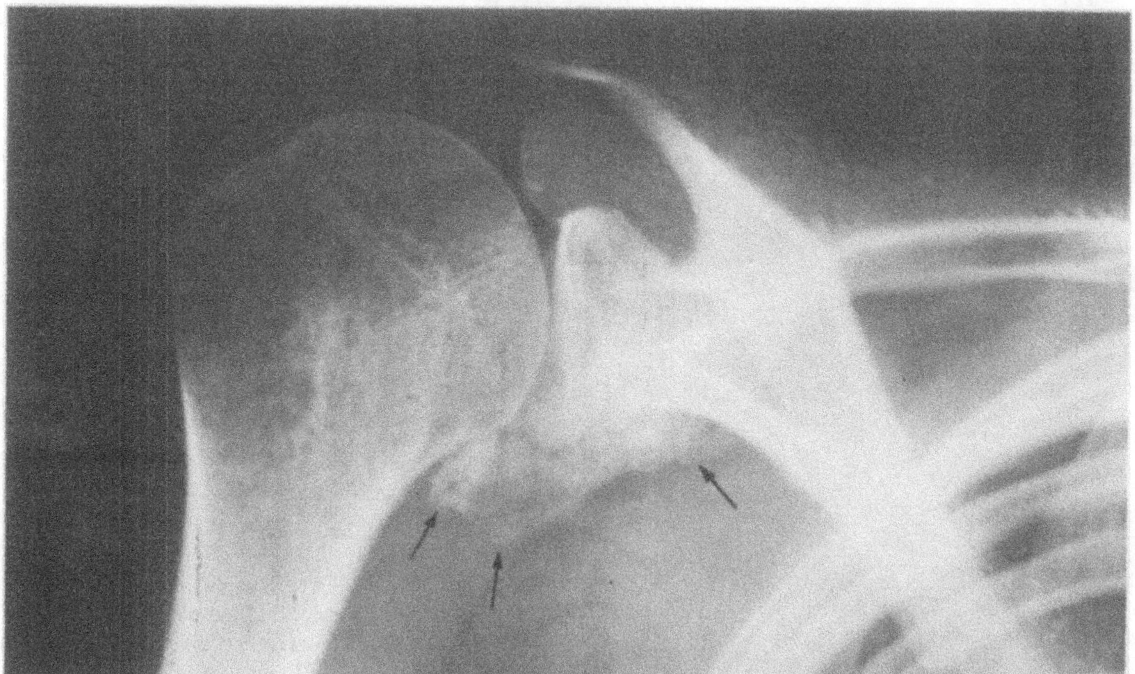

Fig. 16

Fig. 15. Sequels of algodystrophy. Note the atrophy of the cortices and the dense appearance of the bone trabeculae with their fibrillar aspect

Fig. 16. Isolated algodystrophy of the shoulder with multiple microcalcifications which seem to concern the synovial membrane or the articular capsule (→)

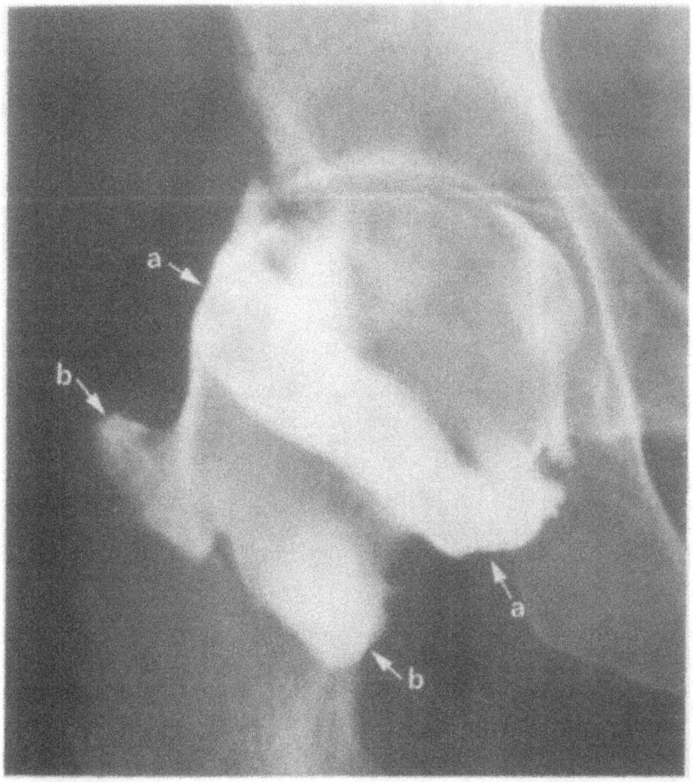

Fig. 17. Retractile capsulitis of the hip. Arthrography: the articular cavity can receive only 5 cm^3 of contrast material. Note the feeble opacity of the medial (*a*) and especially the lateral (*b*) recesses

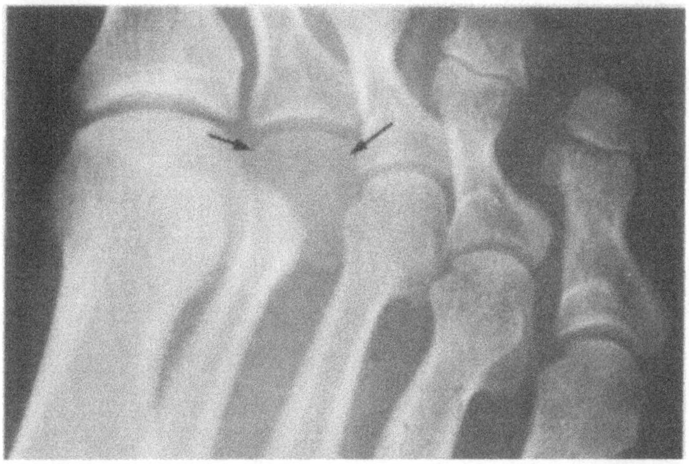

Fig. 18. Partial algodystrophy which manifests itself by homogeneous demineralization of the head of the second metatarsal (→)

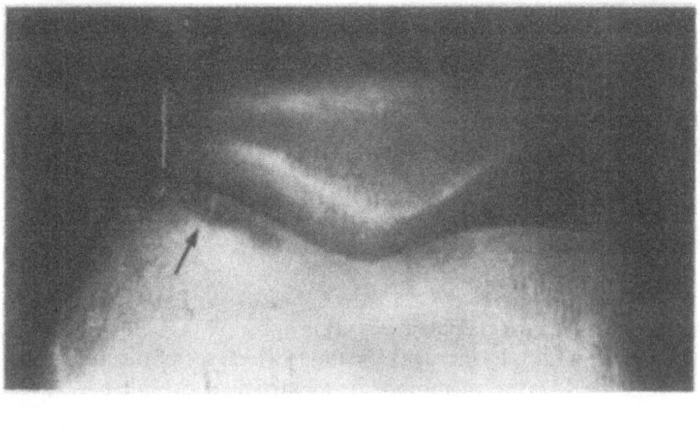

Fig. 19. Parcellar algodystrophy of the right knee. Demineralization with unsharp limits, involving a very confined area of the lateral femoral condyle (→). The subchondral bone lamina is unaffected. This demineralization is only visible on the femoropatellar projection, with the knee flexed at 90°, whereas all other films were strictly normal

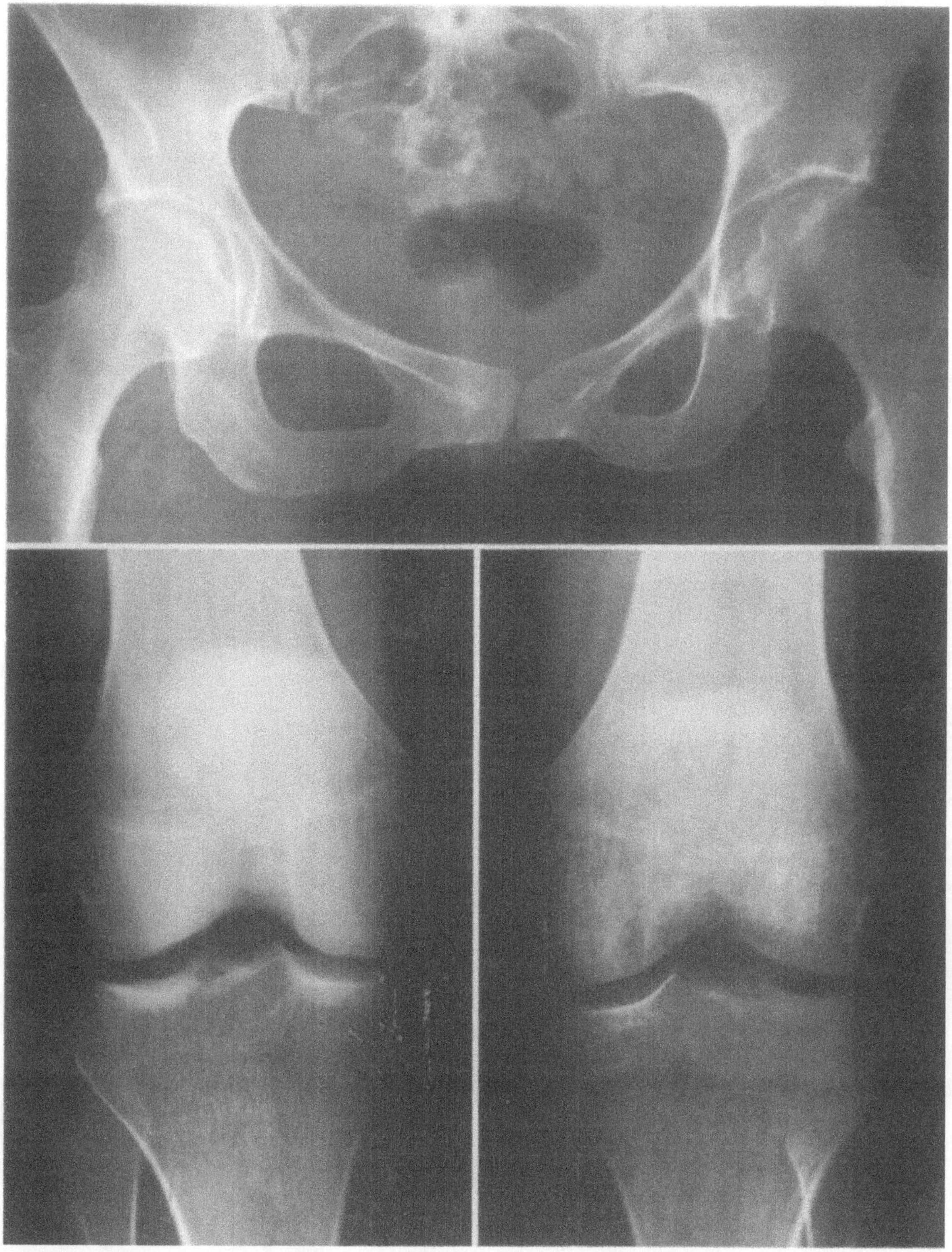

a

b

Fig. 20a, b. Algodystrophy of the left knee. **b** Heterogeneous demineralization of both femoral condyles and of the tibia. **a** Diffuse demineralization of the femoral head and neck, the acetabulum and the ischion, witnessing a clinically silent algodystrophy of the hip. Note the preservation of the bone trabeculae, and also of the femoral head which is even well outlined

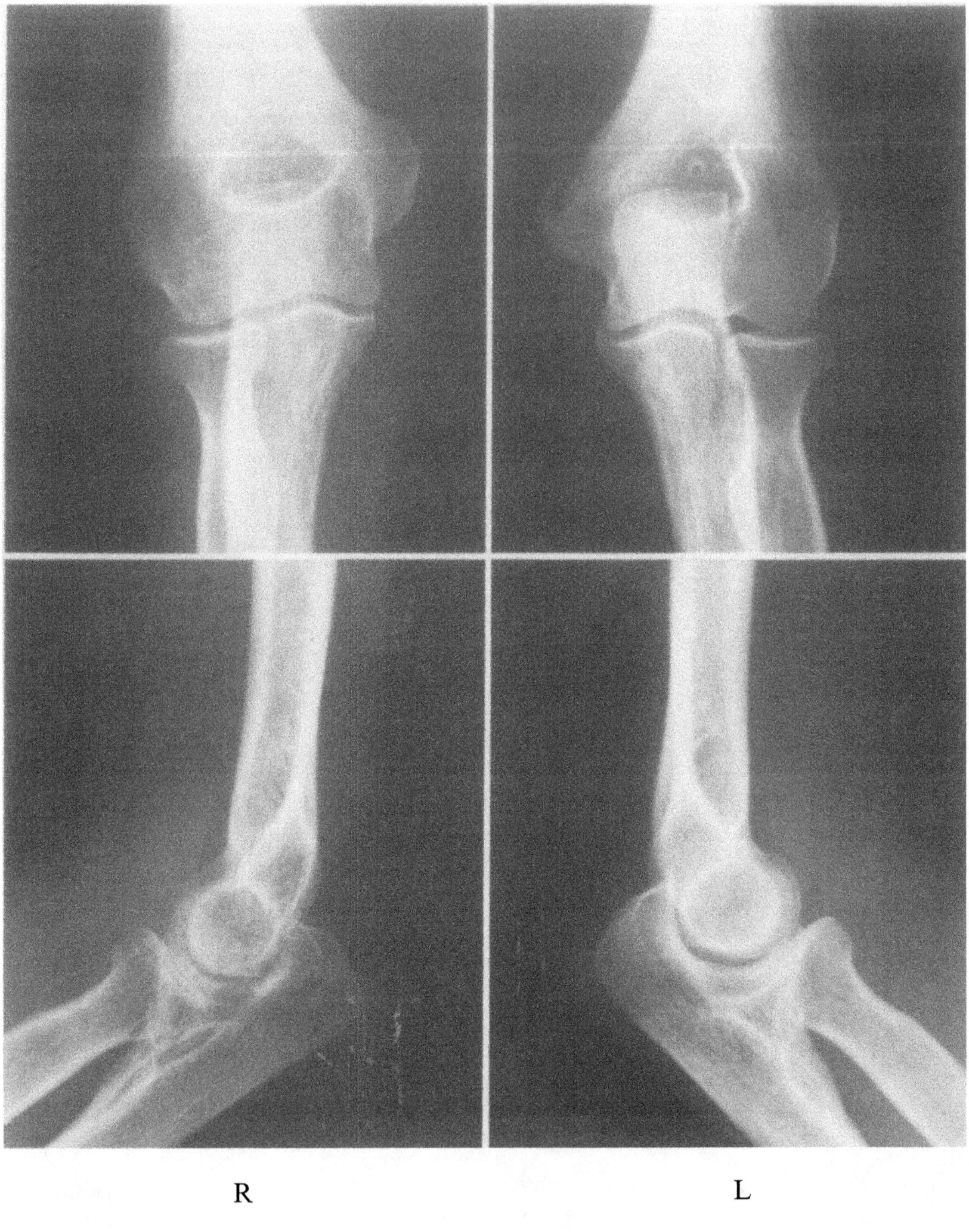

R L

Fig. 21. Frontal and lateral radiograms of both elbows in a case of algodystrophy of the entire right upper limb. Note the heterogeneous demineralization of the right elbow

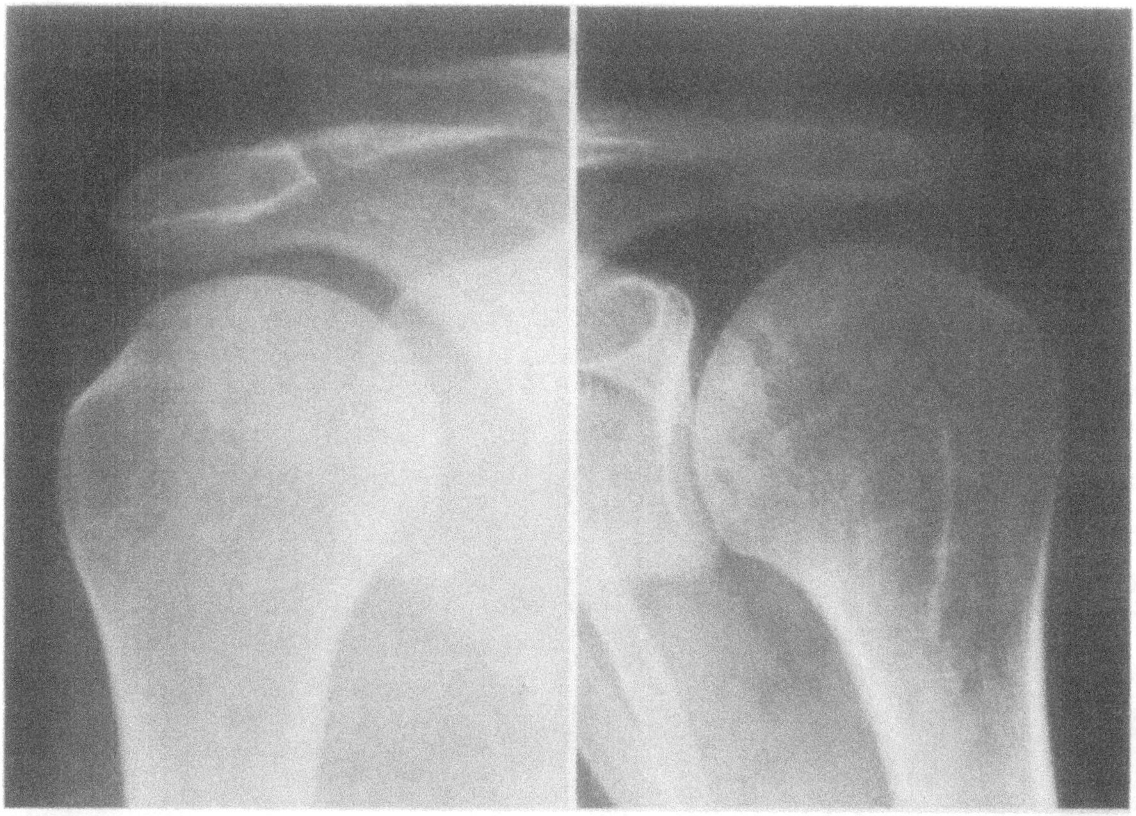

Fig. 22

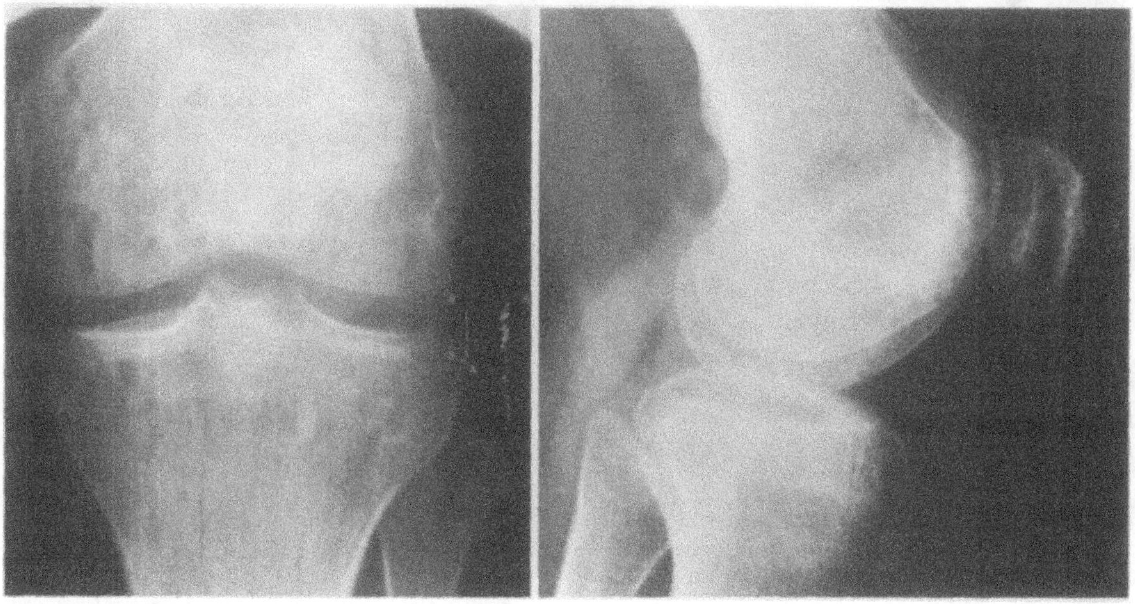

Fig. 23

Fig. 22. Algodystrophy of the shoulder during an inflammatory episode in Reiter's syndrome. Only the humeral head shows heterogeneous demineralization (on the right)

Fig. 23. Algodystrophy of the knee. Note the heterogeneous demineralization involving the femoral condyles, the patella, and to a lesser degree, the tibial plates

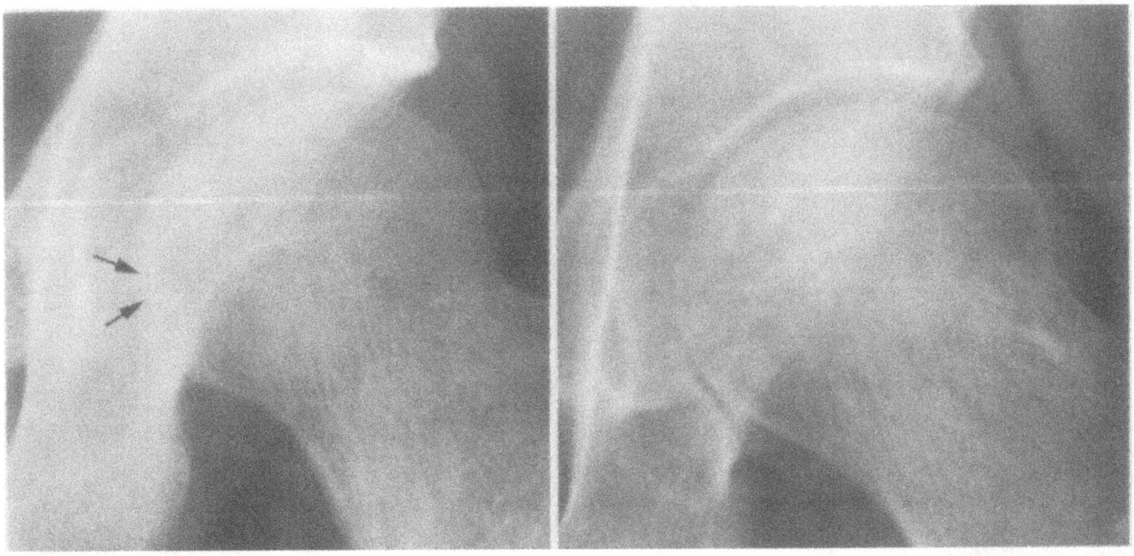

a b

Fig. 24

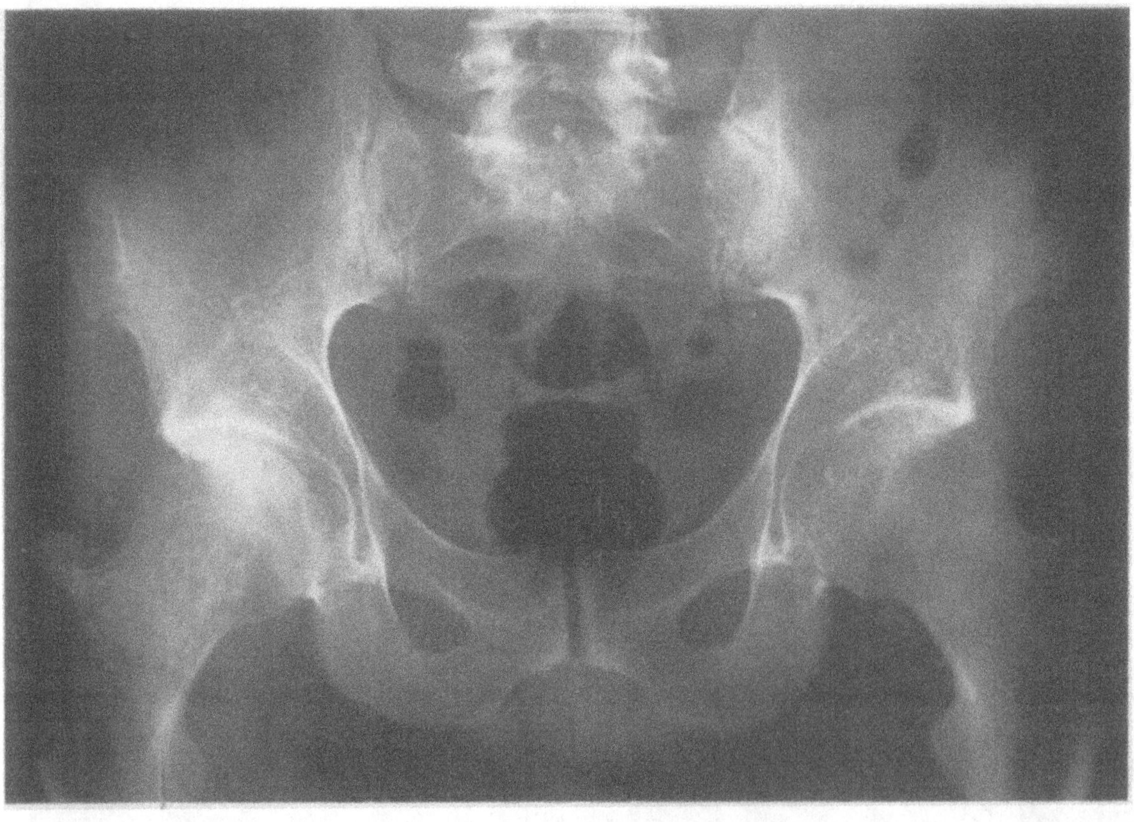

Fig. 25

Fig. 24a, b. Two images of demineralization in algodystrophy of the hip. **a** Complete disappearance of the contours of the medial part of the femoral head (→). **b** Heterogeneous dimineralization of the femoral head with accentuated contours of the medial aspect

Fig. 25. Diffuse rarefaction of the bone trabeculation of the left femoral head and neck and of the acetabulum

Fig. 26. Algodystrophy of the left hip. Note the importance of the heterogeneous demineralization of the femoral head which extends to the femoral neck and to the ischiopubic ramus (→). Note also the demineralization of the upper pole of the femoral head producing a pseudo-eggshell image which is to be differentiated from the image of aseptic osteonecrosis (>→) ►

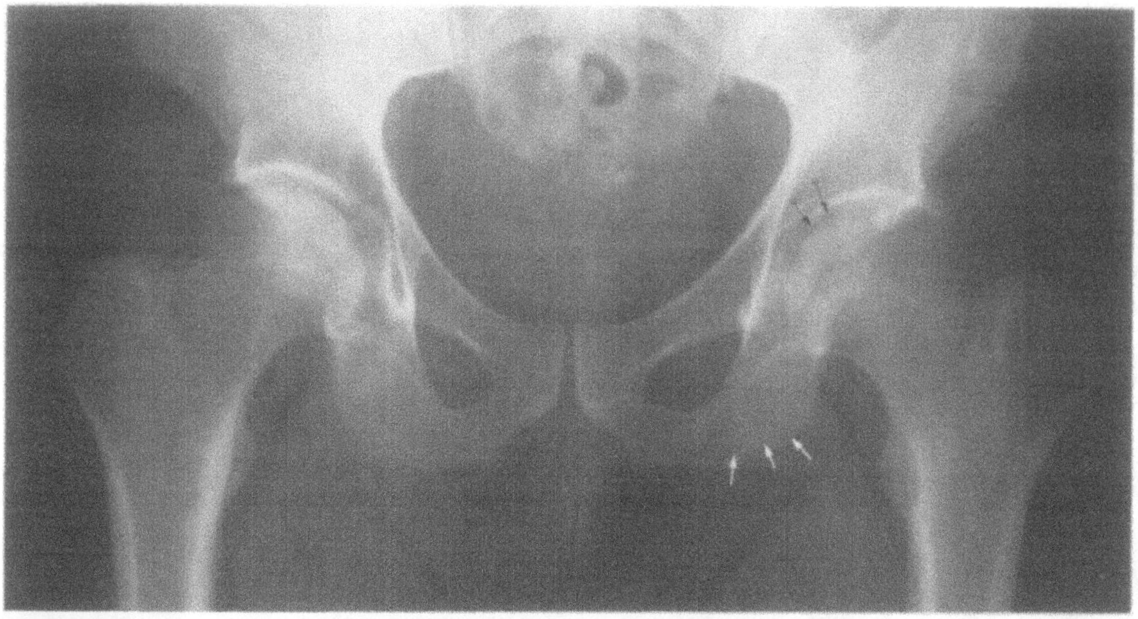

Fig. 26

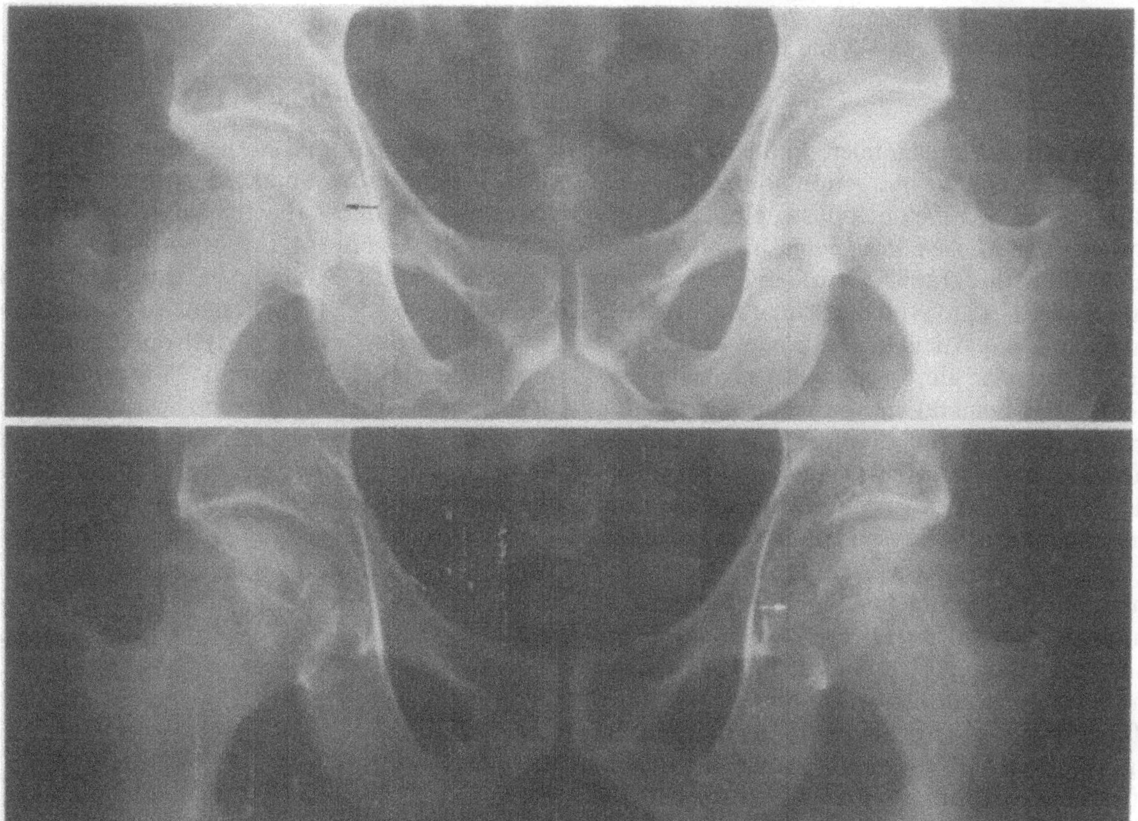

a

b

Fig. 27

Fig. 27 a, b. Bilateral alternative algodystrophy of the hip. **a** 12 October 1972: involvement of the right hip characterized by diffuse demineralization of the femoral head and neck. The outline of the femoral head is no longer visible (→). **b** 1 year later on 13 November 1973: complete healing of the involvement of the right hip and algodystrophy of the left hip evidenced by an unsharp outline of the femoral head (complete disappearance of the medial part of the femoral head contour (→)

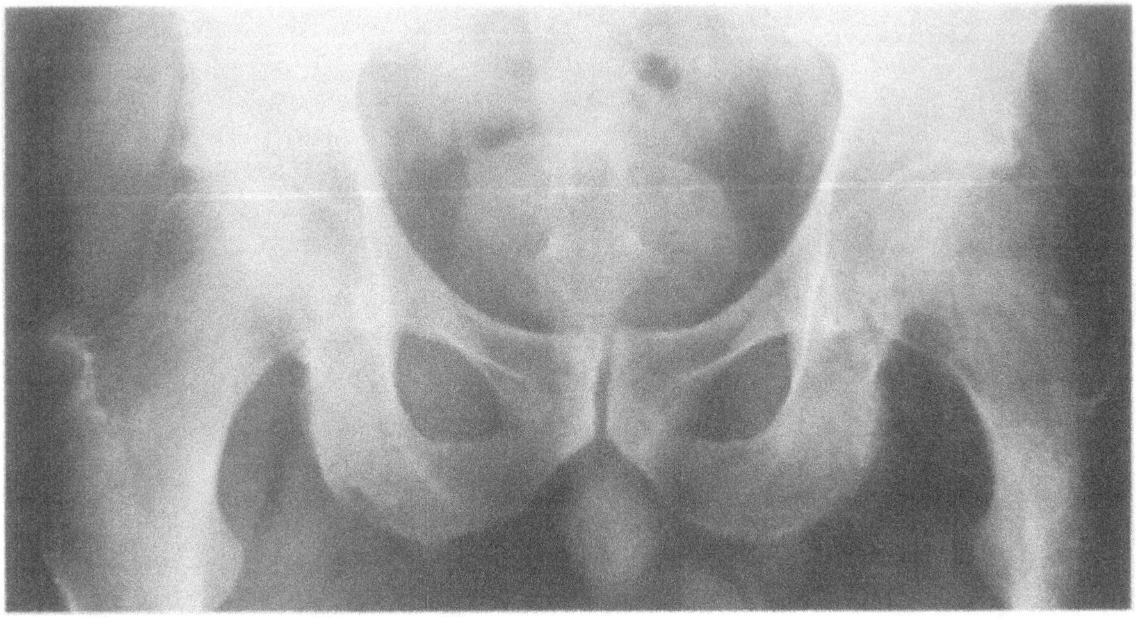

Fig. 28. Algodystrophy of the left hip. Note the heterogeneous demineralization in the femoral head and neck, the acetabulum, the ilio- and ischiopubic rami

As concerns the shoulder, Caillens [113] believes that capsular retraction is probably always related to reflex algodystrophy. He deals only with the *frozen shoulder* in his book, and thinks the arthrographic picture to be characteristic. There is a global reduction of the articular cavity and, in particular, effacement of the axillary recess, with almost no contrast on the surface of the humeral head. According to him, arthrography of the shoulder would also be therapeutically beneficial; he notes improved mobility in the scapulohumeral articulation subsequent to the investigation. He considers it an easy, noninvasive, outpatient treatment, capable of shortening strikingly the course of the frozen shoulder syndrome.

Caroit et al. [118] reported, in 1963, under the term *retractile capsulitis of the hip,* cases of stiffening of the hip without radiological signs, in which arthrography provided evidence of retractile capsulitis. In algodystrophy of the hip, they feel arthrographic images, which have not often been studied yet, would sometimes be normal or show a certain degree of capsular retraction. In one of our cases with clinically, radiologically, and scintigraphically typical algodystrophy of the hip, arthrography showed retractile capsulitis (Fig. 17).

Moreover, anatomic studies (Part 2, Chap. 8) show a more or less marked synovial fibrosis. It seems very likely that capsulitis of the hip and algodystrophy of the hip are diseases of the same nature. Although Caroit et al. [118] and Lequesne et al. [478] hesitate to classify capsulitis of the hip with algodystrophies, according to Coste [149] it represents "a form of reflex dystrophy of this articulation." Study of the various cases published, and our own cases, lead us to consider including capsular retraction of the hip within the algodystrophy group, since it seems to be only a peculiar form of algodystrophy.

G. Arteriography

This examination has only rarely been carried out, and even then not with the technical sophistications of recent years. As with standard radiography, it is necessary to investigate both sides so as to be able to compare the affected side with the unaffected. This requires simultaneous bilateral injection.

Arteriography is strictly normal, as a rule. Soulié et al. [772] have however reported a case of diffuse, filiform narrowing of the arterial network. Schiano et al. [727] have carried out arteriography of both lower limbs in a patient with stage II algodystrophy, and both sides proved to be strictly similar. Guntheroth et al. [337] have carried out a bilateral femoral arteriogram in a 12-year-old child, which demonstrated considerable dilatation of the dorsalis pedis, posterior tibial arteries, and small plantar vessels of the affected side, in contrast to the other side without specific vascular anomalies. The transit time was one-eighth that for the normal foot. Finally, we have performed an arteriography of the upper limb in one of our patients: it was strictly normal.

H. Pertrochanteral and Intra-Femoral Head Phlebography

For functional investigation of the intraosseous circulation, Ficat and Arlet [257] have developed a certain number of paraclinical methods which are simple and harmless and allow the long bones, and more particularly the femoral extremity, to be investigated. The bulk of this section is borrowed from those authors, who have the best experience with this subject.

Injection of 10 ml contrast into the greater trochanter permits opacification of the drainage veins. Radiographs are taken successively at the end of the injection, 5 min later, and 15 min later. Sometimes additional films are taken after 1 h, after 6 h and even the following day, if necessary. The contrast medium is normally evacuated rapidly via the normal efferent veins of the metaphysis.

For intrafemoral head phlebography, 10 ml contrast medium is injected into the femoral head. The X-ray technique is the same. There is, however, an additional efferent vein, the vein of the round ligament. There thus exists the problem of choosing between the two methods. According to Ficat and Arlet's experience, pertrochanteral phlebography provides better images and is usually sufficient in pathologic cases. However, if this method does not give evidence of an anomaly, it is advisable to perform a second injection into the femoral head.

In reflex algodystrophy, the phlebography is almost always abnormal, and gives evidence of diaphyseal reflux and medullary stasis, witnessing congestion in the venous return and drainage disturbances. The authors also report cases in which a systematic hemodynamic investigation of the side unaffected by algodystrophy showed medullary hyperpressure and phlebographic disturbances in otherwise clinically and radiologically normal hips. In these cases one is dealing with *purely hemodynamic forms of algodystrophy*.

Chapter 3 Scintigraphy

Only recently have isotopic investigations been used for algodystrophy. Almost all studies published about isotope investigations in algodystrophy concern the bone. In the chapter on physiopathology we shall see that algodystrophy is in fact a condition resulting from local or locoregional blood circulation disturbances involving the vasomotricity and producing variable effects on the tissues, ranging from involvement of the teguments to more or less extended osseous involvement. The extent and intensity of the process are also very variable both superficially and in depth.

We shall consider successively bone scanning, dynamic isotope investigation of the vascular areas, study of the extravascular interstitial compartment, and joint scanning.

A. Bone Scanning

The use of radioactive agents to investigate osseous diseases has attracted growing interest in the past decade; numerous studies have been

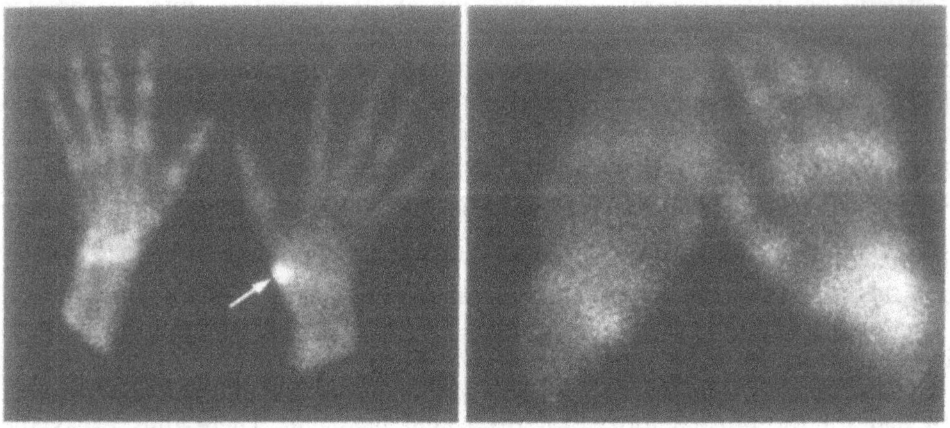

a b

Fig. 29a, b. Bone scanning in two cases of radioclinically typical algodystrophy. **a** Increased uptake over the left wrist and hand. Note in the right wrist an area of increased uptake confined to the point of injection of the radioactive tracer (→). **b** High uptake of the tracer over the right wrist and the metacarpophalangeal and proximal interphalangeal articulations

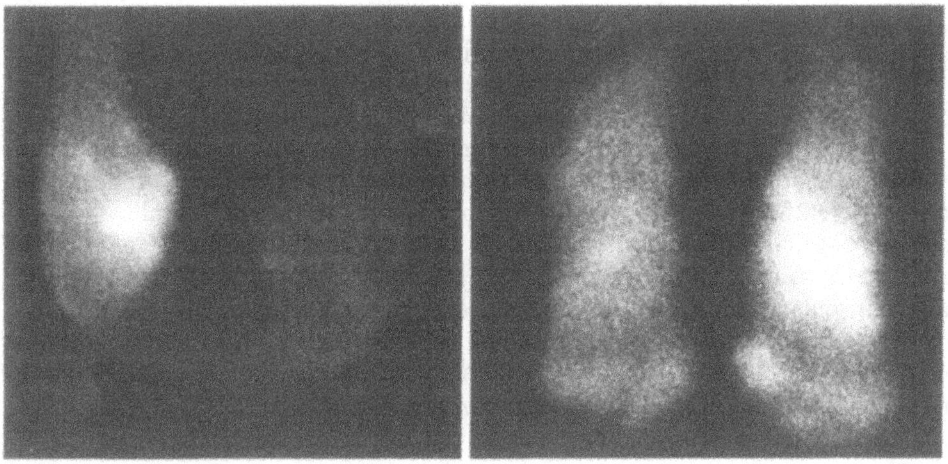

a b

Fig. 30a, b. Two cases of radioclinically typical algodystrophy. **a** Bone scan of the right knee showing high uptake of the tracer over the medial femoral condyle. **b** Left foot: markedly increased uptake of tracer

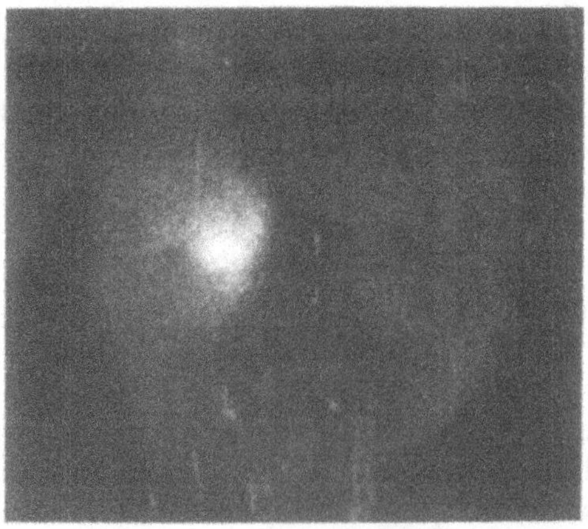

Fig. 31. Parcellar algodystrophy of the medial femoral condyle of the right knee. Note the marked high uptake confined to the region of demineralized bone visible on a single axial projection of the knee.

published, of which only a few concern algodystrophy [212, 215, 220, 294, 383, 430, 610, 698, 712, 756].

I. Technique

The investigation of bone lesions has greatly benefited from the introduction of radioisotopes. Bone scintigraphy utilizes either radioactive tracers which fix onto the bone crystal by substitution (strontium in place of calcium, fluorine in place of hydroxyl), or tracers which fix by absorption on the hydroxyapatite crystal, for example, phosphate labeled with technetium 99m. At present we use mainly technetium 99m labelled pyrophosphates.

The dose injected for one investigation is 15–20 mCi. The corresponding quantity of pyrophosphates is 20 mg. Recording is made 4–5 h after the injection, simultaneously with Polaroid films and computerization. It is possible to obtain either the image of the entire skeleton in AP or PA projection, or segmental views chosen in the light of the clinical data or any pathologic findings seen on the global image. The information can be processed later to provide quantitative data showing the amount of uptake in relation to the topography.

II. Results

1. Increased Uptake

Algodystrophy is one of the osseous diseases for which bone scanning shows the most intense foci of hyperactivity (Figs. 29 and 30). Hyperfixation is a frequent but not absolutely constant feature. It appears very early. In the chapter on radiology, we pointed out that increased uptake at bone scanning can be seen before the radiographic changes become evident.

The intensity of isotope hyperfixation is quite remarkable in algodystrophy; but, like the other manifestations, it varies greatly from one case to the other.

The topography of the isotope hyperfixation is also very variable. The hyperactivity focus can extend to an entire articular area (Fig. 29), sometimes overlapping the adjacent diaphyses; in other cases it may concern only a limited osseous area, or even an extremely small parcella of the bone in an epiphysis (Fig. 31). There exist forms which are localized at their onset, but show the secondary classical locoregional extension described by Lequesne et al. [484], and parcellar forms, described by Doury et al. [210], throughout the course of the disease without subsequent extension.

The hyperfixation may occur only at the clinically patent focus or it may bring to light a plurifocal involvement (Fig. 32). The multiple foci of hyperfixation can remain clinically and/or radiologically completely silent; they can also be accompanied or followed by radiographic and/or clinical changes, as in the case described below.

A 60-year-old man was hospitalized for pain in the root of the left lower limb, with very marked functional disability preventing walking; paradoxically, he still had a normal range of passive movement of the coxofemoral joint, which was only painful at the extremes of the range. A radiogram taken 1 month after the onset showed a very marked, heterogeneous and patchy demineralization involving the left femoral head, the cotyle, and the ischion with a phantomlike appearance of the femoral head and an unaffected joint space.

The diagnosis of algodystrophy of the left hip was made on the clinical, radiologic and biochemical signs (the sedimentation rate was normal), and confirmed by the clinical course. Bone scans showed increased uptake over the left hip, involving the femoral head, the cotyle, and the ischion. There was also an area of increased activity over the left knee without any clinical or radiological anomaly. Healing of this episode was obtained within a few days by calcitonin treatment. $1^1/_2$ months later a new episode occurred with pain in the right knee, demineralization apparent on the radiograms, and increased uptake over the right knee at bone scanning, whereas the scintigram of the left knee was again normal. There was obviously increased activity over the left foot, without clinical and radiographic anomalies (Fig. 32).

This case shows that there is not always a strict parallelism between the clinical, the radiological, and the scintigraphic data.

Increased uptake of the tracer can also reveal forms with clinical signs but without radiologic anomalies throughout the course of the disease, as in the case reported below.

A 63-year-old woman was hospitalized for a sudden pain in the root of the left lower limb which had occurred 2 weeks earlier without any apparent cause. There was complete functional disability and the patient could not walk, but paradoxically, the clinical examination showed a normal range of passive movements of the coxofemoral joint. These movements were

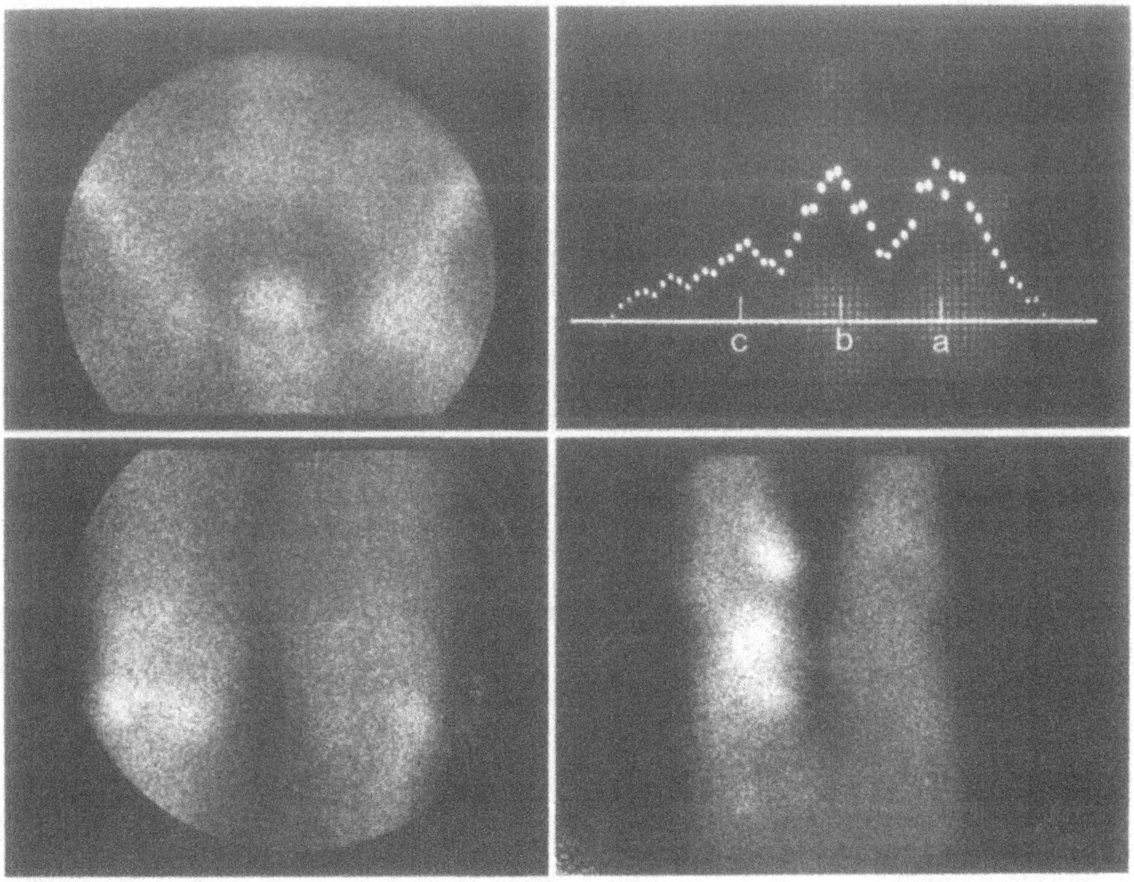

Fig. 32a–d. Bone scans of the two lower limbs. Algodystrophy of the left hip. Plurifocal involvement affecting also the right knee and the right foot. **a** Markedly increased uptake over the left hip. **b** Curve of uptake at the level of the hip. Note on the right the peak of high uptake over the left hip (*a*), in the center the peak of normal uptake of the bladder (*b*) and on the left the peak of normal uptake over the right hip (*c*). **c** Increased uptake over the right knee. Radiologic and clinical signs of this involvement are seen $1^1/_2$ months later. **d** Increased uptake over the right foot. Clinical and radiological signs appear only 3 months later

painful only at extremes of range. Radiograms of the pelvis were strictly normal and remained so throughout the course of the disease. Bone scanning showed significantly increased uptake over the left coxofemoral joint, even at the first examination. The diagnosis of algodystrophy was then advanced and confirmed by the rapid regression of the symptoms after calcitonin treatment. A control examination 3 months after the onset showed that the scintigraphic anomalies had disappeared (Fig. 34).

Duration of hyperfixation is also variable from case to case. No systematic study has been made to determine the evolution of hyperfixation, but the cases in the literature, namely those of Kutzner et al. [429] and our own [215], show that hyperfixation may last 3–12 months or even more.

2. Iso- and Hypofixation

In some rare cases bone scanning can show a normal scintigraphic pattern although the diagnosis of algodystrophy has already been established on the basis of clinical, biochemical, and radiological signs. Thus one of our cases had three clinically evident sites and only one focus of increased activity. Isofixation of the tracer is also frequently seen in algodystrophy of the shoulder.

Some very rare cases also show hypofixation at bone scanning [214]. We have observed one case of algodystrophy of the right foot in which bone scans showed, from the beginning, a very marked hypofixation confirmed by several re-

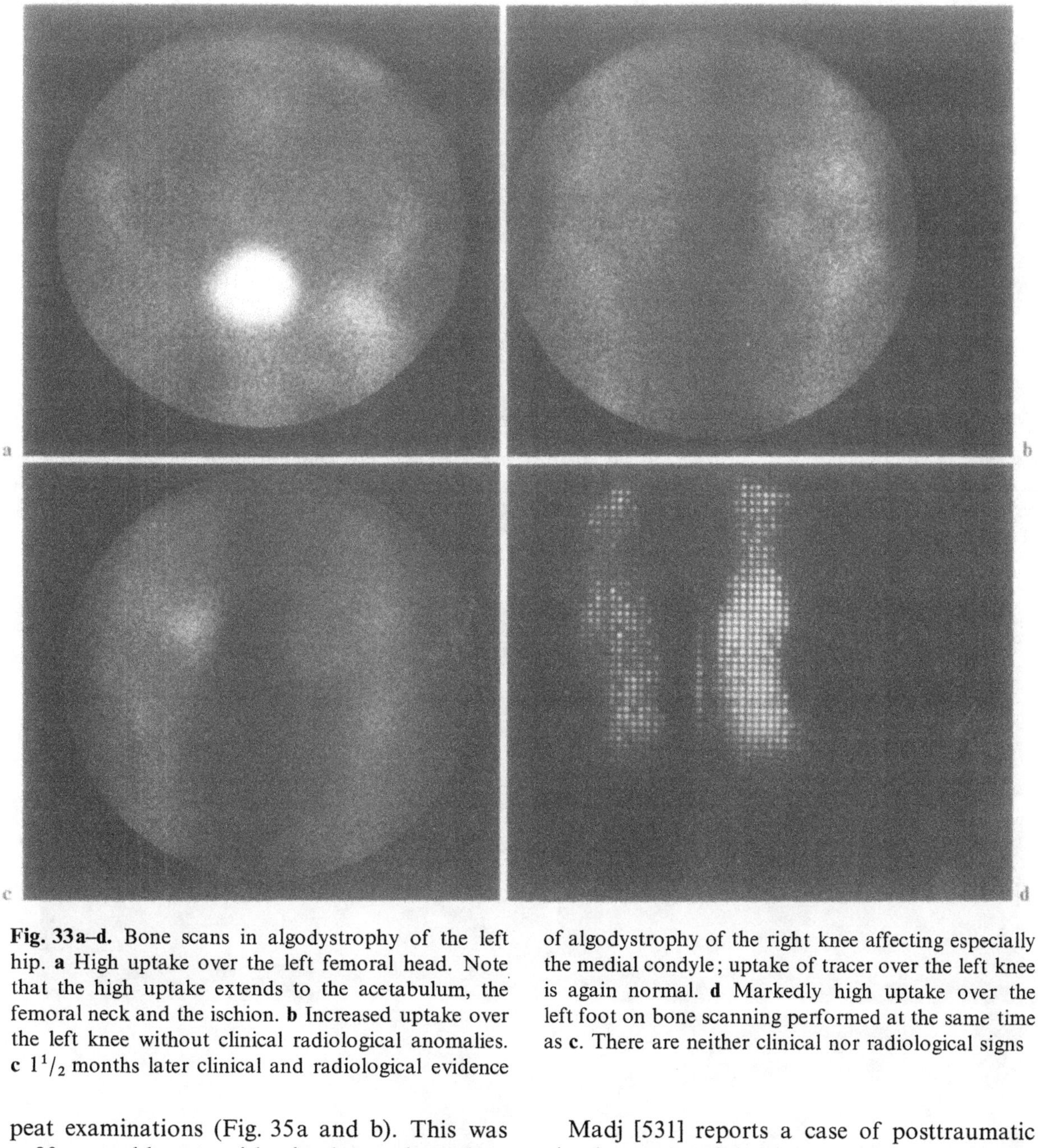

Fig. 33a–d. Bone scans in algodystrophy of the left hip. **a** High uptake over the left femoral head. Note that the high uptake extends to the acetabulum, the femoral neck and the ischion. **b** Increased uptake over the left knee without clinical radiological anomalies. **c** $1^1/_2$ months later clinical and radiological evidence of algodystrophy of the right knee affecting especially the medial condyle; uptake of tracer over the left knee is again normal. **d** Markedly high uptake over the left foot on bone scanning performed at the same time as **c**. There are neither clinical nor radiological signs

peat examinations (Fig. 35a and b). This was a 20-year-old man with algodystrophy subsequent to trauma (a fall on the soles of the feet, without fracture or skin wound). After a very short pseudoinflammatory phase (a few days), the foot took on an ischemic appearance, with decreased warmth of the skin, absence of edema, and patchy demineralization on radiograms. Bone scanning revealed marked hypofixation. The patient improved very slowly. Healing without sequels occurred within 10 months; the scintigraphic pattern was normal by that time (Fig. 35c).

Madj [531] reports a case of posttraumatic algodystrophy of the right ankle in a 9-year-old child, with decreased blood flow and diminished tracer uptake at bone scanning; a sympathetic lumbar block with percutaneous injection of a local analgesic produced increased blood flow and increased activity over the foot and the ankle. The author points out that he observed 4 other cases of algodystrophy in children with lowered activity at bone scanning. This hypofixation corrected with the sympathic block is in contrast to hyperfixation which is usually seen in algodystrophy in adults; the author does not

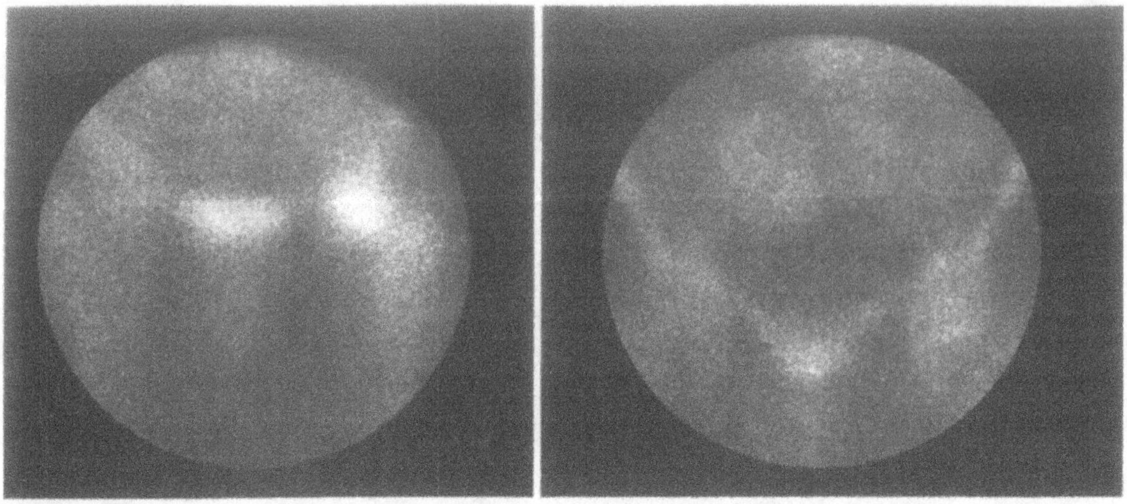

a b

Fig. 34a, b. High uptake of tracer over the left coxofemoral articulation in a clinically typical algodystrophy without radiological signs throughout the course of the disease. **a** 1 February 1977: very high uptake over the left coxofemoral joint at bone scanning. **b** 26 April 1977: the increased uptake has almost disappeared within less than 3 months

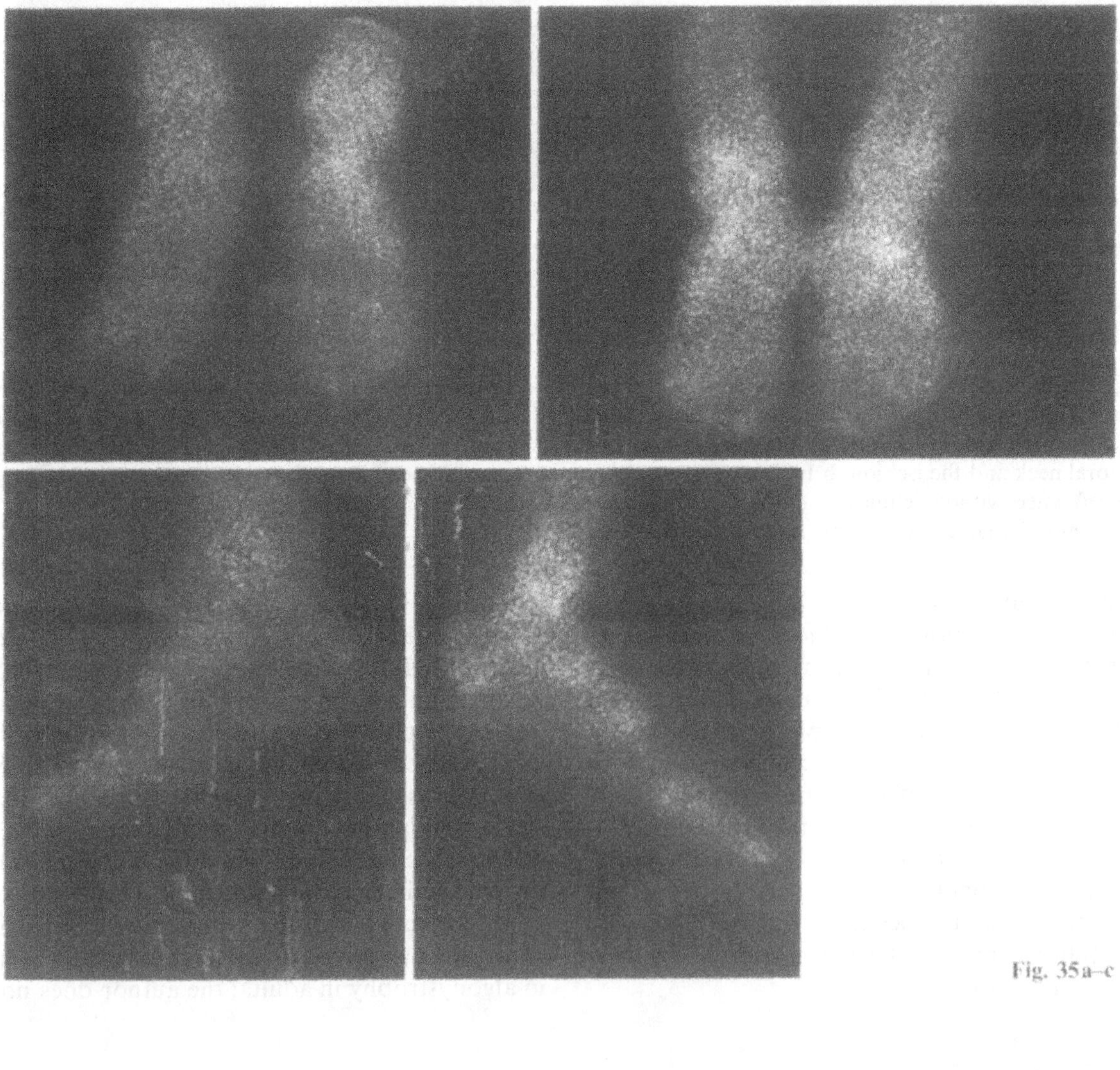

a c b

Fig. 35a–c

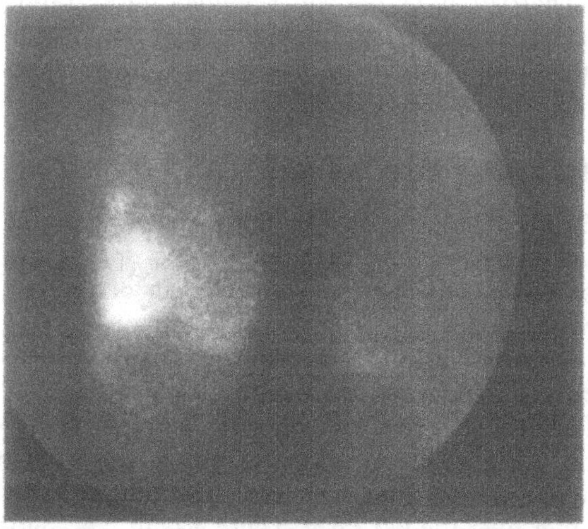

Fig. 36. Bone scans of both knees in anterior projection in a patient with an arthropathy of the right knee suggesting synovitis. Increased uptake confined to the lateral condyle is an argument in favor of algodystrophy

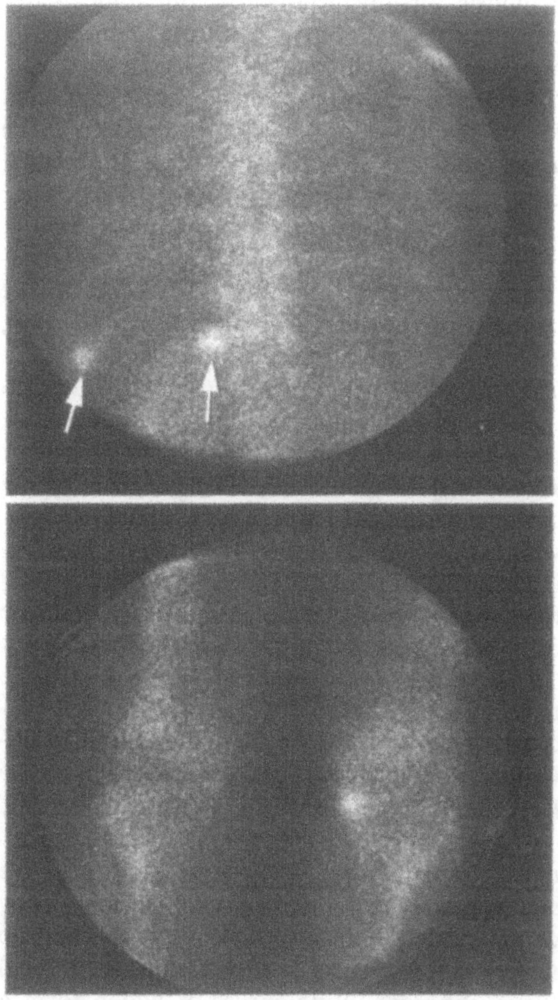

Fig. 37a, b. Algodystrophy of the left knee in a patient with a past-history of a breast cancer. Note (**b**) the high uptake over the medial plate of the left knee, and (**a**) the two foci with high uptake over the right ribs which suggested the presence of metastases (→). These foci were in fact due to recent fractures of the ribs

provide an explanation for the frequency of isotope hypofixation in algodystrophy in children.

3. Usefulness of Bone Scanning for Diagnosis of Algodystrophy

It should be pointed out that increased activity at bone scanning is not specific. But hyperfixation is seen very early, at the time as the first clinical signs. Hyperfixation is correlated to bone remodeling and is thus seen at about the same time as the algodystrophic process, whereas the radiologic pictures witness the calcium loss which is only appreciable when it reaches 15%–30% of the normal bone calcium content. This explains why the radiologic signs of demineralization appear only after a delay of weeks or months, or even never become visible.

These notions are stressed by all authors, in particular Hunder and Kelly [383] and O'Mara and Pinals [610].

The topography of the hyperfixation – localized or locoregional – and its eventual extension to other areas, contribute in about half of the cases to the diagnosis. Among our 74 personal cases [215] increased uptake at bone scanning served, in 38 cases, merely to confirm the

Fig. 35a–c. Bone scan in algodystrophy of the right foot. **a** Marked low uptake over the right foot on 30 January 1979, recorded frontally. **b** Low uptake over the right foot on 30 January 1979 recorded from lateral. **c** Return to normal isotope uptake on 8 September 1979

diagnosis already established on clinical and paraclinical data, but it was the determining argument in the 36 remaining cases.

Increased activity at bone scanning contributed to the diagnosis of algodystrophy before the appearance of radiological signs in 2 cases. Others [295, 672, 685, 756] have made similar observations. In cases that showed no radiologic anomalies during the entire course, the diagnosis of algodystrophy was made only on the strength of the scintigraphic features (6 cases, including 1 occurring in Lobstein's disease).

The site of the increased activity contributed to the diagnosis of algodystrophy in 14 cases of parcellar algodystrophy (Fig. 31), in 2 cases of algodystrophy mimicking Dupuytren's disease or scleroderma, and in 2 cases of algodystrophy with congestive reaction of the synovia mimicking arthritis of the knee (increased activity confined to the medial condyle counted in favor of algodystrophy; (Fig. 36).

The locoregional extension of the hyperfixation may, in some instances where aseptic osteonecrosis is suspected from the clinical and radiological point of view, lead one to consider the hypothesis of algodystrophy (Fig. 33).

Using technetium 99 m labeled diphosphonates, Gaucher et al. [295] made a quantitative and topographic study of the fixation. They demonstrated that algodystrophy of the hip produces an intense, homogeneous epiphyseal focus, the isocounting curves of which form a targetlike image situating the maximal fixation at the center of the femoral head, and locoregional extension overlapping onto the cotyle and the femoral neck, whereas in osteonecrosis of the femoral head there is pure hypofixation at onset, directly related to bone necrosis, followed by perilesional reactive hyperfixation.

Extension of the isotope hyperfixation to another joint adjacent to or at a distance from the affected articulation, whether or not the latter is the site of clinical and/or radiological signs of algodystrophy, allows one to determine the extent of the algodystrophic process, and sometimes even to affirm the diagnosis of algodystrophy (Figs. 28 and 29), as some authors have pointed out [295, 672, 685, 756].

The evolution of the hyperfixation. In some difficult cases, the regression of the increased uptake of tracer, within 3–12 months in our cases and up to 15 months in Gaucher's cases, establishes the diagnosis of algodystrophy (Fig. 34).

Hypofixation by the bones is much more rarely seen than hyperfixation, but it may also contribute to the diagnosis, as in one of our cases reported above (Fig. 35).

4. Limits of Bone Scanning

Besides the lack of specificity already pointed out, we have seen that the isotope uptake can be normal during the entire course of the disease.

In some instances, foci of hyperfixation related to other causes can also be rather misleading. In one of our patients who had had breast cancer 11 years earlier, bone scanning showed two hyperfixation foci, one over the ribs and the other over the left knee. There was in fact algodystrophy of the left knee, confirmed by other features, particularly the clinical course, and posttraumatic rib fractures which had not been mentioned by the patient (Fig. 37).

Finally, a distinction is to be made between images of pathologic isotope hyperfixation and certain asymmetrical patterns of fixation. Note, however, that these physiological hyperfixations are usually very moderate. When there remains a doubt, repeat scintigrams should be performed.

5. Significance of Scintigraphic Data

Hyperfixation is an indicator of the speed of restoration of the calcium pool; it is thus conceivable that hyperfixation could be very marked in algodystrophy. But what is the explanation for cases with isofixation or hypofixation?

It must first be pointed out that algodystrophy does not necessarily involve the bone: in such forms the radiographs as well as the bone scans remain normal throughout the course of the disease.

On the other hand, it is not inconceivable that a more or less prolonged phase of hyperfixation could be followed by isofixation, and then hypofixation preceding the return to a normal uptake of the tracer. Scintigraphic investigation thus provides evidence of one of these three phases, the durations of which may be very variable.

In conclusion, bone scanning is an essential investigation for algodystrophy and the scintigraphic changes deserve to figure among the criteria of this disease.

B. Isotopic Exploration of the Vascular Sector

Rénier et al. [671, 674] have recently studied the vascular compartment by means of a dynamic gamma-angiographic technique: an embolus of 10 mCi of red cells marked with technetium 99 m is injected, and the activity in the area of the joints affected with algodystrophy and of the unaffected joints is then recorded for 45 min by means of a gamma-camera connected to a minicomputer. Following the injection of labeled red cells, the activity-time curves show an increased rate of diffusion at the site of the algodystrophy in 24 cases out of 26, which is consistent with an increase in the vascular volume in the area of algodystrophy (the investigation is carried out about 1.4 months after the clinical onset).

C. Isotopic Exploration of the Interstitial Area

Rénier et al. [674] have also studied the interstitial compartment by means of an identical technique of dynamic gamma-angiography with ^{99m}Tc-pertechnetate, which diffuses rapidly in the interstitial spaces and becomes fixed in the tissues.

Activity-time curves obtained following an injection of ^{99m}Tc-pertechnetate showed an increase in the rate of diffusion at the site of algodystrophy in 23 cases out of 25, which corresponds to an increase of about 80% in the vascular and extravascular interstitial compartments taken together. The increase in the interstitial compartment, i.e., the edema, was above 80%.

D. Joint Scanning

The first scintigrams of the joints were performed after intravenous injection of radioactive serum albumin. Technetium-labeled serum albumin and iodine 131 were also used, and more recently joint scans with sodium pertechnetate have been carried out.

The isotope, particularly technetium injected as pertechnetate, concentrates in the richly vascularized areas: it fixes especially on inflamed synovia, but not exclusively there, so that in the case of algodystrophy it is almost impossible to distinguish what part of a hyperfixation is produced by the synovia and what part by the extravascular interstitial tissues.

Chapter 4 Densitometry

Numerous methods for *indirect radiodensitometry* have been proposed since 1920 but none of them could be used in day-to-day practice. There is considerable divergence in the results published by the different authors and the measurements are very complex [401, 434, 849].

The method is based on the comparison between the radiographic picture of a bone segment and that of a reference object of known composition, which are X-rayed simultaneously. The intensities of blackening of the film produced by the reference object – usually an aluminum scale – and by the bone are compared by means of a photometer. A reference curve permits the bone density to be determined. The method is quite simple and attractive in theory, but in fact there are numerous sources of error depending on the technique of X-raying, the utilization of a film and the photometric measurement [451].

Computer tomography being by definition a densitometric method, some authors have thought of using it for this purpose. Unfortunately it is a very complex method which would have to be adapted to permit routine utilization, but the results so far obtained seem quite interesting.

There are two *isotope densitometry methods*. The first is aimed at measuring the total body calcium [132, 143] or the calcium content of a segment of a limb by *neutron activation*. This technique requires extremely sophisticated equipment so that it is unlikely ever to become a routine technique.

Direct measurement of bone mineral in vivo, introduced in 1963 by Cameron and Sorenson [114] seems suitable for routine use after some improvement. A source of radioactive iodine 125 emits a monochromatic beam of low energy photons (27.6 keV). This beam traverses the bone where it undergoes a certain attenuation; the transmitted beam is measured with a scintillation counter. The radioactive source and the scintillation counter are held rigidly together by means of a mechanical joint. This arrangement is set in motion by a motor in a direction perpendicular to that of the bone under study. Measurements are made every millimeter across the cross section of the bone. A curve is thus traced representing the attenuation of the photon beam resulting from its passage through the tissues during scanning. The attenuation shifts the curve at each point by an amount proportional to the mass of calcium phosphate traversed by the beam. Thus, the area enclosed by the attenuation curve and the baseline is proportional to the amount of calcium phosphate contained in the slice of bone scanned by the beam. This surface can be calculated by planimetry or by computer; the value obtained, expressed in grams per square centimeter, is called the "bone mineral content."

This index is valuable insofar as it indicates the mechanical resistance of the bone, but it does not adequately represent the degree of bone mineralization. The same figure can in fact correspond to a bone of small section which is strongly mineralized and a bone of larger section which is poorly mineralized. For more accuracy this index should be divided by the cross-sectioned area of the bone under study. Unfortunately the equipment does not permit measurement of this area. Therefore we content ourselves with dividing the index by the width of bone marked off by the beam during scanning, so that we obtain a parameter called the "mineral index," expressed in grams per square centimeter.

Direct densitometry is thus a simple method and has an accuracy of about 2%–3%. It is quick and harmless, allowing follow-up of decalcification in man.

We chose to study the radius at the point of junction of the middle and distal third. First we studied a reference population of 73 women and 50 men whose ages ranged from 20 to 81 years [543]. All subjects were whites of the caucasian type. We excluded from this series all patients who could have had an abnormal calcification rate. Account was taken of sex, age, and occurrence of menopause in the women.

When we started this study we were not interested particularly in algodystrophy but rather in diffuse skeletal demineralizations, mainly those related to hyperthyroidism [847]. This is why we measured the bone density at the level of the radius.

In 1971 Goldsmith et al. [316] carried out a study of the bone density measurements in several distinct areas of the limbs (radius, cubitus, humerus, calcaneum, phalanges) and compared them to the density of the vertebral column measured by indirect radiodensitometry [315]. This study showed that measurement of the bone density of the distal extremity of the radius allowed accurate follow-up of the variations in mineralization of the thoracic spine. Cohn's work [144] led to the same conclusions.

Our study concerning the measurement of mineralization of the radius in algodystrophy of the lower limbs is not far enough advanced, and the number of cases studied is too small, for there to be intrepretable results. Moreover we have to adapt our method so as to permit measurements of the bone density of the calcaneum, the metacarpals, the metatarsals and the phalanges, of the hands and the feet. As a matter of fact, demineralization predominates in the epiphyses and eventually in the metaphyses, so that measurements in the lower third of the radius are almost always normal.

Genant et al. [305] have studied bone mineral determinations by photon absorptiometry in 6 patients. "For all the 6 patients examined, the involved hand, when compared with the uninvolved hand or with age- and sex-matched control values, showed evidence of decreased values. Significant progressive loss by serial measurement was demonstrated in all 4 patients having this determination. As a group, the mean bone mineral content of the involved extremities was 1.40 cm^{-1}, as compared to 1.89 for the uninvolved extremities and 2.94 for the controls. Bone loss demonstrated by this technique results from increased porosity and thinning of cortical bone and, to a lesser extent, loss of intramedullary trabecular bone, since all three components lie within the periosteal envelope measured by this method. Both quantitative techniques indicate that the clinically less involved contralateral extremity was in fact mildly demineralized."

Chapter 5 Thermography

Thermography is a method of graphically demonstrating the pattern of local heat emission of a body. The variations of skin temperature are shown as gradations of blackness or whiteness of a film or variations in color. The main advantage of thermography is that it does not require any injection material or irradiation of the patient, but actually measures the heat radiation emitted by the patient.

Up to now thermography has not been used in algodystrophy. In a publication about thermography in rheumatic pathology, one of us [93, 329] reported a few cases. Schiano et al. [727] used the method in 4 patients.

An area of localized or generalized warmth or coolness in the hand can be detected by thermography. But the investigation should always be carried out on both sides to permit comparison with the unaffected side. Theoretically there are three possibilities: the affected side may be warmer than the unaffected (Figs. 38 and 39), or both sides may be identical, when the disease

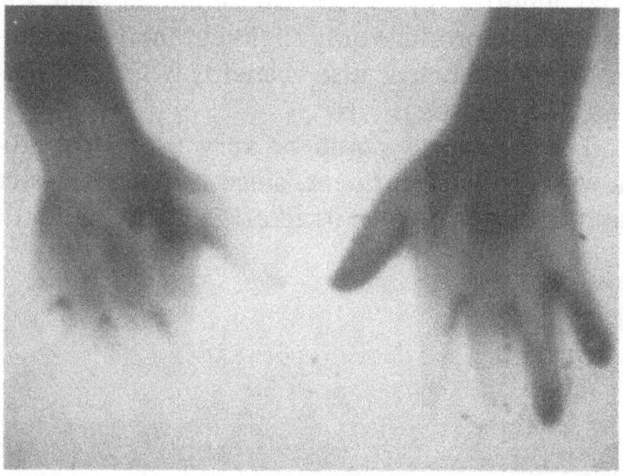

Fig. 38. Thermography gives evidence of hyperthermia of the left hand in a case of posttraumatic algodystrophy. Note the irregular distribution of the hyperthermia, the thumb and the two last fingers being much hotter than the index and the medius

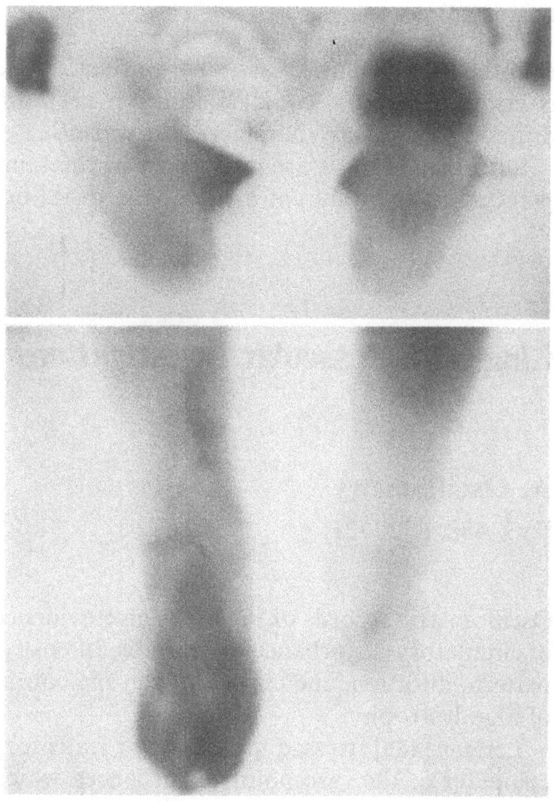

a

b

Fig. 39 a, b. Thermographic investigations in two cases ► of algodystrophy of the lower limbs. **a** Note the marked hyperthermia ($\Delta = 7°$) of the metatarsophalangeal area of the left foot on a recording of the plantar aspect of both feet. **b** Significant hyperthermia predominating on the medial aspect of the right foot in another case of algodystrophy

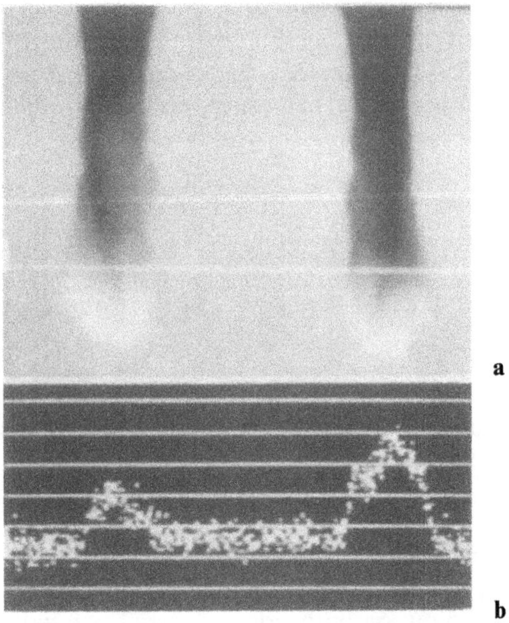

Fig. 40a, b. Thermogram of both feet and legs in a patient with reflex algodystrophy of the right foot, in the ischemic phase. **a** The patient presented with ischemic algodystrophy without hyperemic phase. That accounts for the right foot being colder than the left. **b** Quantification of the temperature deviation recorded at the base of the metatarsals. Note on the left the temperature is 1° above that on the right (deviation of 0.5° per line)

is in the intermediate phase, or the affected side is cooler (Fig. 40); coolness is however more difficult to measure than increased warmth.

Surprisingly there are differences in the temperature of the different areas of the distal extremity of a limb. In algodystrophy one or several fingers or toes can be warmer, whereas the others remain normal. The same irregularity in thermic distribution is also seen in the normal hand or foot. These findings confirm the irregularity in the distribution of the algodystrophic process, which may involve only some areas of the distal extremities. The hyperthermic area most often overlaps the region showing radiologic or scintigraphic evidence of algodystrophy, but coincides rather accurately with the clinically involved area.

In patients in whom thermography had been performed prior to any treatment, Schiano et al. [727] found that the temperature of the diseased side and of the unaffected side had become about similar after 1 week's treatment, and identical after 2 weeks' treatment. According to these authors, thermography would be an easy means of following up the evolution of the disease.

The new technique of thermography with microwaves will perhaps allow the temperature of various deeper structures (muscles, joints) to be measured, rather than merely their thermic effect on the skin. Temperatures of muscles and joints will be recorded independently, so that algodystrophies of the shoulder and the hip, which produce only slight cutaneous thermic changes, could also benefit from thermographic investigations.

Thermography could be very useful for following-up the treatment, since it is noninvasive and does not involve irradiation of the patient.

Chapter 6 Vascular Investigations

A. Oscillometry

[293, 488, 672, 723]

Oscillometric records of the limbs give evidence of circulatory disturbances of variable intensity, pattern, duration, and chronology in the course of algodystrophy.

Leriche [488] stressed the lasting or transitory character of the vasomotor disturbances which almost always accompany open or closed injuries to the extremities. According to him, there is usually an appreciable reduction in the oscillations in the distal segment, and this vasoconstriction persists for days, weeks, or even months after the original trauma. In other cases, the vasoconstrictive phase is followed by an increased amplitude of the oscillations, which may last a very long time. The oscillometer demonstrates vasomotor disturbances before any evidence of clinical signs, but these disturbances may be of very short duration.

According to Rénier et al. [672], in algodystrophy the oscillometer shows an increased index proximal to the diseased joint during the first months of the disease, followed by a return to normal or even a diminution of the index. The increased index in the proximal segment would be secondary to the peripheral microcirculatory barrier with capillary stasis related to venular constriction and to the opening of arteriovenous anastomoses. In algodystrophy the oscillometric curve in the segment proximal to the affected articular area varies with the evolution of the disease, which accounts for the contradictory findings reported in the literature.

B. Capillaroscopy

The authors who studied the capillaries in microcirculatory disturbances, particularly algodystrophy, report venular stasis with marked opening of arteriovenous anastomoses.

C. Doppler Effect

Velocimetric study using the Doppler effect proves to be, at present time, one of the best methods for atraumatic investigation of the blood flow. Its reliability and accuracy, and the quality of the data provided render it valuable for investigating all stages. It is based on measurement of the variations in frequency of ultrasound received and transmitted by the red cells. This frequency difference is proportional to the velocity of the blood flow in a vessel. It thus becomes possible to determine the instantaneous and the average velocity of the blood flow, as well as its direction.

The investigation is in several phases: the Doppler method allows the vessel to be identified by means of an audible Doppler signal; the velocity curves are then recorded on a patient at rest, for each vessel segment being studied. The direction of the flow is assessed. Analysis of the velocity curves allows objective appreciation of the vascularization in the areas under study, and thus assessment of acceleration or deceleration of the blood flow, and hence of venous stasis.

It was thus an attractive prospect to analyze, by means of the Doppler effect, the distal circulation of an affected limb compared to the unaffected, in a disease related to vasculosympathetic disturbances, such as algodystrophy.

We have analyzed with the Doppler method the vascularization in 25 patients with algodystrophy of the limbs at different stages. Fifteen of these investigations gave normal results. In 10, the following anomalies were recorded: in 1 case the distal artery of the lower limb of the affected side was not perceptible; in 3 cases the capillary pulses were not perceived on the diseased side; in 4 cases there was diminished flow velocity in the artery on the diseased side but no evidence of stenosis; in 1 case the flow velocity was increased on the affected side; and in 1 case, finally, the flow velocity was diminished on the diseased side. These results are apparently contradictory, but we must keep in mind that the vascular disturbances in algodystrophy have a variable chronology. Accurate appreciation of these perturbations would require repeat studies.

As was pointed out by Leriche [494], "the blood circulation pattern regulated by a traumatized or perturbated sympathetic system is very difficult to define; it is mainly out of balance, at times it is of the vasoconstrictive type, at others of the vasodilatative type, at still others of the stagnative type. We only record the condition at the precise moment of the examination and nothing more."

This accounts for numerous interpretation errors. Only in 1 case were we able to perform repeat examinations at different stages of the disease: the first examination, at the onset of the symptoms, was normal; the second, during the third month, showed insufficiency of the artery on the diseased side; the third examination, in the fifth month, was again normal.

It would be interesting to use the Doppler method for repeat examinations at short intervals in the course of algodystrophy. Such repeat studies would very likely give evidence of the blood flow disturbances that are characteristic for algodystrophy.

Chapter 7 Electromyography

Variable but usually moderate degrees of muscle atrophy are frequently seen in algodystrophy. In Chap. 8 we give an account of the few studies which mention muscle involvement in algodystrophy.

Meissner and Sieber [559] conclude that nervous dysregulation produces muscle degeneration.

Schiano et al. [727] found a primary involvement of muscle fiber in two cases of algodystrophy, stage I–II shoulder-hand syndrome, in whom muscle biopsy had been performed. Kirsch [411] refers to muscular changes involving both the muscular vessels and fibers.

Interpretation of such contradictory findings is not easy.

Louyot et al. [522] report their experience with electromyography in 16 cases of algodystrophy, including 9 involvements of the lower limbs and 7 involvements of the upper limbs, in whom the symptoms had been lasting more than 3 months at the time of the examination. The electromyographic investigation was performed with coaxial Bronck needles inserted on muscles in the affected areas; it showed characteristic neurogenic changes which were quite marked in two cases, with anomalies in the morphology and increased frequency of the potentials, discreet or dissociated in 7 other cases, with fibrillation potentials at rest, and a normal contraction pattern in two cases, polyphasic potentials in 5 cases, and decreased conduction speed in 1 case; in the 7 remaining cases the records were normal or almost normal with only discreet changes in the morphology of the potentials.

McCord et al. [554] report a case of regional migratory algodystrophy of the lower limbs followed over a 9-year period, with a clinical muscular involvement characterized by muscle atrophy. The investigations included an electromyogram of the muscles affected by the algodystrophic process, which demonstrated spontaneous activity with fibrillation potentials and reduced number of motor units, consistent with partial acute denervation. The authors interpret these findings as an inflammatory involvement of the nerve endings either associated or not with a radiculopathy provoked by ischemia.

Dumoulin [226] has also made electromyographic investigations of the muscles in the affected areas in 22 patients presenting with posttraumatic algodystrophy of the limbs. He observes that the distal latency is increased by 15%–25%, and that there are polyphasic potentials with a reduced number of motor units, without signs of denervation. According to the author, these abnormal findings are not due to lesions of the nerve trunks but witness the inflammatory pattern of the muscle involvement associated with increased neuromuscular irritability.

We have performed electromyographic investigations in 17 patients with algodystrophy, comprising 2 involvements of the upper limbs and 15 of the lower limbs. In all 17 the disease had lasted at least 3 months at the time of the first electromyogram. In 8 cases the electromyogram was strictly normal and in 9 cases it showed anomalies characterized by a peripheral neurogenic process in the diseased areas with diminished sensory conduction velocity in 3 cases, and decreased motor conduction velocity in 2 cases. In the two remaining patients (both diabetics) the anomalies were bilateral.

Electromyographic investigations in algodystrophic patients give contradictory and inconstant results. It seems very likely that the involvement of muscles subsequent to the algodystrophic process is variable from one case to the other, sometimes producing a predominantly primary muscle involvement, sometimes affecting the nerve roots or the nerves, and sometimes even causing a simultaneous muscle, and nerve involvement, all these changes being probably dependent on circulatory, or more precisely vasomotor distubances, whereas in other cases the muscles remain unaffected by the algodystrophic process.

Besides McCord's study [554], which concerns only a single case, no sequential electromyographic investigations have been made, to our knowledge.

It seems quite possible and even very likely that sequential, and especially early, electromyograms would show anomalies, if not constantly then at least more frequently than in the studies so far performed.

Chapter 8 Pathology

The pathologic examination should be able to shed light on the physiopathogenesis (Part 7) of algodystrophy. Unfortunately, since its description in 1901 by Sudeck, this condition has not been submitted to investigations concerning its pathology and bearing on larger series, on all localizations, on all tissues, and on all stages. The more or less spontaneous healing certainly does not encourage one to perform systematic biopsies. Moreover after Leriche [492] pointed out the underlying vasomotor imbalance, most authors admitted that biopsy would not be as harmless as had been thought. One may well hesitate to add the trauma of a biopsy when the factors provoking algodystrophy are supposed to be of the reflex sympathetic type. To our knowledge, however, nobody has ever shown that surgical biopsy performed in algodystrophy during the evolutive phase has aggravated the condition or delayed healing; but neither has the contrary been demonstrated.

The two only substantial series of pathologic examinations which are available, although bearing only on the bone, are Rieder's in 1936 [680] and Rutishauser's in 1956 [708]. The first worker reports only bone biopsies, whereas the second also provides some incomplete findings on the skin, muscles, periarticular structures, cartilage, and bone. According as the authors thought that the origin of the disease should be sought in bone, synovia, or muscles, their works have concerned one or other of these tissues. Algodystrophy has very likely the same pathologic pattern regardless of the site affected. If earlier studies have mainly concerned autopsy or amputation specimens, the more recent ones have mainly been performed in the coxofemoral joint. Since algodystrophy of the hip is a recently recognized condition, the biopsies have mainly been aimed at providing clues for the diagnosis and at ruling out osteoarticular tuberculosis or neoplasia [382]. According to Arlet et al. [16], who report the results of histopathologic studies in 9 cases of hip involvement, drill biopsy of the femoral head is not only of diagnostic interest but also relieves pain and leads to healing or at least marked clinical improvement. Although it is impossible to assess whether the recalcification rate in these cases was different from what it is spontaneously, no aggravation is reported as having occurred subsequently to the biopsy.

Although some authors do indicate at what point in the clinical course they carried out the biopsy, they do not always give details of the clinical, radiological, or scintigraphic stage. Since algodystrophy has a very variable course, the date of the biopsy with regard to the clinical or radiological onset is not really significant, especially since transitional features can exist between the different pathologic stages.

One may also ask whether the biopsy really was taken from the part affected by algodystrophy. For instance, the drill biopsies performed by Arlet et al. [16] never included the subchondral bone; Hunder and Kelly [382] indicate neither the site where their biopsies were taken, nor the technique they used. In our two histomorphometric examinations we took the biopsy specimen from the iliac wing. Given the irregular topographic distribution of algodystrophy, it is not surprising that the results can be so different.

Are there differences in the pathologic pattern related to the etiology of algodystrophy? Rutishauser et al. [708] and Rohner [691] have shown the pathologic changes to be similar regardless of their etiology.

A certain number of experimental studies in animals have been devoted to algodystrophy [68, 273, 343, 410, 436, 665, 680, 731, 812, 820]. Various means have been employed to produce algodystrophy, not all successful. One may moreover wonder whether the histologic pattern thus obtained is really close to the features in humans. By sectioning a nerve, for instance, it has been possible to produce certain of the features seen in algodystrophy in man. Bircher calls the condition thus obtained "*Sudeck-ähnliche Verhältnisse*" and not true algodystrophy. In spite of this essential distinction, experimentation in animals has certainly provided very valuable data.

We shall consider successively the findings of different authors in analyzing biopsies from various tissues: synovia, cartilage, bone, and periarticular tissue, also the vessels, which seem to play a particularly important role in determining algodystrophy.

A. Synovia

As with bone biopsies, there are no substantial series of synovial biopsies, apart from the study of Hunder and Kelly [382] which comprises 9 specimens, the series of Genant et al. [305] of 7 synovial biopsies and that of Blauth [76], of 8 cases.

In almost all cases biopsy had been performed to rule out another disease and to establish the diagnosis. Note that most biopsies concern the hip.

We would also like to quote the publications of de Marchi et al. [191] (2 biopsies of the hip), of Lequesne [474] (1 biopsy of the hip), of Rénier et al. [676] (2 biopsies of the hip and 1 of the knee), of Hasche and Meyer [354] (1 biopsy of the hip), and of Arlet et al. [16] (2 biopsies of the hip). We have already pointed out that in our opinion, retractile capsulitis of the hip as described by Caroit et al. [118] and by Lequesne [478] should not be classified separately.

As concerns the shoulder, the pathologic examinations are probably more numerous and always concern retractile capsulitis. As we have included them as algodystrophic processes, we shall also describe in this chapter the lesions of the synovial occurring in these capsular involvements. Neviaser [597] noted the presence of a thickened and fibrous capsule. Later, Welfling [854] also studied this type of lesion. Some fragmentary case reports have been published following surgery in cases of "frozen shoulder" syndrome.

We report below the observation and iconography of the synovial biopsy of the knee in one of our patients:

In July 1978 a 76-year-old man experienced a sudden arthropathy of the right knee without apparent cause. The diagnosis of arthritis (or of congestive attack of arthrosis) of the right knee with intra-articular effusion was considered on the basis of the clinical findings. The sedimentation rate was normal. There was neither hyperleukocytosis nor polynucleosis. The joint fluid was paucicellular (12 leukocytes/mm^3). The radiographs of the knee showed demineralization of both condyles; the subcondral bone lamina was preserved and was seen as a thin border. Bone scanning showed marked high uptake of tracer, predominantly over the lateral condyle (Fig. 31). Since the diagnosis of algodystrophy could not be definitely established, *synovial biopsy* was carried out. The histologic examination (Dr. Thabaut) showed a normal amount of synovial villi. The synovioblastic lining was partly hyperplastic and partly normal. The underlying connective tissue contained congestive vessels, but little or no inflammatory infiltration (Fig. 41). Complete healing without sequels was rapidly obtained by treatment with calcitonin.

We have also found in the literature a few other isolated cases in which synovial biopsies were made.

Macroscopically, we saw the same features as Hunder and Kelly, namely "grossly, the synovial membrane appeared abnormal (injected, or thickened, or both) in five of the nine cases." Microscopically, the findings of all workers can be summarized in four characteristics: apparent *integrity of the superficial layer* of the synovial membrane, without hyperplasia; discreet presence or *absence of cellular infiltration* of the inflammatory type; *hypervascularization* with unchanged vascular walls, depending on the stage of the disease, sometimes with a pseudoangiomatous appearance; and development of *fibrosis* in the deep synovial layers.

B. Cartilage

An even smaller amount of data is available on the cartilage than on the synovial membrane.

In Chap. 2 we pointed out that the integrity of the cartilage is a cardinal feature for the diagnosis. Some rare cases with changes in the cartilage have however been reported. We consider changes in the cartilage to be most often due to complications which are only exceptionally related to algodystrophy.

Some authors report finding, at surgery, a normal articular cartilage. Hunder and Kelly [382] examined the cartilage in six of their nine cases. In just one case "the cartilage was normal except for one area at the base of the head that seemed partially destroyed." Langloh et al. [446] describe thus their findings in case 7: "microscopic examination of the specimen showed normal fibrocartilage."

We must however, point out Rutishauser's et al. [708] findings. These authors found the cartilage to be sometimes superficially invaded by the pannus and its osseous aspect to be infiltrated by a connectivo-vascular bud of medullar origin. This may cause complete erosion of the

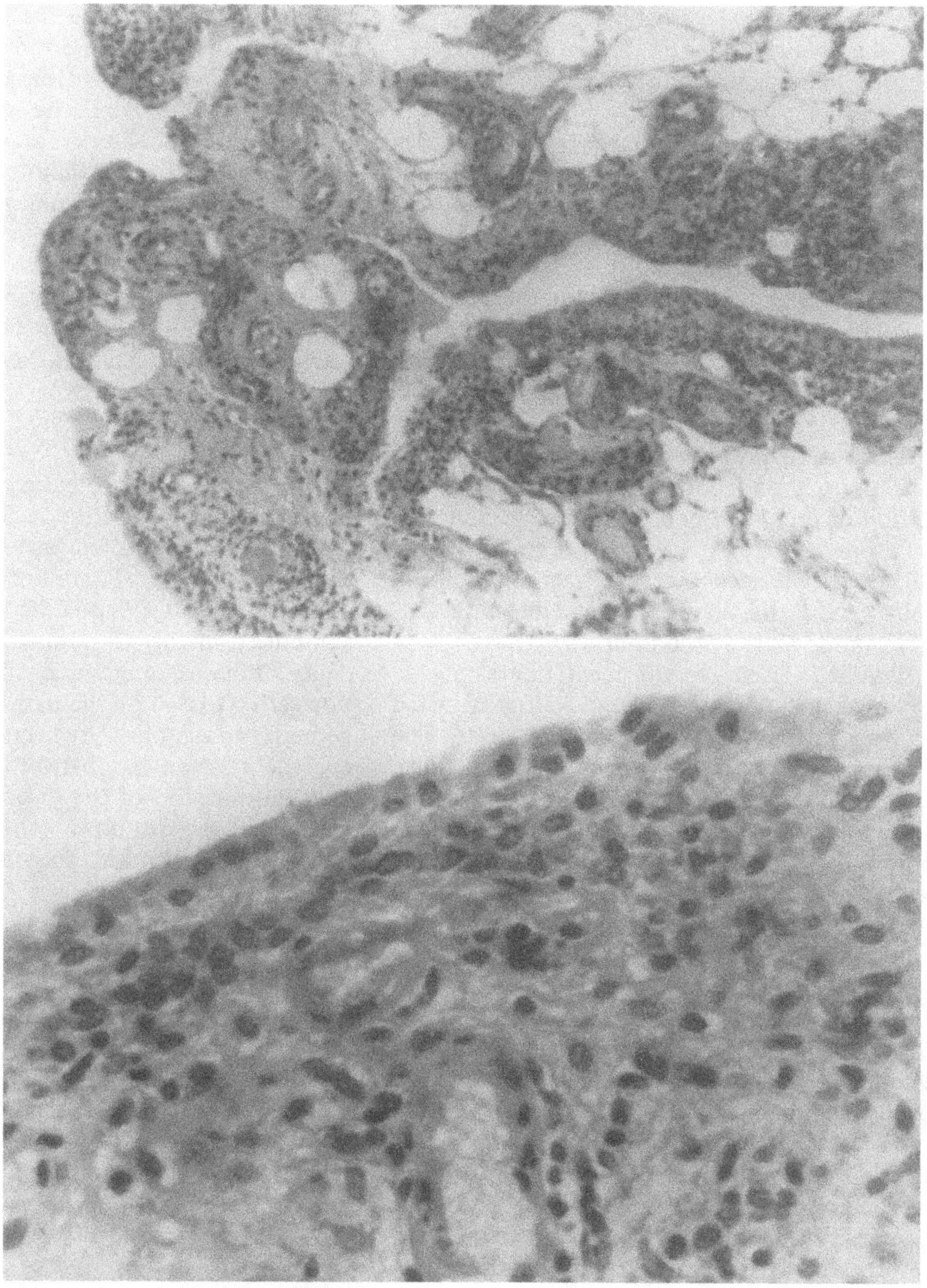

a

b

Fig. 41 a, b. Synovial biopsy. Normal synovial villi with partly hyperplastic, partly normal synovioblastic lining. The connective tissue contains congestive vessels but little or no inflammatory infiltration. **a** Low magnification. **b** High magnification cartilage which is replaced by fibrotic adherences resulting in loose ankylosis. Rutishauser can thus conclude that "the pannus and even fibrotic ankylosis belong to the Sudeck's syndrome".

In his publication, Rohner [691] provides more complete data. In his case 3, which includes a description of the radiologic appearance of the knee on the 30th, 50th, 84th, and 116th days and during the 9th and 14th months, he notes from the beginning that the cartilage becomes atrophic, is destroyed, and is later on repaired. The articular surfaces reappear but remain irregular with a tendency to develop osseous bridges.

The author notes marked destruction of the articular margins, in opposition to the classical notion of preserved bone contours in Sudeck's syndrome. There is however no reason to be surprised that such a marked atrophy should bring about irreversible significant modifications in the articular contours.

Case 4 is certainly the most interesting as concerns the joints. Severe algodystrophy lasted 6 years, involving the foot and the ankle. The first specimens were taken from the tibia, talus, and calcaneum. At the junction of the posterior and middle thirds, the tibial articular cartilage bore a deep notch on its medullar aspect. The terminal bone lamina remained continuous and stretched like a bridge accross this cavity. More anteriorly, the elements of the articular plate were again separated: whereas the bone lamina kept its rectilinear direction, the underlying cartilage slipped away and became progressively thinner. The talocalcanean joint undergoes fibrous ankylosis.

The last two cases have similar features, but they are less marked. Note, in case 5, a small marginal pannus on the inferior edge of the talonavicular joint, with only very superficial resorption of the cartilage. The remainder of the cartilage shows superficial transformation into fibrocartilage.

The authors ask "whether a preexistent change in the cartilage is responsible for the organization of medullar vessels, or whether the medullar buds provoke secondary changes in the cartilage which they infiltrate. Why does this penetration, which occurs superficially, become parallel to the articular spaces instead of progressing in depth and producing articular synostosis, which is only seen in some rare places? For the time being, we must content ourselves with gathering the facts, and among them we can say that we did not find splitting of the articular plates in the Sudeck syndrome of the upper limb which we have examined."

More recently, Lagier and Van Linthoudt [439, 440] presented 5 radiologic investigations in algodystrophy concerning the posterior part of the foot, of which 4 also had a histologic examination. These authors note that "longstanding and severe algodystrophies can show cartilaginous and articular changes i.e. dissection in depth with 'duplication' of the subchondral bone lamina; superficial dedifferentiation with fibrotic and even bony ankylosis. In addition there may be capsulo-ligamentous ossification and cortico-periosteal remodeling... If the Sudeck syndrome is responsible, at least indirectly, for articular changes, the origin of these should be searched for in a dystrophic element affecting the soft tissue of the joint. The authors attribute it mainly to immobilization. The incidence of these changes depends on the articulations affected and on the patients. It would thus be useful to establish, by means of further studies, the relationship between these ankyloses and the duration of the disease or the clinical features of the disability... The therapeutic interest of mobilization does not only concern bone rarefaction."

Even more recently, Arlet et al. [15] reported similar findings.

The observations are not in absolute contradiction with our clinical and radiological data. Articular complications are indeed seen in longstanding algodystrophic processes, although Rutishauser et al. [708] report a case of bone algodystrophy with 20 years' duration at stage III, in which the cartilage appears remarkably well preserved.

We do not agree with the authors from Geneva as concerns the frequency of such an articular involvement in algodystrophy. But this is probably due to a different selection of patients. Finally the explanation which seems to us the most satisfactory is that the rare cases of algodystrophy with evidence of lesions in the cartilage concern patients who had severe traumatisms. Now such traumatisms are known to be responsible for changes in the cartilage subsequently inducing arthrosis.

As concerns the case reports of the Geneva authors, nothing prevents us from thinking that the severe traumatism might have induced both the algodystrophic process, and, unrelated to this, the lesion of the cartilage.

C. Bone

I. Macroscopy

All authors, both the pathologists and the surgeons, point out the lack of hardness of the affected bones, and how easily they are sectioned, even with the operation knife. Ficat et al. [258] speak of bone with the consistency of "wet sugar" and with liquefied bone marrow resembling yellowish, grayish, or salmon-colored mash.

The comparison between a bone specimen looked at through a magnifying glass and its radiologic appearance is very instructive. It is mainly the Geneva school – Rutishauser et al. [708], Rohner [691], Lagier and Van Lindhout [439, 440] – who have made this kind of study. Rarefaction of the bone trabeculae is seen and, at stage III, thickening of some of them, producing a heterogeneous distribution of the spongy network; some of the trabeculations are thickened and others are atrophic. In one case of Lagier and Lindhout, 8 years after the onset of the disease there were still areas with thickening of some trabeculations of the spongy bone. This thickening of some trabeculations is sometimes responsible for a more or less filamentous appearance, reflecting "hypertrophic osteoporosis," as Kienböck calls it [408].

II. Microscopy

In 1902, Exner [251] performed a histological examination in 3 of his 28 cases. He compared these specimens with specimens from controls of the same age and sex. In the pathologic specimens the number of bone trabeculations was diminished and their thickness was also reduced. The subchondral bone was very thin; it measured only a few micrometer, so that it was hardly visible with a low magnification. The author noted also some groups of cells contiguous to the bone trabeculae, but he did not say whether they were osteoblasts or osteoclasts. The three biopsies were taken in chronic cases (lasting 1, $1^1/_2$ and 11 years).

From Exner's study until 1936, when Rieder [680] published his well documented paper "Acute bone atrophy," there was a lack of systematic histologic examinations in acute forms. To his 16 cases in man, where biopsies were taken between the 9th day and the 39th week, Rieder adds an experimental material of 9 rabbit calcanea. Summarizing his work, he draws the following conclusion: "Contrary to the radiographic appearance which gives evidence of bone atrophy only after a delay of 3 to 4 weeks, histology already shows signs of atrophy after 8 days. At this early stage osteoporosis is characterized by a decreased thickness of the bone trabeculae, and increased medullar volume. There exists also, although to a lesser degree than at a later stage, hyperemia of the intraosseous and periosteal vessels. There is intense osteoclastic resorption and proliferation of thin, fusiform mononuclear or giant osteoclasts. Besides the more or less marked resorption, there is also, in all cases, a proliferation of osteoid tissue. This osteoid substance is however only rarely calcified, conveying the impression of a perturbated normal bone formation process." Rieder believed that in very acute forms, in particular those of infectious origin, resorption begins in the giant osteoclasts. On the other hand, in less acute processes, especially noninfectious ones, there would be vascular resorption combined with osteoclastic resorption, one or other type of resorption being predominant.

The vessels, especially those in the medullar spaces, have increased volume and are engorged, so that there is hyperemia.

Finally, Rieder concludes: *patchy acute bone atrophy is the consequence of a more or less early cellular reaction leading to a transformation (apposition of resorption) with marked apposition of osteoid seams.* In spite of extended and often multiple rows of osteoblasts, the calcification of the large osteoid seams is perturbated. There is thus a qualitatively defective apposition of new bone (dystrophy). What is striking at the acute stage is that there is no decreased cell formation as in atrophy but on the contrary extraordinarily dramatic remodeling. In spite of the degree of osteoclasia, Rieder wonders if this suffices to explain acute bone atrophy. He has an idea that there are chemical processes which also contribute to produce atrophy. We shall consider this problem again later. Rieder's histological observations were confirmed in

1938 by Sudeck [795] and in 1943 by Remé [665]. More recently, in 1956 and 1957 Rutishauser et al. [707, 708] and Rohner [691] confirmed the existence of stages II and III of posttraumatic osteoporosis. According to them the bone tissue, during the dystrophic stage, is the site of bone remodeling and of quite irregular atrophy. The remodeling produces a regular mosaic pattern. This appearance results from a disturbance in remodeling which is less deep and much more orderly than in the Paget's disease. At the same stage, according to these authors, the bone marrow is reticulate, oligocellular, and devoid of fat cells. As concerns the vascularization, muscular hyperplasia of the arteries, intimal hyperplasia, neoformation of the capillaries, and sinusoid ectasia are observed. The hemodynamic disturbances are evidenced by intracapillar plasmostasis and later interstitial edema, and often also globular stasis in the capillaries. At stage III the epiphyseal atrophy is characterized by "atrophy with marked remodeling of the trabeculations; there is no more trabecular metaplasia. The adipose marrow contains only rare hematopoietic islets. The cortical layer is thin and has a striated appearance. The vascular walls are again normal."

These same Geneva workers have made studies on posttraumatic osteoporosis, and also osteoporosis with other etiologies; there was no evidence of morphologic characteristics specific to each etiology.

Lacroix and Ponlot [436] made experimental studies on posttraumatic osteoporosis in dogs, using microradiography and historadiography of bones labeled with calcium 45. In their conclusions these authors affirm that experimental posttraumatic osteoporosis of compact bone produces a more extended remodeling than is normally the case. Fontaine et al. [271] used an analogous histochemical technique and came to similar conclusions: the specific activity of the bones increases proportionally to their degree of osteoporosis. Bone scanning confirms these findings. The anatomo-scintigraphic studies performed by Tilden et al. [815] on anatomic specimens of the femoral head showed that ^{99m}Tc-polyphosphates became fixed linearly at the junction between bone tissues of different maturity, with a marked affinity for young and still poorly mineralized bone tissue. The precise histological site where technetium-99m fixes is discussed; it is probably of a mixed type, and concerns both the mineral substance (hydroxyapatite crystals) and the intercellular protein. Rosenthal and Kaye [697] demonstrated the role of the intercellular substance and particularly of immature collagen in the fixation of ^{99m}Tc-phosphates. As was pointed out by Genant et al. [305] and by Siegel et al. [764], there is indisputably a vascular factor, but hypervascularization intervenes mainly to facilitate the exchanges between the tracer and the bone tissue. Capillary permeability also plays a nonnegligible part [292].

Active resorption with osteoclasts present is one of the mechanisms of osteoporosis, especially of subchondral osteoporosis (subchondral resorption).

Another hypothesis raised to explain decalcification concerns *osteolysis*. Until now, the presence of a phenomenon of osteolysis has not been proved. Leriche and Policard [502] thought this phenomenon was the main factor in bone resorption, but the idea has not often been considered subsequently. All components of the fundamental substance of the bone trabeculae are resorbed by an acellular phenomenon; osteolysis takes place close to the cellular interspaces. Meyer [566], whose work is reported in another part of this book (Chap. 8), has demonstrated that entire trabeculations are the site of a demineralization phenomenon due to a reduction in the volume of the crystallites, i.e., a true reduction in the calcium charge of the bone trabeculae. Moreover, the components of the fundamental substance at the periphery of certain trabeculations are resorbed, resulting in a quantitative diminution of the bone tissue.

Other studies refer to bone biopsies [191, 228, 252, 382, 439, 446, 472, 570, 607, 696, 763].

Arlet et al. [16] took drill biopsies of the femoral head. They are quite aware that a specimen taken by drill biopsy of the hip does not include the subchondral bone, i.e., the site where osteoclastic resorption would be most marked. They do however report marked active reconstruction, which in 6 of 9 cases they observed to be sometimes very considerable. Osteogenesis occurs either peripherally, along already present trabeculations, or within the medulla, developing within the connective tissue and showing deformed neotrabeculations which are poorly anastomosed if at all. Finally, osteogenesis can also develop buds at the edges of the trabeculations, as pointed out by Rohner.

The early occurrence and intensity of the osteogenesis can at least partly account for the increased uptake of tracer at bone scanning; but high uptake can also be due to consolidation of microfractures.

Arlet et al. stress the marked changes occurring in the medullar interspaces. They are often devoid of hematopoietic tissue, and of part of the fat tissue. Stasis is a constant feature. The spaces between the fat cells are almost always distended, being filled with an amorphous substances. This is the plasmostasis described by Rutishauser. It is almost constantly seen in cases with disturbed intraosseous circulation. Sometimes the sinusoids and the venules themselves are dilated. Finally, there exists a pseudotelangiectasic proliferation. The walls are thickened and abnormally fibrotic, and the lumen is narrowed. The various features can be schematized as follows: Phase I, or acute phase: simultaneous evidence of the following phenomena occurring in the bone trabeculae: osteoclastic bone resorption, peripheral osteolysis (?), diffuse demineralization, increased osteoblastic apposition. Phase II: a phase of slow remodeling, with predominence of apposition and remineralization phenomena. Phase III, the stage of the sequels: the remaining and the newly apposed bone tissue have a normal structure, but the apposition phenomena, which are again normal, cannot compensate the loss of tissue that occurred in the first phases; normally structured bone substance may thus remain in an atrophic condition and be quantitatively diminished, while medullary spaces remain fatty.

It seems important to report the findings of Rutishauser et al. [708]. They noticed that stage II and stage III can coexist, so that a division into different stages seems rather artificial.

III. Electron Microscopy

To our knowledge, only Meyer [566] has made an electron microscopic study in algodystrophy. His study concerns a posttraumatic involvement of the knee of 14 months' duration. The radiograms show diffuse hypertranslucency of the patella and absence of the trabecular pattern: there is evidence of more or less translucent areas, which are ill-delimited and have an unsharp appearance. According to the author, these features are consistent with a stage II condition.

The histologic examination gives evidence of marked, nonspecific chronic synovitis and of exceptionally marked osteoporosis of the patella. Atrophic trabeculae are scattered through the adipose bone marrow. There is also important bone remodeling with a very clear predominance of osteolysis. In contact with the spongy bone trabeculations there are numerous dilated and congestive blood capillaries. Very rare osteoclasts are present. Some trabeculae are surrounded by a series of osteoblasts and there is osteoid tissue between the preexistent bone and the osteoblasts. The arteries have thickened walls, without endarteritis, and are always congestive. This appearance is consistent with a stage II condition as described by Rutishauser et al. [708] and by Rieder [680].

According to Meyer, there are two types of change involving the ground substance. At the periphery of certain trabeculae occurs an *acellular osteolysis phenomenon.* All components of the ground substance undergo resorption. This osteolysis leads to a quantitative diminution in bone tissue. The trabeculae have no peripheral area formed by nonmineralized collagen fibers as is normally the case, but are seen to be bordered by mineral fibrillar elements, suggesting dislocation or disaggregation of the mineralized ground substance. The morphology of these elements identifies them as fragments of the mineral sheaths of the collagen fibers. Meyer thinks he can reasonably conclude that resorption of the matrix takes place, all its constitutive elements disappearing. This resorption occurs at the periphery of the trabeculae, in contact with the medullary spaces. Meyer recognized this mechanism as osteolysis according to the definition given by Leriche and Policard [502].

The second type of lesion of the ground substance observed by Meyer consists in the *diminution in the size of the crystallites.* The crystallites of a normal patella are better outlined and larger than those of an osteoporotic patella. This lesional process extends to entire trabeculations without, however, involving them all. There are areas with normal matrices, others with an intermediate appearance, and still others with complete demineralization. The organic ground substance keeps its normal appearance.

These studies have not however been confirmed up to now.

IV. Microradiography

In his thesis, Meyer [566] compares the patella of a 22-year-old healthy man (a) with that of a 61-year-old patient suffering from senile osteoporosis (b) and with the patella in an algodystrophic process (c). The examination shows a diminished thickness of the trabeculations from (a) to (c), but it mainly demonstrates the differences in the mineralization. Whereas the radiotranslucency, i.e., the mineralization, of (a) and (b) is almost similar, (c) has a clearly increased translucency with regard to (a) and to (b), thus witnessing *marked mineral loss.*

V. Static and Dynamic Histomorphometry

The quantitative histologic appreciation of bone specimens appears as a well-adapted method for direct study of normal and algodystrophic bone tissue. As a matter of fact, it permits precise evaluation of the rarefaction by measurements of the thickness of cortical compact bone, and of the absolute bone volume of spongy bone. It also allows evaluation of the precise importance of the main factors of bone remodeling by quantifying osteoclastic and periosteocytic resorption, and osteoblastic apposition. Tetracycline labeling of the calcification fronts make it possible to determine the calcification rate of the preosseous tissue. Finally, by comparing the calcification rate with the value of the osteoid thickness index, one can deduce the osteoblastic appositional rate.

Unfortunately, only a few cases have been studied with this method. Farkas and Nemes [252] published a case of posttraumatic reflex algodystrophy with a histomorphometric study. The bone samples were taken at the moment of the traumatism, at stage I, i.e., 2 months after the traumatism, and finally at stage III.

In relation to the normal specimen taken right after the traumatism, the bone volume was diminished by 15% after 2 months, whereas at stage III there was again an increase in the bone volume, since the diminution relative to the normal specimen was only 9%.

We report below our only two bone biopsies analyzed by the Bone Histodynamics Research Laboratory, Lyon. The specimens were taken from the iliac bone, after we had verified by bone scans that there was increased uptake of the tracer in this area.

A 25-year-old woman presented on 5 February 1976 with a butterfly wing shaped fracture of the lower extremity of the right tibia, which was treated by extension and plaster until 15 May. As soon as the plaster was removed, there appeared edema of the ankle, pain in the foot, ankle, and knee, slightly reduced plantar flexion of the ankle and flexion of the knee, and, above all, total disability, We saw the patient for the first time on 29 July 1976. The clinical diagnosis of posttraumatic algodystrophy was made then, and confirmed by radiographic and scintigraphic findings. The radiographs show demineralization of the right hemipelvis and hip, and marked demineralization of the lower extremity of the right leg and of the ankle and foot. Bone scanning evidenced a clear focus of high uptake over the right hemipelvis, the medial part of the right knee, and over the malleolus and metatarsus on the right.

The laboratory findings were normal. Calcitonin-induced hypocalcemia showed the blood calcium level to be decreased from 2.28 mmol/l to 2.21 mmol/l. The 24-h hydroxyprolinuria was 141.16 μmol.

The patient was given a treatment of 50 units porcine calcitonin, at a rate of 2 injections per day for 6 days, then 1 injection every day for the following 6 days, and then 3 injections per week for another 8 weeks, i.e., a total of 42 injections.

Rehabilitation was undertaken, but on 23 September 1976 a fall caused a new fracture on the same site as the first. The patient was hospitalized for treatment of this second fracture and bone biopsy was considered. Radiologically, the demineralization was just as marked and extended as it had been in July, and so was the high uptake of tracer. Again the biochemical findings were normal, but there was a paradoxical response to the calcitonin test (2.38 mmol before and 2.5 mmol 6 h after injection of 100 units synthetic salmon calcitonin). The 24-h hydroxyprolinuria was 119.79 μmol.

Decalcified and undecalcified iliac bone specimens taken by biopsy after tetracycline labeling were analyzed (Dr. C. Edouard and Prof. P. Meunier, Bone Histodynamics Research Laboratory, Lyon). The sample comprised the two cortices, which had normal thickness but were very notched with voluminous resorption lacunae and numerous haversian lumina lined by thin osteoid seams (Fig. 43). For the patient's age, the spongy bone was markedly rarefied with a low trabecular bone volume of 14.7% (normal values: 22.9 ± 4.5). The osteoclastic resorption surfaces were normal and little extended, with very rare osteoclasts in the spongy bone (3.6% on the decalcified section, and 1.9% on the nondecalcified section; normal values: 3.6 ± 1.1).

The cross-sectional area of the periosteocytic lacunae had increased to 59 μ^2, (normal: 50.7 ± 5.5). The relative osteoid volume of the spongy bone had increased to 6.2% (normal: 2.1 ± 1.4). The osteoid seam thickness index was normal at 18.3 (normal: 19.3 ± 3.1). The double labeling with tetracycline was clearly readable with fluoroscopy; the double labelings were quite extended. The calcification rate was normal: 0.93 μm/day in the cortical bone, and 0.89 μ/day in the spongy bone (normal: 1.2 ± 0.6).

To conclude: this was a case of *osteoporosis* involving both the cortical and the spongy bone, which had reached the reconstruction stage. There was no trabecular osteoclastosis but the intracortical hyperosteoclastosis seemed to persist. There were also signs of extended trabecular apposition. Finally, there was also evidence of enlarged periosteocytic cavities.

Complete healing was obtained by July 1977, i.e. 16 months after the first accident. Follow-up radiographs of the right limb and of the pelvis were taken in February 1979 and proved quite normal.

It should be pointed out that in this case bone biopsy was taken in an area distant from the fracture focus, which had shown radiologic features of demineralization and high uptake on bone scanning. The biopsy was taken 7 months after the first fracture and 1 month after the second, after almost complete immobilization for 7 months, and finally after the patient had been treated with large doses of calcitonin.

The second case report including a biopsy is the following:

A 22-year-old man suffered contusion of the right hip subsequent to a road accident in July 1972. Immediately after this traumatism he stopped working for 1 month.

When he had been working again for 2 months, disability of the right lower limb set in. He was then hospitalized in the department of Prof. J. Arlet in Toulouse. The clinical examination performed at that time showed evidence of painful limitation in the hip motion, especially abduction and internal rotation. There was also indisputable muscle wasting of the quadriceps. X-rays performed on 20 January 1972 show definite osteoporosis of the upper extremity of the right femur and of the femoral head (films taken before that date were all normal). Bone scanning showed a high uptake of strontium 87 over the right hip. Pertrochanteral phlebography showed increased venous pressure (above 30 mm Hg).

All these findings are consistent with reflex algodystrophy. The clinical course followed a chronic pattern. Pain and limitation in articular mobility persist.

The range of movements at different dates is summarized in the table below:

	31.7.73	23.7.74	13.5.75
Flexion	90°	80°	70°
Abduction	0	25°	30°
Adduction	–	20°	30°
External rotation	0°	20°	10°
Internal rotation	0°	5°	0°
Extension	–	5°	0°

Radiographs carried out on 30 April 1975 still show bone rarefaction in the femoral head and in the cotyle, and subchondral resorption without deformation of the femoral head. Bone scanning with ^{99m}Tc-diphosphonates showed discreet increased uptake of the tracer over the coxofemoral joint. Opaque arthrography of the coxofemoral head, performed at the same time, showed a moderate retraction of the capsule of the coxofemoral joint and a lower articular recess still present.

Between 1972 and 1976, pain and functional disability persisted and the patient walked with two crutches.

We saw the patient for the first time on 6 August 1976. There was then a marked amyotrophy of the glutei and of the quadriceps muscle (diameter of the thigh 15 cm above the patelly 45 cm on the right, 49.5 cm on the left). The coxofemoral mobility was markedly restricted: flexion 60°, abduction 10°, adduction 10°, lateral rotation 10°, medial rotation 10°, extension −40°.

On account of this aggravation, surgery was decided upon and the operation performed on 15 September 1977 (by Dr. R. Anger). After a Watson Jones incision of the right hip, the anterior aspect of the hip was cleared. As soon as general anesthesia had taken effect, the movements of the hip, particularly extension, became possible. Since the capsule seemed narrowed and retracted, H-shaped capsuloplasty of the anterior aspect of the hip was performed. When the capsule was sectioned, there was a gap of 3 cm between the edges of the section. There were numerous intra-articular free bodies of the size of wheat grains, some of which were attached to the synovial membrane and witness the existence of chondromatosis.

The straight and the reflected tendon of the rectus femoris, the psoas tendons and the tensor fasciae latae were sectioned. An iliac bone biopsy was performed.

The pathologic examination of the *articular capsule, the synovial membrane, and the chondromes* (by Dr. C. Guiraudon) showed that the articular capsule was fibro-hyalin or most often normal, the synovial membrane had congestive capillaries; there were some subsynovioblastic cartilaginous nodules under formation; the chondromas were formed of juxtaposed cartilaginous nodules, of which some were voluminous with some calcium deposits and covered with a lamellar connective wall with a thickened synovioblastic margin. It was a synovial chondromatosis. The histologic examination of the bone sampled on the iliac crest (by Prof. P. Meunier, Dr. C. Alexandre, and Dr. C. Edouard) showed, on the decalcified and undecalcified fragments, cortices of 2,250 and 900 μ thickness. The trabecular bone volume was markedly lowered for the patient's age: 11.5% (normal: 23.1 ± 4.1% in sex- and age-matched controls). The osteoclastic resorption trabecular surfaces were increased to 6.8% (normal: 3.6 ± 1.1), but the Howship lacunae were most often devoid of osteoclasts.

The cross-sectional area of the periosteocytic lacunae was normal at 50.1 μ^2 (normal: 50.7 ± 5.5).

The medullary adipose volume was increased to 34.1% (normal: 24.1 ± 5 in age-matched controls).

The relative osteoid volume of the spongy bone was normal at 3.4% (normal: 2.1 ± 1.4). The osteoid surfaces were normal at 16.4% (normal: 11.0 ± 6.8). The osteoid seam thickness index was normal at 20 (normal: 19.3 ± 3.1). Under fluorescence the double tetracycline labeling was clearly visualized. The calcification rate was normal: 0.71 μm/day in the cortical bone, 0.62 μm/day in the spongy bone (normal: 0.72–0.13). In cluclusion: this was a case of *pure osteoporosis with hyperosteoclastosis* compatible with the diagnosis of algodystrophy or of immobilization osteoporosis.

In July 1979, there was still a very marked bone demineralization in the right hemipelvis and in the upper extremity of the right femur, and bone scanning still gave evidence of high uptake of radioactive tracers. The clinical state was about the same as before the operation, i.e., pain in the right coxofemoral joint, necessitating use of two crutches, and a walking range of about 100 m. Moreover, the mobibility of the coxofemoral articulation was still extremely restricted.

We are aware that publication of this case report is open to criticism. Some will consider it a case of synovial chondromatosis with capsular retraction and osteoporosis of the pelvis revealed by a traumatism. We consider it a case of posttraumatic algodystrophy with a chronic course, with synovial chondromatosis as a second factor provoking and maintaining the algodystrophy.

VI. Attempt at a Histodynamic Interpretation of the Algodystrophic Mechanism

In the light of the concepts of Frost [288, 289], and on account of the findings of the Bone Histodynamics Research Laboratory, Lyon, directed by Meunier [564], we would propose the following interpretation. Besides the reduction in volume of cortical and trabecular bone (Fig. 42) we also observed a marked multiplication of the osteoclasts in both the spongy and the cortical bone. The cortex is very anfractuous, similar to what is seen in hyperthyroidism, in hyperparathyroidism, and in immobilization osteoporosis (Fig. 43). This hyperosteoclastosis is followed by intense multiplication of the osteoblasts (Fig. 44) with extended osteoid seams, contrary to what is seen in immobilization osteoporosis, where apposition is much more diminished [574].

Bone remodeling is a cellular phenomenon occurring throughout one's lifetime at the level of the spongy bone, endosteum, haversian bone, and periosteum. In the adult the remodeling determines the rate of renewal of the bone tissue, the total amount of osteoids in the skeleton, the existence of bone gain or bone loss in certain parts of the skeleton, and the balance between resorption surfaces and bone formation. A cardinal point is that remodeling is not the summation of the activities of a certain number of dispersed, unconnected osteoblasts and osteoclasts [288]. It is the sum of the activities of a certain number of units of microscopic size: the "basic multicellular unit" (BMU), which is the site of three interrelated cellular mechanisms: activation (A), osteoclastic resorption (R) and osteoblastic apposition (F). The last never entirely compensates for the resorption, so that there is a small tissue deficit (d) after each cycle. The result is a sequence $A \rightarrow R \rightarrow F$. According to the "stair-graph" proposed by Meunier, various mechanisms can increase the loss of bone:

1) The multiplication of the basic multicellular units (BMU) by an increase of their birth rate (situation B, Fig. 45). The individual minute deficits (d) of the BMUs are then also multiplied. Under these conditions, resorption surfaces, number of osteoclasts, osteoid surfaces, and osteoblastic surfaces are all increased, and this is characteristic of high remodeling osteoporoses.

2) A depression of osteoblastic productivity without change in the activation of BMUs can also increase the loss of bone. The osteoblastic depression magnifies the tissue deficit at the level of the BMUs (situation C, Fig. 45).

3) A combination of both mechanisms described above is encountered in a few instances, for example in corticosteroid-treated patients in whom serum parathyroid hormone is high, or in disuse osteoporosis (situation D, Fig. 45).

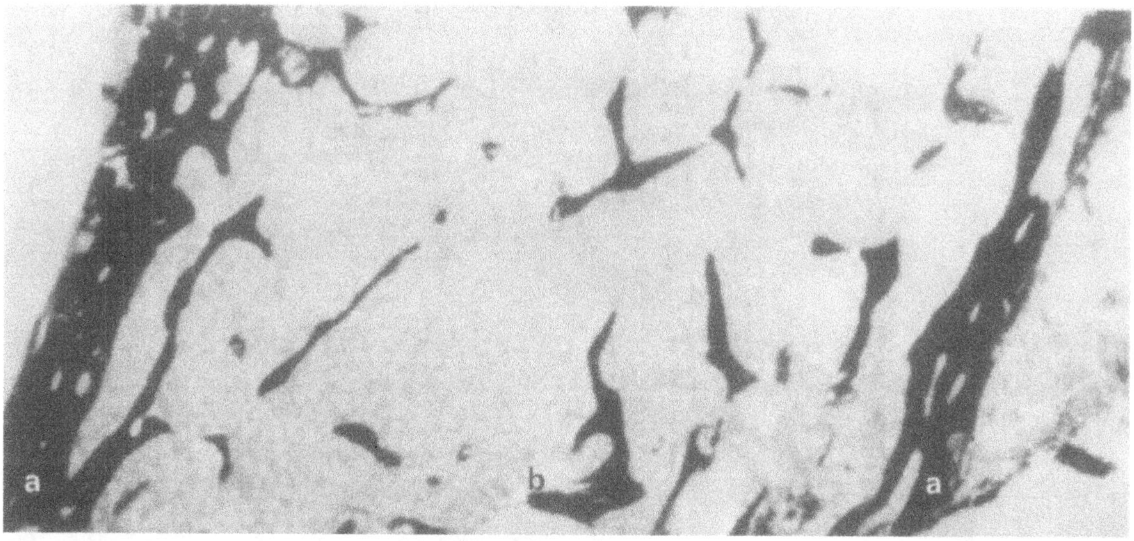

Fig. 42. Section of an undecalcified iliac crest specimen obtained by transiliac biopsy with an 8 mm inner diameter trephine in a case of algodystrophy of the lower limb. Note the reduced trabecular bone volume (Stain: Solochromecyanin R). **a,** Cortical bone; **b,** Trabecular bone. (Courtesy of M. Megard and P. Meunier, Lyon)

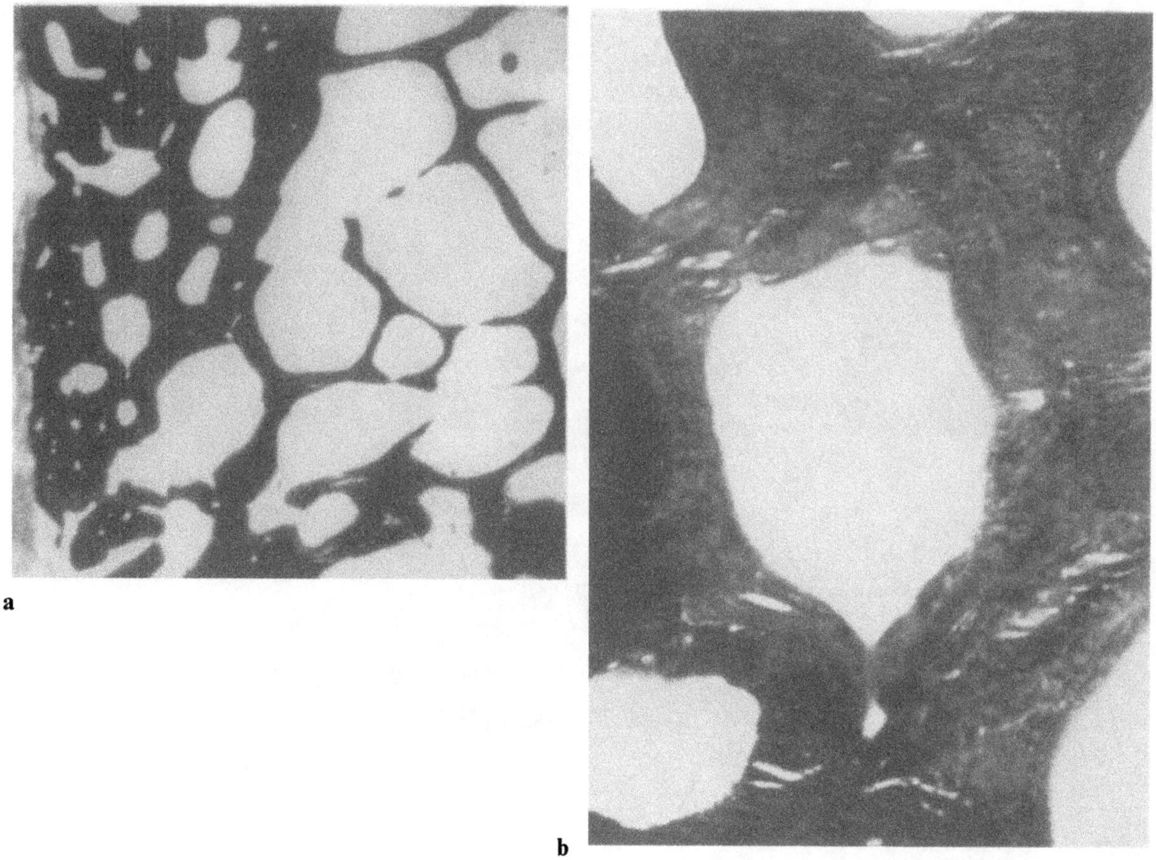

a b

Fig. 43a, b. Right iliac crest biopsy in a case of post-traumatic algodystrophy of the right lower limb, 8 months after a fracture of the tibia and about 3 months after the clinical onset of algodystrophy. The thickness of the cortical bone is normal, but it is very anfractuous with voluminous resorption cavities that are incompletely filled. **a** Cortical bone. On the right spongy bone. **b** Closeup of the cortical bone

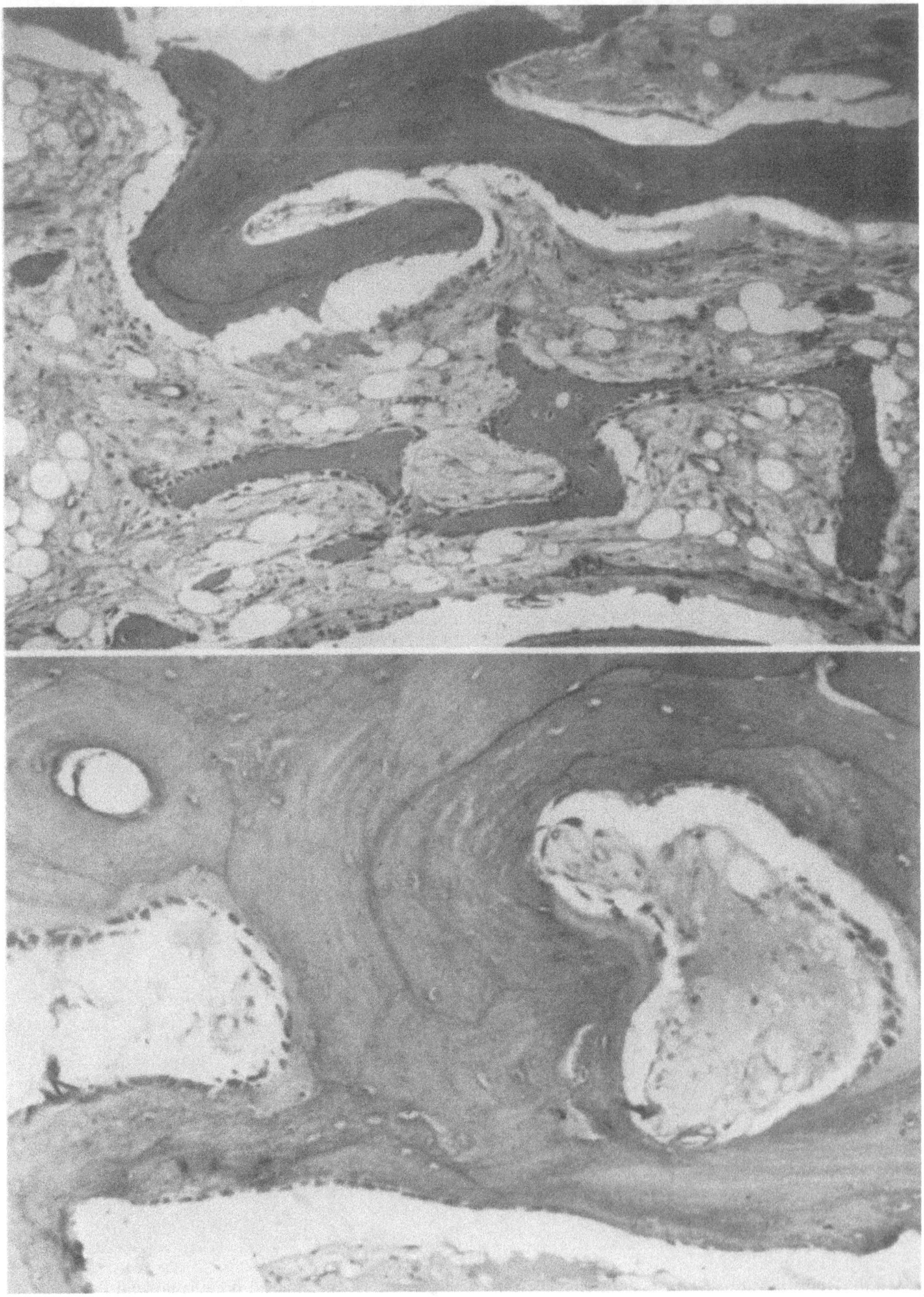

a

b

Fig. 44a, b

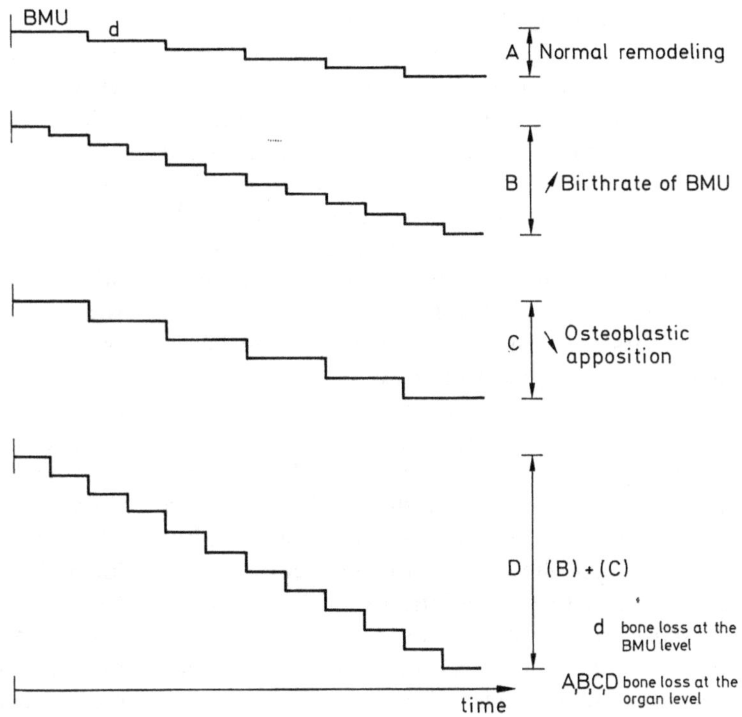

Fig. 45. Diagrammatic representation of the loss of bone tissues in normal aging (*A*), in high remodeling osteoporoses by thyroid hormones or parathyroid hormone (*B*), in osteoporoses with osteoblastic depression such as corticosteroid-induced osteoporosis (*C*), and in situations where A and B are combined, as in corticosteroid osteoporosis with high parathormone or in disuse osteoporosis (*D*). *d* represents the bone loss at the BMU level or the individual minute deficits. (*A, B, C,* and *D* represent the bone loss at the organ level. Algodystrophy falls into situation *B* with increased resorption surface, number of osteoclasts, osteoid surfaces and osteoblastic surfaces, but it is only a locoregional mechanism. (From P. Meunier)

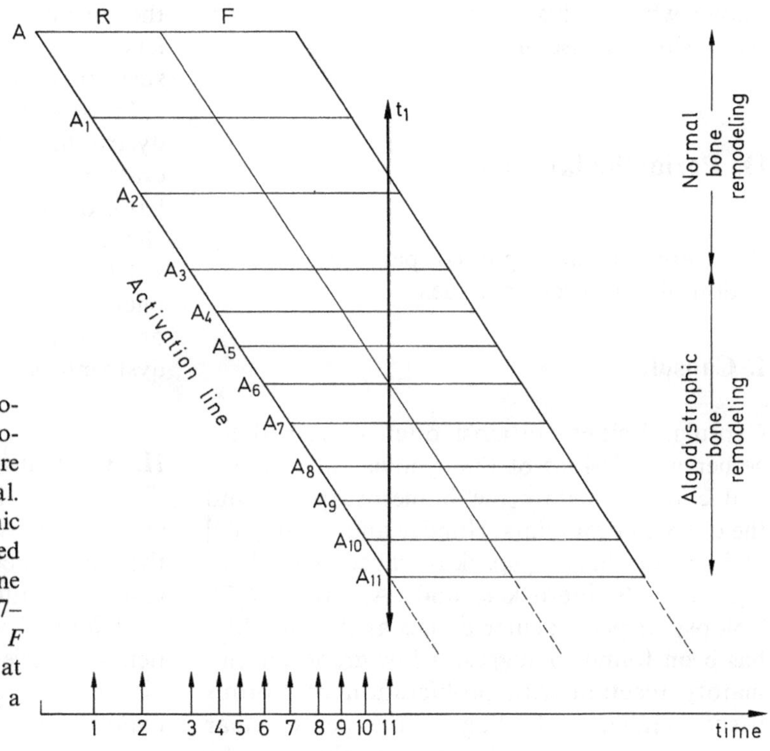

Fig. 46. Ladder graphs (from Frost, modified). Algodystrophy starts at the moment A_3. A larger number of BMUs are activated in a shorter time than usual. The vertical line t_1 forms the graphic equivalent of a biopsy done and analyzed at that moment. It includes normal bone (*2*) algodystrophic bone at phase *R* (*7–11*) and algodystrophic bone at phase *F* (*3–6*) with a larger number of BMUs at the active phase, algodystrophy being a disease of the activation

◄ **Fig. 44 a, b.** Marked osteoblastosis in two cases of algodystrophy of the hip. Bone specimen obtained by drill biopsy of the femoral head. **a** Specimen taken during the second month of the clinical course. **b** Specimen taken after $3^1/_2$ months of the disease. (Courtesy J. Arlet, Toulouse)

It seems to us that algodystrophy would fit into the category of high remodeling osteoporoses, and could thus be depicted by the scheme in Fig. 45. There exist extended active remodeling surfaces (situation B, Fig. 45). There would also exist a sudden activation of these remodeling foci, but these changes would remain locoregional, and we would like to stress this point. For Frost [290] the regional traumatism is a local activator of BMU formation, the other activators concerning the entire skeleton being parathormone, growth hormone, thyroxin, and some vitamin D metabolites.

If we adopt this interpretation for bone remodeling in algodystrophy, the histological findings are coherent with the biochemical data (calcitonin-induced hypocalcemia, calciuria, hyperhydroxyprolinuria), with the scintigraphic data, and with the evolution of the condition. *In short, algodystrophy would be a locoregional disease of the BMUs*. During the initial osteoclastic phase, which is related to a sudden excess of activation, there is bone loss and then subsequent osteoblastic reconstruction. It is still unknown whether this reconstruction is not abnormally slow in case of algodystrophy.

D. Periarticular Tissues

There are only rare reports of pathologic examination of periarticular tissues.

I. Capsule

Capsular lesions are most often described together with lesions of the synovial membrane, and concern mainly the humeroscapular and the coxofemoral joints. Hunder and Kelly [382] and de Marchi [191] speak of capsular thickening. For Steinbrocker and Argyros [777], "biopsy of periarticular tissues at the shoulder has been found to suggest a low-grade inflammatory reaction with proliferation of fibrous tissue, similar to finding in the periarticular structures of non-specific periarthritis, or the frozen shoulder."

Louyot et al. [523] published a case of retractile capsulitis of the shoulder subsequent to treatment by isoniazid in a case of Pott's disease.

At the autopsy of this patient, who died from a mesenteric infarction, the shoulder was dissected, disclosing a thickened and adherent capsule of which a specimen was taken. The sample was a piece of capsulosynovial tissue prolonged at one extremity by a striated muscle insertion. There was no evidence of alteration of the fibers in the muscular area, but a moderate interstitial adipose or collagenous hyperplasia and, on some sections only, some discrete infiltrations of peri- and intervascular round cells. As concerns the capsule itself, there was no evidence of degenerative or dystrophic alteration of the ground substance or of the collagen. On the contrary, the capsule appeared thickened and there were also some discrete inflammatory infiltrations of round cells, which are sometimes located around the vessels, sometimes parallel to the surface, but situated within the vascular walls, sometimes accompanied by moderate amounts of fat tissue. Finally, there was a discrete subendothelial hyalin deposit in the walls of some small arterioles. There were moreover, occasional granules of hemosiderin dispersed in the capsular tissue. There were a few nerve fillets in the paravascular areas; they were often surrounded by dense collagen.

In conclusion: this was an apparently nondystrophic capsular involvement, but with moderate nonspecific chronic inflammation. On the basis of this case, the authors feel entitled to eliminate iatrogenic capsuloligamentous involvements either secondary to treatment by phenobarbital, isoniazid, or radioactive iodine, or occurring in diabetes, from the group of algodystrophies.

II. Aponeuroses, Bursae, and Tendons

Once more we would like to point out that the data which we possess concerning aponeuroses are quite incomplete.

Steinbrocker reported: "In two of our patients, biopsies of the skin, subcutaneous tissue and muscle of the finger in advanced shoulder-hand syndrome gave no distinctive information. Fascial tissue from a palmar contracture in a shoulder hand syndrome was not distinguishable microscopically from the histology of classical Dupuytren's contracture."

In their work on phenobarbital-induced rheumatism, Arlet et al. [17] give details of the biopsy of an aponeurotic nodule of the hand, and of the subjacent tenosynovial sheath. The nodule had a fibrotic structure, as in Dupuytren's disease, and contained a small lymphocytic infiltration nodule. The tenosynovial sheath was abnormally thick and fibrotic: the intima was slightly edematous and there was a lymphocytic cellular infiltration nodule in the thickness of the fibrous sheath.

The serous bursae are most often unaffected, but they may also undergo retraction and become adherent.

The tendons can also be affected by an algodystrophic process. The frequency of this involvement is certainly underestimated.

III. Muscles

In 1942 Sudeck [796] stated: "As concerns the cutaneous and the muscular changes, we know nothing."

The work of Sieber and Meissner [763] concerning muscle biopsies, affords some data on the histological changes observed in the muscles in algodystrophy, although none of these changes is specific.

As concerns the muscle vessels, there may be active hyperemia, whereas other patients show arteriolar constriction and venous dilatation. In some cases there is a perivascular cellular infiltration. Muscular degeneration is evidenced by absence of cross striations, muscle bundles arranged in clods, granulations in the sarcolemma and vacuolization; these features are seen in 7 of 11 cases. In three, there is interstitial edema. Finally, the fibrosis of the interstitial substance which is observed in the most advanced cases, represents for these authors the terminal stage of the Sudeck syndrome.

After jointly studying the urinary elimination of creatine and creatinine, as well as the quantity of oxygen required by the muscle, the authors think that there are two types of lesion. The first form, which is accompanied by an increase in muscular metabolism and can rapidly lead to healing, is an active vasodilatation. The second form shows a diminution in the metabolic exchanges and should be interpreted as a nervous dysregulation responsible for muscular degeneration. But the two forms could equally well be only two successive evolutive stages.

In a case of shoulder-hand syndrome subsequent to treatment by phenobarbital, Schiano et al. [727] took a biopsy of the deltoid muscle. They observed disappearance of the double striation of the fibrils and hyperplasia of the sarcolemmal nuclei, disposed in peripheral or central columns. All these muscular changes were clear and diffuse and suggested a primary involvement of the muscular fibers.

In some cases, particularly in isoniazid-induced algodystrophies, lesions of the muscle fibers have been found but they could have been related to the associated polyneuritis described by Brouet and Marche [104].

We do not know the exact number of cases studied by Kirsch [410], but he reports muscular changes with passage from the functional state to a state of irreversible morphologic changes involving both the muscular vessels and the muscular fibers. Between muscle fibers, perimysium, and connective tissue, there is marked edema.

At stage II of algodystrophy, the affected vessels show vacuolar swelling of the intima, perivascular edema, and edema of the vessel walls. These lesions are not all reversible. It is known that vacuolization of the endothelial cells can be reversible, whereas swelling leads almost always to sclerosis of the vascular walls. This state is similar to the state described in hypoxia.

IV. Cutaneous Tissues

Although it would be very easy to sample a fragment of skin while performing an operation, very few histologic examinations of skin have been made in algodystrophy. We shall quote first the observation of Moriame et al. [585]. Their patient had been hospitalized owing to suspicion of incipient systemic scleroderma. "The pathologic examination of a skin biopsy taken on the forearm, shows evidence of an atrophic epidermis, associated with dermal sclerosis. The collagen fibers are markedly thickened and there are very few fibroblasts. The thickness of the adipose tissue is reduced. There are rare pilosebaceous appendages and the sweat glands are within the collagen tissue." Unfortunately we have no details of the clinical history, but we suspect it was a matter of an atrophic state.

In one of his observations Rutishauser et al. [708] point out the marked atrophy of the epidermis and of the hair follicles, and the presence of irregular and often follicular hyperkeratosis. The dermis is edematous and the subcutaneous tissue has almost disappeared.

The capillaries of the fat tissue show marked endothelial swelling.

The rare cases of algodystrophy reported by dermatologists do not include cutaneous or subcutaneous biopsies, which is surprising, to say the least.

V. Vessels

While studying the pathology of the various structures, we have already referred to the state of the vessels. This point however seems important enough to deserve a few paragraphs of its own.

There is great confusion concerning the physiopathology of algodystrophy: vasodilatation subsequent to an initial phase of vasoconstriction, according to Leriche [494], who spoke of hypervascularization on account of the pseudoinflammatory appearance of the affected articular area; reflex capillary stasis, according to Huet and Hugier [381]; ischemia due to diminished blood flow in the intraosseous arteries, according to Rohner [691]; and finally, slowed circulation and drainage difficulties evidenced by medullary stasis and blockage of the efferent osseous vessels, according to Ficat and Arlet [257].

We would subscribe to Rohner's conclusions. The disease seems to be characterized by dystrophic foci of osteomedullary activation combining slowed circulation, sinusoidal distension, fibrosis, and accelerated osteoclastosis soon followed by reconstruction. It is moreover known that moderate reduction of the blood flow in bone stimulates osteogenesis. The focal and disseminated character of these lesions accounts very likely for the irregular dappled appearance of decalcification on roentgenograms.

We would like to recall here the four types described in the classification of medullary lesions of vascular nature proposed by Ficat et al. [258]:

Type 1 comprises vascular changes, ectasia of the sinusoids, plasmostasis, hemorrhages, parietal thickening of the arterioles, xanthomatization, and fibrosis, all these disturbances being factors of ischemia.

Type 2 is medullary necrosis with dislocation, fragmentation, or confluence of the adipocytes and eosinophilic reticulate necrosis.

Type 3 is trabecular necrosis (disappearance of the osteocytes, oncosis, microfractures), associated with medullary necrosis.

Type 4, finally, consists of necrosis associated with signs of bone apposition along the dead trabeculae.

To our knowledge, there has been no publication concerning changes in the lymphatic vessels in algodystrophy.

VI. Nerves

Rutishauser et al. [708] report the median nerve to be the site of numerous foci of fatty degeneration of isolated myelinic fibers.

To our knowledge, however, the only case report including a histological examination of the nervous system is that of Soulié et al. [772]. This concerns a shoulder-hand syndrome in a case of fatal syphilitic aortitis. Histologically there was an endothelial proliferation in the territory of the last two cervical and first thoracic roots. The meninges, at the point where the roots emerge, the sheaths of the roots (mainly of the dorsal root), and the ganglionic pole were the site of an infiltration which in some places forms a continuous layer and in others, small nodules between the displaced nerve fibers. It was a proliferation of endothelial elements which formed a syncytium and cells with a large clear nucleus, poor in protoplasm, which took on in some areas the characteristics of fibroblasts. Dilacerated connective fibers, stained red-brown by silver methods, were intermingled with the reactional cells. In the meningeal cul-de-sac, the appearance was more that of granulation, and the vessels had undergone changes.

The topography of these findings is rather peculiar. At the level of the third thoracic root, the curious appearance of micromeningioma is no longer seen, but there is now moderate reactional infiltration. The tenth thoracic and second lumbar roots were sampled as controls and seen to be normal.

The spinal ganglions corresponding to the infiltrated roots were affected, especially at their medial pole and in their juxtaradicular prolongation. Besides the normal cells there were also features of chromatolysis and liquefaction, and signs of sclerosis and thickening of the capsule, and some glial nodules of substitution, marking the place of the cells which had disappeared.

The roots themselves, on the other hand, were only moderately affected. The myelin was roughly normal. Some degenerated axons were seen on the sections stained according to the method of Gros.

The medulla was studied at different levels and seen to be practically normal. The lateral horn was not modified. The cervical spinal cord showed some axonic degeneration of the posterior columns and a slight microglial reaction. The meninges, vessels, myelin, and cells had here their usual appearance.

In the peridural space the vessels were normal. There was no leukocytic infiltration but a sclerosis of the interstitial tissue and of the connectivo-fatty spaces, with some calcospherites.

In conclusion: this was an endothelial reaction of a peculiar type and topography. The spinal cord was normal, but the thoracocervical roots showed degenerative changes of a certain number of cells of the spinal ganglions, and especially infiltration of submeningeal cells forming in places true small meningiomas. The changes were mainly localized on the distal part of the posterior roots. The last cervical and first thoracic roots are electively involved: this is exactly the place one would have expected, given a knowledge of anatomy and the relations of the nerves, to be affected in a case of shoulder-hand syndrome.

The localization at the distal, juxtaganglionic part of the roots is that of the infiltrates and inflammatory reactions encountered in some chronic intoxications, in arterio-sclerosis, in cancer, and in tabes. Now the patient under study was syphilitic, but the scarcity of the clinical signs and the absence of changes in the cerebrospinal fluid had ruled out tabes. Further anatomic verifications are however needed if definite conclusions are to be made.

Part 3 Clinical Forms

Chapter 1 Topographic Forms

The topographic forms have already been described in Part 1, Chap. 3.

Chapter 2 Evolutive Forms

The potential evolution of an algodystrophic process is at present still unpredictable, but it is certainly significant: both as concerns its extent, considering the size of the area that may be affected, and considering the long duration of the disease and the possibility of successive episodes over several years in a single subject. This polymorphism allows a certain number of evolutive forms to be distinguished.

A. Initial Plurifocal Forms

These are characterized by the simultaneous or almost simultaneous involvement of two or more articular areas by about the same stage of the disease. Besides the forms with obvious clinical signs, we would mention the frequent plurifocal forms with only radiologic and/or scintigraphic manifestations.

I. Patent Forms

1. In the Upper Limb

In the upper limb the bipolar form is responsible for the classical shoulder-hand syndrome (see Part 1, Chap. 3), which has a very evocative appearance but is relatively infrequent (10 cases in our series of 250).

The associated involvement of shoulder, elbow, and hand constitutes the tripolar form, the frequency of which varies with the authors: according to Ravault [645] it is found in one-third of cases; May et al. [549] found its clinical manifestations 3 times in 20, and Schiano et al. [727] in 4 of 34 shoulder-hand syndromes. In our series it was seen once in 10 shoulder-hand syndromes. Involvement of the elbow is usually transient and recovers without sequels.

The bilateral forms of the shoulder-hand syndrome are rather frequent: Ravault [645] found them in more than one-third of cases (19 out of 52); in their series, Schiano et al. [727] note bilateral involvement 11 times in 34. In our material, we found only 2 cases. It is exceptional for bilateral involvement to occur simultaneously, as in our two cases. Most often there is an interval of several weeks between the involvement of the two limbs, so that really an alternating shoulder-hand syndrome is seen. Sometimes the two hands only are simultaneously affected; this occurred in three of our cases.

These bilateral forms are more frequently encountered in algodystrophies with a metabolic etiology: 6 of the 11 cases of Schiano et al. [727] belong to this group. Of the 6 bilateral forms of our series, one concerns a diabetic and two have a phenobarbital origin.

2. In the Lower Limb

In the lower limbs simultaneously occurring plurifocal forms are relatively rare. Harif [351] reports a foot-knee involvement in 12% of cases, a tripolar form in 5%, and a bilateral form in 8% of cases. Among 188 cases, Serre et al. [754] noted 5 foot-knee involvements (of which 1 was bilateral), 1 knee-hip involvement, 14 bilateral involvements of the feet, 2 bilateral involvements of the hips, and 1 bilateral involvement of the knees. In their series of 48 algodystrophies of the lower limbs, Schiano et al. [727] found involvement of foot and knee 8 times, of knee and hip 2 times, and only one tripolar involvement (foot-knee-hip). In our statistics bearing on 168 algodystrophies of the lower limbs, our findings were the following: foot-knee involvement in 10 cases, bilateral involvement of the feet in 7 cases and of the hip in one case, and a single tripolar form.

3. Simultaneous Involvement of the Four Limbs

Simultaneous involvement of the four limbs is relatively rare. Usually these polyarticular algodystrophies associate a bilateral shoulder-hand syndrome and involvement of the hip, or even the knee and/or toes, and may cause diagnostic problems in distinguishing them from rheumatoid arthritis or polymyalgia rheumatica. This form can be seen during diabetes or may be provoked by chemotherapies (ioniazid – ethionamid – phenobarbital). Compared to algodystrophies of classical locoregional cause, these iatrogenic polyarticular algodystrophies are usually fibrotic rather than demineralizing, and stiffening rather than edematous, justifying the term "polycapsulitis" proposed by Lequesne [483].

Numerous publications deal with these polyarticular forms. In 1956, Ravault and Durant [648] reported a case of algodystrophy affecting both shoulders, both hands, and both hips in a 50-year-old male suffering from angina pectoris and diaphragmatic hernia.

In 1967 Arlet et al. [17] reported 15 cases of rheumatism caused by phenobarbital and involving all four limbs.

Lequesne [470] proposes calling these polyarticular forms "extended shoulder-hand syndrome." In 1969, Deshayes et al. [198] noted 12 cases of extensive algodystrophy out of 22 cases secondary to tuberculotherapy. In 1970, Lequesne [476] reported 12 cases of algodystrophy in patients with diabetes mellitus, of which one was a case of "quadricapsulitis." In 1972, Louyot et al. [523] described a case of "capsuloligamentous involvement" due to isoniazid, combining a bilateral shoulder-hand syndrome and moderate stiffening of the left hip and right knee.

In 1973, David-Chaussé et al. [177] reported 3 cases of algodystrophy affecting all four limbs. The first case concerned a 75-year-old man operated for an angioma of the middle cerebral artery, who had been treated with phenobarbital; the second case concerned a 70-year-old woman who had also been treated with phenobarbital for epilepsy of vascular origin; the third case concerned a 64-year-old man who had had severe coronaritis for 10 years.

In 1976, Lequesne and Dreiser [483] report two cases with simultaneous polycapsulitis in cardiac patients: one case of coronaritis and one of operated mitral valve affection. In one of these cases the condition was fibrotic from the outset, without an edematous or demineralizing stage, deserving thus the term "polycapsulitis"; in the other case, the polycapsulitic appearance followed the more classical edematous picture after the third month.

In 1977, in their series of 103 cases, Schiano et al. [727] noted three forms affecting all four limbs; the first had a phenobarbital origin, the second concerned a diabetic, and in the third there was no known precipitating factor.

II. Latent Forms

Besides the forms with patent clinical signs, there are very often infraclinical forms with purely radiologic and/or scintigraphic signs: these are the latent forms. They may involve the same limb or the contralateral limb. Their clinical course is unpredictable: they may remain entirely asymptomatic or produce delayed clinical manifestations.

Thus in their series Schiano et al. [727] noted, among 34 shoulder-hand syndromes, a purely radiologic involvement of the elbow 2 times; and among 30 algodystrophies of the foot, a radiologic involvement of the contralateral foot 4 times, a radiologic involvement of the knee on the same side 2 times, and a radiologic involvement of the other foot and of both knees 2 times. Out of 8 algodystrophies affecting simultaneously the foot and the knee, Schiano et al. found one case with an associated radiologic involvement of the hip.

In our series of 250 cases, we made the following findings: there was one radiologic involvement with demineralization of both hands and both shoulders, with clinical involvement of one hand only; among 92 algodystrophies affecting the foot we found 4 cases with a radiologic involvement of the ipsilateral knee, 1 case with radiologic signs on the other foot, and two cases with radiologic signs on the knee and the hip on the same side.

Moreover, as has been pointed out by two of us, bone scanning has shown the frequency of increased isotope uptake in clinically normal segments. In such cases it is thus possible to speak about "pure isotopic forms" [215].

B. Secondarily Extensive Forms

These are characterized by the successive involvement of several articular regions, at variable intervals in time, the first site remaining evolutive.

In *the upper limb* the shoulder-hand syndrome is a schematic example of this form. But true extensive algodystrophies of the lower limb begin with the bilateral forms, which are encountered in about one-third of cases. Sometimes an algodystrophy with rapid or dramatic onset also affects both sides at once, but more often there is an interval of several weeks to a few months separating the involvements of the two sides, so that an alternating form is realized. Finally, algodystrophy may overlap the upper limb and migrate to the lower limbs: hips, knees, and even feet.

These extensive forms are more often seen in algodystrophies of chemotherapic origin. Rheumatism due to treatment with phenobarbitals has long been recognized: it would certainly turn out to less rare than is generally thought if it were systematically searched for in all cases of atypical algodystrophy. Algodystrophy subsequent to chemotherapy of tuberculosis has received increasing attention since 1961: isoniazid has been identified as the responsible agent, but the association of this drug with ethionamid seems to increase significantly the risk. Finally, algodystrophies of this type have also been reported in diabetes and hyperthyroidism, especially after treatment with iodine 131.

These iatrogenic algodystrophies have peculiar features in common: there is usually no initial edematous stage, radiologic signs of osteoporosis are mild or absent, capsular fibrosis and stiffness are very marked, and palmar or plantar fibrous nodules are often present.

For all these reasons some workers [482, 523] thought it necessary to distinguish this condition from common demineralizing algodystrophies. This seems to us unjustified, since there are numerous intermediate forms to prove that demineralizing algodystrophies and fibrotic algodystrophies are only extreme conditions, each developing predominantly one aspect of a usually mixed symptomatology.

While extended forms of the shoulder-hand syndrome are relatively rare, *the inferior limbs* are very often the site of extensive forms. The time lapse between the successive episodes is very marked, sometimes being several months, so that the duration of the disease is quite long and discouraging for both patient and physician. The progressive extension has no preferential pattern but is most often ascending, extending to the adjacent articulation, i.e., from the foot to the knee, and from there eventually to the hip. Sometimes however the condition migrates to the other side, preferably to the homologous articulation, resulting in an *alternating form*; this is quite common in the feet, somewhat less frequent in the knees; in the hips bilateralization is not exceptional, although not very frequent.

In their series, Serre et al. [754] found 54 extensive forms among 188 cases (28%), distributed as follows with regard to the initial site: 18 extensive forms from the knee (10% of the cases), of which 15 were to the homolateral lower limb and 3 to the contralateral lower limb; 32 extensive forms from the foot (25% of the cases), of which 25 were to the homolateral lower limb and 4 to the contralateral lower limb; 4 extensive forms from the hip, of which 3 were to the homolateral lower limb and 1 was an alternating form.

Schiano et al. [727] note among their series 6 extensive forms, of which 5 affected the lower limbs. Among about 60 demineralizing algodystrophies of the hip, Lequesne and Maurer [485] note the extensive form in one-fourth, but they do not indicate the precise topography.

We found 16 alternating forms, of which 6 affected the feet and 4 the hips, in our series of 250 cases.

Contrariwise, algodystrophy of the lower limbs extending to the upper limbs is possible but exceptional: we found only one convincing case in Riera's thesis [682].

Finally, *extension to the spine* may occur, as described by Gougeon and Moreau-Hottin [320] in 1966, and by Serre et al. [747, 753] in 1968 and 1974 (see Part 1, Chap. 3).

A final proof of the expansive potential of algodystrophies of the lower limbs is provided by the occurrence of successive episodes in the same patient's life: these are the *forms with multiple episodes* reported for the first time by Gougeon and Moreau-Hottin [320]. Recently several French and American publications have pointed out observations of the same sort [228, 446, 670, 743, 801]. Two of us described in 1973 three cases of "*plurifocal recurrent algodystrophy*" [216].

The intervals between two episodes vary from 6 months to 10 years and these intervals are entirely symptom-free; some radiologic signs, such as a rough appearance of the bone structure, may however persist. The algodystrophic episodes proper have no significant peculiarities: they are perhaps more often polyarticular than the average, but their clinical course and recovery have the usual duration.

C. True Recurrent Forms

These forms are characterized by the occurrence of algodystrophy confined to the same articulation and are exceptional. Gougeon and Moreau-Hottin [320] report one case, Langloh's series [446] has two, and 3 cases concerning the hip have been recorded respectively by Hasche and Meyer [354] Temesvari et al. [806], and Lequesne [474]. In our series we have 3 cases, two affecting the foot and one the hip.

Remarkably, an articulation affected with algodystrophy is usually spared during subsequent episodes, as if protected; there are however some exceptions to this rule. As stressed by Rénier [669] one cannot explain why "a disturbance in the regional neurovegetative regulation seems to be able to occur only once in the same territory."

D. Partial Forms

These forms were described in 1976 by Lequesne and Bensasson [479], who also gave their precise characteristics in 1977 [484].

Analogous facts had also been reported in 1972 by Damman [170] with reference to 3 cases of algodystrophy confined to 2 or 3 fingers of one hand.

Two forms can be distinguished: the radial type, which affects only one or two metacarpo-metatarso-digital rays, and the zonal type, in which decalcification is confined to the femoral head, to a condyle of the femur, or to a tarsal bone.

I. Radial Forms

These affect only one or two carpo-metacarpo-phalangeal or tarso-metatarso-phalangeal rays. The clinical signs consist of pain and edema confined to one or two fingers, or to one or two toes.

As is usual in algodystrophy, the radiological signs are seen only 3–6 weeks after the onset of pain; they consist of hypertranslucency of one or two fingers, predominantly the epiphyses, which regresses tardily. It may remain partial throughout the course of the disease, as in Lequesne's case 1 [484], but it may also spread, as in Lequesne's case 2, where it extended from the third ray to the entire foot by the third month. We have observed 2 cases of radial algodystrophy involving only the head of a metatarsal and, in one of the cases, extension to the second and third rays of the foot.

II. Zonal Forms

In this type demineralization is confined to a restricted area of the knee or hip: patella [146], lateral or medial condyle, superolateral quadrant or posterior part of the femoral head. Of Lequesne's seven cases, four involved the knee and three the hip.

The clinical picture does not greatly differ from that of the classical form, but, as concerns the knee, pain is confined to the patella or to the lateral or medial condyle of the femur.

The radiological evolution is however quite peculiar: normal appearance during the first month, then partial demineralization during the second month, and finally widespread extension with the classical picture of algodystrophy, on the average by the fourth month. Lequesne has pointed out a migrating form in 2 cases out of 7 with simultaneous global demineralization.

The main interest of this peculiar form of algodystrophy lies in the difficulty of its diagnosis during the 2–3 months when demineralization remains zonal and infectious, acute inflammatory, and above all, tumoral processes enter into the discussion.

E. Parcellar Forms

Two of us described this peculiar form of algodystrophy [211] with reference to 7 cases, of which 6 affected the knee.

Clinically this form was characterized by an elective punctual pain at the level of a femoral condyle or of a tibial plate. The radiologic investigation showed an extremely confined demineralized area with unsharp limits, always sparing the contours of the cortical bone. Bone scanning with technetium 99m showed a more or less localized and more or less marked increased activity in the 7 cases. The clinical course was quite particular, since in 6 of the 7 cases the involvement remained strictly confined and recovery occurred within a few weeks or months without locoregional extension. In the 7th case the involvement of the cuboid bone was initially very restricted but extended subsequently to the entire foot as in Lequesne's cases.

Chapter 3 Incomplete Forms

A. Clinical

One of the characteristic features of algodystrophy is its very broad clinical polymorphism including both the most dramatic and the most incomplete forms. We would also like to stress that the hyperemic phase is sometimes very short or even absent, so that the patient is seen only at the ischemic phase.

Algodystrophy of the foot is very often responsible for a misleading clinical picture characterized by painful disability with a strictly normal clinical examination. As was stressed by Serre et al. [754] the discrepancy between the absence of objective signs at the clinical examination and the painful disability on walking is strongly evocative of algodystrophy of the foot which may subsequently be confirmed by roentgenograms and bone scans.

The same considerations hold good for *algodystrophy of the hip,* which often causes total functional disability, usually with few clinical signs.

B. Radiological

In the same way as there are painless algodystrophies, there are also algodystrophies without radiological signs. Harif [352] found 3 cases among 85 without radiologic signs during the entire course of the disease (see Part 2, Chap. 2). In our series of 250 cases we had 8 cases without radiological features during the entire course; one of these cases concerned an involvement of the foot in a Lobstein's disease. Very recently, Lequesne and Spartien [487] reported 5 such cases, including 2 which affected the hip. In these cases bone scanning is most informative and may be the main basis for the diagnosis.

C. Scintigraphic

In algodystrophy increased activity at bone scanning is very frequent but not absolutely constant.

In some rare cases, bone scanning can show *normal uptake,* as in one of our cases with three clinically involved sites, but only one increased activity focus. In algodystrophy of the shoulder, the common finding is isofixation.

Finally, in some exceptional cases, there may even be *isotopic hypofixation*; this was stressed by Majd [531], and we have seen it in a case of algodystrophy of the foot (see Part 2, Chap. 3).

Chapter 4 Atypical Forms

Unusual clinical features may raise difficult problems of diagnosis.

A. Hyperinflammatory Forms

In some cases the pseudoinflammatory clinical syndrome is particularly intense and characterized by marked swelling of the soft parts, significantly red skin with increased local warmth and severe spontaneous pain interfering with sleep. These various signs may suggest the possibility of septic or infectious arthritis, this diagnosis being ruled out, however, by the clinical course, the laboratory findings, or even puncture of the articulation at biopsy of the synovia.

B. Pseudophlegmonous Forms

The pseudophlegmonous appearance of algodystrophy is particularly seen on the hand, making it difficult to differentiate from septic tenosynovitis, or from phlegmon of the digital sheaths, as was the case in two of our observations.

C. Fibrotic Forms (Pseudo-Dupuytren)

At the level of the hand, algodystrophy may involve atrophy of the tissues, accompanied by sclerosis and tendinous and aponeurotic retraction, sometimes causing deformations of the fingers, which remain in a semiflexed position producing the classical "neurotrophic claw." There are sometimes also palmar nodular indurations so that the appearance may be difficult to distinguish from that of true Dupuytren disease.

D. Pseudosclerodermic Forms

In these exceptional cases, algodystrophy affecting the hands produces atrophy of the subcutaneous tissue and a clinical picture evoking scleroderma. In two of our cases with involvement of both hands, the diagnosis could not be definitely made, especially since the biopsies were not conclusive.

Finally, study of the clinical forms leads us to stress the *extreme polymorphism* of the clinical manifestations and of the radiologic and scintigraphic signs, and the great variability in the clinical course and severity of algodystrophy. This accounts for the fact that the affection has been described under numerous names and that some authors have described distinct entities.

We believe that all these clinical pictures are only aspects of one and the same disease, which justifies the term *algodystrophy* which we have adopted.

Part 4 Differential Diagnosis

Taken separately each clinical or paraclinical sign may lead one to consider several diagnoses.

As we have already said, algodystrophy may present with incomplete or atypical forms, sometimes very misleading forms suggesting very different diagnoses. Thus, the pseudoinflammatory clinical syndrome can simulate inflammatory or infectious osteoarticular processes; the radiological syndrome can mimic inflammatory, infectious, tumoral, or dystrophic bone diseases; the isotopic syndrome may sometimes be reminiscent of certain bone diseases.

Chapter 1 Inflammatory Processes

A. Synovitis

The pseudoinflammatory clinical syndrome involving an articular region, sometimes accompanied by marked swelling, red skin, increased local warmth, spontaneous pain or pain provoked by active and passive movements, leads quite naturally to the diagnosis of arthritis, i.e., synovitis.

Examination may give evidence of an intraarticular effusion. In this case, removal of the fluid is advisable; if analysis shows it to be paucicellular, rich in mucin, and poor in fibrin, then the diagnosis can be corrected.

Synovial biopsy performed with a trephine when the joint is accessible, will rule out the diagnosis of synovitis. It demonstrates the absence of cellular infiltration, the marked vascular congestion, and the absence of abnormal synovioblastic lining.

In certain cases scintigraphy helps to rule out synovitis by giving evidence of a localized increased uptake, while synovitis would show diffuse hyperfixation.

Sometimes, however, it is very difficult to establish the diagnosis, although there are usually no biochemical signs of inflammation in algodystrophy.

Inflammatory or infectious *monoarthritis* as well as tuberculous arthritis may be confusing.

Oligoarthritis may also be responsible for a clinical picture mimicking a plurifocal form of algodystrophy.

Rheumatoid arthritis may be simulated by algodystrophy, as in one of our cases reported in Part 6; the case concerns a man with a polyarticular involvement of the wrists and the metacarpophalangeal and proximal interphalangeal articulations, resulting in bilateral and symmetrical stiffness in the morning with a clinical picture strongly evocative of rheumatoid arthritis.

The involvement of the shoulders, the absence of biochemical inflammatory signs, the ineffectiveness of anti-inflammatory drugs, and above all the fact (difficult to elicit) of regular phenobarbital intake, were all clues for the diagnosis, which was moreover confirmed by the patient's rapid and complete recovery after suppression of the phenobarbital.

Another of our cases concerns a patient with algodystrophy of the hand following synovectomy of the metacarpophalangeal articulations for rheumatoid arthritis. In this case it is difficult to know what part was played by the rheumatoid arthritis, taking into account the surgical trauma.

But rheumatoid arthritis may raise other problems. In a case of arthritis which is well controlled by the therapy, there may occur an arthropathic episode which is not directly related to the rheumatoid process, but rather to algodystrophy, as in the case reported below:

A 72-year-old woman had a definite rheumatoid arthritis (according to the ARA criteria) which had evolved for 25 years with bilateral and symmetrical involvement of the wrists, the metacarpophalangeal and proximal interphalangeal articulations on both hands, both shoulders, and the cervical spine. For several years 6 mg deltacortisone per day had kept the disease well under control, when in March 1978 there suddenly occurred pain in the medial aspect of the right knee, although the rheumatoid process had never affected the knee up to then.

The pain in the right knee was spontaneous, interfered with sleep and prevented walking and weight-bearing.

At examination there was moderate swelling confined to the medial aspect of the right knee (the perimeter of the knee was increased by 1 cm) and the local warmth was clearly increased.

Palpation did not reveal intra-articular effusion, but a localized tender spot was found on pressure on a very confined area of the medial condyle, whereas the other areas of the tibial and femoral epiphyses where absolutely painless on palpation. The mobility of the joint was normal apart from pain at the end of the flexion range. The alignment of the limb was normal, and there was no abnormal motion or any sign of meniscus involvement. The erythrocyte sedimentation rate was 30 mm after 1 h (previous laboratory data had been similar, in keeping with the rheumatoid disease).

The radiographs were normal. The clinical picture ruled out the first hypothesis to come to mind, namely an episode of the rheumatoid disease of the knee. The possibility of aseptic necrosis of a femoral condyle or of algodystrophy was also considered.

Bone scan with technetium 99m showed significantly increased uptake confined to a "parcella" of the medial condyle of the right knee.

Calcitonin therapy produced rapid and complete recovery without clinical, radiological or scintigraphic sequels, thus confirming the diagnosis of parcellar algodystrophy of the right knee in a quiescent rheumatoid arthritis.

In 1954 Coste et al. [155] had reported a case of algodystrophy of the upper limb occurring in rheumatoid arthritis. They pointed out that treatments which improve arthritis (gold, deltacortisone) did not produce any changes in the algodystrophic syndrome (shoulder-hand type).

Recently, Barraud et al. [34] reported two cases concerning patients aged 55 and 58 in whom an algodystrophic condition had developed after a traumatism and then evolved into rheumatoid arthritis; according to these authors, posttraumatic algodystrophy would favor the development of rheumatoid-type inflammatory arthropathy in certain predisposed subjects.

Algodystrophy in other inflammatory rheumatisms may also cause diagnostic problems. We have observed a case of posttraumatic algodystrophy of the foot in a patient suffering from quiescent *ankylosing spondylarthritis,* two cases of typical algodystrophy of a shoulder and a knee during a *Reiter's syndrome,* and one case of algodystrophy of the shoulder during *polymyalgia rheumatica.*

With regard to these cases it seems possible that the impact of the inflammation on the articulation in question constituted a factor initiating algodystrophy, in the same way as a traumatism to the joint.

Gout and other forms of microcrystalline arthritis can predispose to algodystrophy. In a patient suffering from gout or chondrocalcinosis, it may be that the articulation is affected by microcrystalline arthritis or it may be a case of algodystrophy. These forms of arthritis are very likely favoring factors, as are hyperlipidemia and diabetes mellitus, frequently encountered in patients with gout.

B. Phlebitis

Phlebitis of the lower or the upper limbs can be mistaken for algodystrophy. The clinical picture can be very similar, making diagnosis difficult, especially since algodystrophy may complicate a true phlebitis; the clinical signs of both affections are then present successively or intermingled.

But, contrary to what is seen with phlebitis, in algodystrophy the cardia rhythm remains normal, the sedimentation rate is not elevated, the bone scan shows early signs of hyperactivity, and the roentgenograms show demineralization. Moreover, there is usually an indurated vein in cases with phlebitis.

Chapter 2 Infection

A. Osteitis

Algodystrophy may present with acute pain and bone involvement characterized by a heterogeneous demineralization, suggesting osteitis.

In some of their cases of partial demineralizing algodystrophy, Lequesne et al. [484] point out the difficulty of the differential diagnosis with an infectious process, osteitis, or even osteoarthritis.

But there are no biochemical inflammatory signs in algodystrophy, and above all the regressive course of algodystrophy finally rules out osteitis.

B. Abscesses

The pseudophlegmonous appearance of algodystrophy is mainly seen on the hands, in which case the differential diagnosis with septic tenosynovitis and with phlegmon of the digital tendon sheaths can be very difficult.

In one of our cases a phlegmon of the sheath of a flexor tendon had been diagnosed. Surgery had shown absence of suppuration: there was only a paucicellular fluid. In such cases the evolution is often longer-lasting, carrying the risk of sequels, e.g., increased fibroaponeurotic retraction.

In the case described below, we hesitated for a long time over whether or not to undertake surgery.

A 54-year-old very anxious man consulted us in October 1979 with a very acute inflammation of the third finger on his right hand, which had occurred very suddenly. The finger was significantly swollen, the skin was warm, red, glistening, and tense; the pain was very severe, preventing the slightest movement. The clinical picture was that of a phlegmon of the flexor sheath of the right third finger. Over the next few days the inflammatory manifestations were still greatest in the third finger and also extended to the hand; the sedimentation rate remained normal; there was no hyperleukocytosis.

Uricemia at the upper limit of normal caused us to suspect gout, but this diagnosis was ruled out by the failure of colchicine therapy. The laboratory data showed a hyperglycemia of 9.3 mmol/l and hyperlipidemia of 11 g/l, with hypertriglyceridemia of 3 mmol/l.

Finally, we decided not to operate, and recovery without sequels was obtained within 4 months after a phase of stiffness and sclerodermiform appearance of the hand.

C. Septic Arthritis

A diagnosis of septic arthritis suggested by the clinical features is rapidly abandoned after study of the articular fluid removed by puncture, whenever this is possible – in algodystrophy this fluid is always paucicellular – and on the grounds that there is no hyperleukocytosis and that the sedimentation rate is not increased. In addition, the subchondral bone lamina is almost always spared: the roentgenogram shows it delineating the contours of the demineralized bone. Nevertheless, true septic arthritis may accompany or be followed (after healing) by an algodystrophy provoked by the septic agression.

We have come across two cases with septic arthritis of a metatarsophalangeal articulation treated with antibiotics which first recovered and later showed recurrence of the clinical and inflammatory symptoms. In both cases it was a matter of algodystrophy affecting the entire foot, which healed entirely within a few months, without sequels other than a rough and fibrillar appearance of the bone trabecula on radiograms.

Chapter 3 Tumors

A. Benign Tumors

The differential diagnosis with some benign tumors, particularly *osteoid osteomas,* of certain forms of algodystrophy, such as the parcellar form, is very difficult. Very localized pain, very confined hyperactivity at bone scanning, and absence of biochemical inflammatory signs are seen in both conditions. The roentgen examination does not always provide clues in favor of one or the other diagnosis. The regressive evolution of the algodystrophy or even biopsy will sometimes allow the diagnosis to be confirmed.

According to Lesquene et al. [484] a *giant-cell tumor* may be responsible for an osteolytic appearance very similar to that seen in partial demineralizing algodystrophy of the knee or, more rarely, of the hip; however, as we have seen, in algodystrophy the osteolysis affects the subchondral bone selectively and only spares the subchondral bone lamina, which is not the case with giant-cell tumors.

B. Malignant Tumors

Again, it is with partial osteoporosis, which Lequesne particularly emphasized, that differential diagnosis with *primary malignant tumors,* such as *reticulosarcomas, fibromas,* or *lymphosarcomas,* is considered, especially when there is involvement of the femoral condyle or the femoral head, both of which can be partly or totally destroyed.

In algodystrophy, however, the subchondral bone lamina is spared, as has already been pointed out. The contours of the bone are thus clearly visible, the more so since the subchondral bone may have almost disappeared. It should however be kept in mind that in some rare cases, even the subchondral bone lamina may be interrupted, so that the differential diagnosis with a malignant tumor becomes very difficult and may necessitate bone biopsy.

Bone metastases may also be considered, although the same radiologic arguments usually allow a malignant process to be ruled out.

In bone syndromes suggesting a primary or a secondary malignant tumoral process, sucessful treatment by calcitonin or beta-blocking drugs with rapid and definite healing, is strong evidence in favor of algodystrophy, as in the two cases reported in Part 2, Chap. 3: one case concerns a very incapacitating involvement of the hip in a woman who had had a uterine cancer, and the other an involvement of the knee in a woman with breast cancer; in both cases bone scanning had shown markedly increased uptake, which entirely regressed within 4 months.

Chapter 4 Bone Necrosis

The early stage of aseptic necrosis, particularly of the femoral head or of a femoral condyle in the knee, is very difficult to differentiate from algodystrophy. The clinical picture is the same in both conditions, i.e., pain on weight-bearing or even at night and a discrepancy between the severe functional incompetence, sometimes interfering with walking, and the relatively well preserved passive mobility, with pain occuring only at the limit of range of movement. Neither condition has biochemical inflammatory signs. The biological background is often the same, and according to certain authors, the physiopathologic mechanism is similar in the two diseases. The roentgenograms are not very informative; at the onset the pattern is almost normal, or sometimes there is an inhomogeneous dappled appearance, very difficult to interpret. Even the phlebogram or the histologic study performed on a trephine biopsy specimen do not always permit differentiation of these two conditions [14]. One may also observe, as in one of our cases, necrosis of the femoral head and contralateral algodystrophy of the hip 6 months later.

Bone scanning shows increased activity in both conditions but extension to the acetabulum, the femoral neck, the ilio- and ischiopubic rami, and sometimes to the femoral diaphysis, or even to one or several articulations of the lower limbs count in favor of algodystrophy.

Analysis of the increased uptake by selective counting is particularly rewarding in weighing these alternative diagnosis, as was demonstrated in the study of Gaucher et al. [295]. In algodystrophy of the hip the increased uptake is very marked from the onset; it has its own site and is homogeneous; the isodensity curves form a "targetlike" image. Within a few months there is no more abnormal uptake. Contrariwise, in necrosis of the femoral head the tracer uptake is normal at the onset; there may even be hypofixation as direct evidence of bone necrosis. Later, there is a "halo" or a crescent-shaped hyperfixation delineating the necrotic area. Sometimes the reactional increased uptake may extend and mask the low activity of the necrotic area.

Osteonecrosis of the condyles of the knee may be responsible for a clinical picture very similar to that of parcellar algodystrophy. Here too, regression without clinical or radiologic sequels confirms the diagnosis of parcellar algodystrophy. In 50% of cases recovery is considerably accelerated by calcitonin therapy; it is thus quite legitimate to use it as a test therapy. Of course it is valuable as such only when it is very rapidly effective.

Chapter 5 Arthrosis

Arthrosis of the articulations of the limbs usually causes mechanical-type pains and quite characteristic though not specific radiologic signs. But in some instances and in certain sites the radiological signs appear rather late, as for example in the knee.

Thus, in the case of a painful knee it may be difficult to differentiate gonarthrosis from algodystrophy. Moreover, evidence of arthrosis consists of congestive episodes with a mild inflammatory pattern, increased local warmth, discreet swelling, and paucicellular intra-articular fluid which shows no inflammatory pattern. The roentgenograms may be almost normal. In such cases the differential diagnosis between algodystrophy and an arthrosic episode is almost impossible. Only the evolution will permit a definite diagnosis.

Furthermore, in a patient in whom the diagnosis of arthrosis has been arrived at on clinical and radiological grounds, algodystrophy may occur as well, so that the manifestations of both diseases are mixed up together. Radiologic signs characteristic of algodystrophy and markedly increased activity on bone scans count definitely in favor of algodystrophy.

Chapter 6 Miscellaneous

A. Fatigue Fractures

Fatigue fractures are related to overstraining of joints by repeated microtraumatisms to an unaffected bone, in the absence of an obvious single traumatism. They often present with a clinical picture of the pseudoinflammatory type, very similar to that of algodystrophy. Neither condition shows any inflammatory signs and both have normal radiograms for one or more weeks after the onset of pain. In both cases also, bone scanning with technetium 99m shows increased uptake of the tracer; but in algodystrophy this increased activity is usually more diffuse, whereas in cases of fatigue fracture it is distant from the joint. This may be a clue to the diagnosis, but the radiologic evolution is the main diagnostic factor.

B. Chondromatosis – Osteochondromatosis

Cayla et al. [125] reported in 1965 three cases of a demineralizing form of chondromatosis of the hip.

Lequesne et al. [478] reported four cases of capsular retraction associated with chondromatosis of the hip. In such cases the question arises whether demineralization is directly related to chondromatosis or whether the chondromatosis is associated with algodystrophy; we report a case with such an association in Part 2, Chap. 8.

However that may be, in such instances chondromatosis mimicks algodystrophy, and only arthrography provides more precise data for diagnosing chondromatosis.

C. Dupuytren's Contracture

In the upper limbs algodystrophy may cause atrophy of the tissues: skin, subcutaneous cellular tissue, muscles, tendons, aponeuroses, bone. The atrophy is accompanied by sclerosis and tendinous and aponeurotic retraction, sometimes causing deformation of the fingers and an irreducible semiflexed claw-like position involving mainly the fourth and the fifth fingers. There are also nodular proliferations. The condition may be confused with the true Dupuytren's contracture. Such a confusion is especially difficult to avoid since Dupuytren's contracture may have various causes, e.g., traumatism, microtraumatism, or lesions of the peripheral nerves or of the central nervous system [46, 380, 525].

D. Dupuytren's Disease of the Foot

Dupuytren's disease of the foot, which is associated with Dupuytren's contracture in a non-negligible number of cases, is a nodular fibroblastic proliferation of the plantar fascia. Algodystrophy of the foot results sometimes in retraction of the plantar fascia, which is indistinguishable from Dupuytren's disease of the foot, since the latter may also be subsequent to a traumatism.

E. Scleroderma

It is mainly on the hands that atrophy and sclerosis of cutaneous and subcutaneous cellular tissue may produce a clinical picture resembling scleroderma. When the bone is affected, bone scanning can be very useful for diagnosing algodystrophy.

Skin biopsy does not enable one to make the differential diagnosis, and it remains very difficult in cases of bilateral involvement, as in two of our cases [150, 525].

F. Osteolysis

I. Idiopathic Osteolysis

In some cases of algodystrophy the locoregional demineralization is so marked that idiopathic osteolysis may have to be considered.

Idiopathic massive osteolysis, described in 1838, is rare; in half of the cases it occurs subsequently to a traumatism. It is unilateral and affects the bones of the shoulder and thoracic girdle. It causes mechanical-type pain and partial or complete disappearance of a bone; it extends by contiguity. The condition may become stabilized, but normal bone structure is never restored, which is not the case with algodystrophy.

II. Idiopathic Acro-osteolysis

The possibility of idiopathic acro-osteolysis also has to be discussed, although it is very rare in algodystrophies with massive demineralization of hands and feet. Idiopathic acro-osteolysis, however, is rarely painful. Its slow evolution ends with progressive disappearance of the affected bones and extension to other bones. It is in fact a true bone lysis, starting at the extremity of the phalanges with thinning-out of the bones, which taper like partially consumed candy cone and finally disappear. This is quite different from what is seen in algodystrophy, where the shape of the bone is preserved and the contours almost always remain visible.

III. Secondary Osteolysis

This is usually more easy to diagnose. We have already mentioned the difficulties arising with osteitis and tumors.

Rheumatoid arthritis may be complicated with osteolysis of the metacarpals and of the first phalanges.

Tabes, syringomyelia, and lepra may be responsible for a progressive lysis of certain bones. These lesions are very evocative since they are painless and accompanied by global or thermoalgesic hypoesthesis. Osteolysis may also be encountered in hyperparathyroidism. The hypercalcemia which is usually present orientates the diagnosis.

G. Osteoporosis Following Immobilization

Osteoporosis following immobilization causes very difficult differential diagnostic problems with alogodystrophy stricto sensu, and has given rise to innumerable discussions for about 100 years with no agreement having been reached as to the borderline between immobilization osteoporosis and algodystrophy.

H. Posttraumatic Paget's Disease

In some cases of algodystrophy at the sequellar stage, the rough appearance of the bone trabecula may be so marked as to be mistaken for a case of Paget's disease.

Rohner [691] reports three cases with a pathologic study and compares the posttraumatic pagetoid bone changes with the atrophic stage of algodystrophy.

I. Sprains

The problem of posttraumatic algodystrophy following a sprain may be difficult.

One must first distinguish sprains from the inflammatory signs of primary algodystrophy. Very often the patient with a sprain seeks medical help because he believes the inflammatory symptoms must be the result of a possibly overlooked traumatism. Careful inquiry may sometimes rule out traumatism. When there is obviously a sprain, one must try to elucidate what part is played by the sprain and how much is attributable to a subsequent true posttraumatic algodystrophy, the pseudoinflammatory manifestations of which have taken over where the manifestations related to the sprain left off.

The diagnosis of algodystrophy will be based on clinical, radiological, biochemical, and scintigraphic data and on the clinical course.

K. Somatic Conversion Syndromes: Hysteria

In some atypical forms of algodystrophy it may be difficult to assess the organic nature of the disease. This is the case particularly with algodystrophy of the foot with severe pain preventing weight-bearing but without clinical signs. apart from moderate hypothermia. One may even be tempted to suspect the patient's good faith.

The discrepancy between total functional incompetence and almost complete absence of objective clinical signs could lead one to suspect diagnosis such as pithiatism, somatic conversion syndromes, hysteria, or even simulation. In such instances the clinical examination may give evidence of local hypothermia, supporting the organicity of these manifestations, as has already been reported by Babinski and Froment [28] and as we noted in three cases. Hyperreflexivity may also be present or even inexhaustible epileptoid trepidation. Babinski and Froment [26] went as far as to administer chloroform narcosis, which allowed them to confirm the authenticity of the tendinous hyperreflexivity.

The roentgenograms are usually normal at the onset of the disease but may give evidence of demineralization after one or more months, suggesting algodystrophy. In cases with silent roentgenograms, bone scanning can provide valuable data by giving evidence of hyperfixation or more rarely hypofixation and allowing confirmation of the organicity of the functional manifestations, suggesting the diagnosis of algodystrophy [264, 386, 397, 836].

Part 5 Positive Criteria

In Part 3 we pointed out the great polymorphism of algodystrophy that includes typical and easily recognizable forms as well as the most atypical and incomplete forms. Diagnosis of algodystrophy is based on a number of criteria. Each clinical or paraclinical sign taken separately is nonspecific and is sometimes not even evocative of algodystrophy. It is the association of these different criteria which enables the diagnosis to be made.

Clinical Criteria

Pain may have a sudden or a progressive onset; it can be of the mechanical, inflammatory, or mixed type and involve an articular area or be diffuse, localized, or even very strictly confined to a part. It can be sponteous or provoked by palpation or mobilization. There is, in addition, more or less marked swelling, and increased local heat. There are also changes in the appearance of the skin, which becomes pink or even cyanotic; these changes are aggravated by the sloping position. Sweating is increased to a greater or lesser degree. There is also marked functional disability contrasting with the relatively well preserved amplitude of the articular movements during passive mobilization. Finally, certain localizations are strongly evocative of algodystrophy: e.g., simultaneous involvement of a shoulder and the homolateral hand – the classical shoulder-hand syndrome.

When the patient is seen after a several weeks' or months' more or less spontaneous evolution, there is often no edema. The appearance of the articular area can be quite normal. The skin has a normal coloration, it may be cold and may sometimes have a sclerodermiform appearance. The contrast between this apparently normal articular area and the total functional disability with severe pain, for instance on weight-bearing in the conditions affecting the lower limbs, is now very striking and strongly suggests algodystrophy.

Radiological Criteria

Absence of any radiographic anomaly is a constant finding during the onset of the disease and is not an argument against algodystrophy. After some weeks' evolution, the demineralization may be homogeneous and vitreous, but the most typical feature is heterogeneous demineralization producing a patchy and dappled appearance of the bone with multiple lacunae of variable but usually rather small size, which are poorly outlined and distributed on the epiphyses and even the diaphyses of the articular area. This latter criterion is in itself an argument, if not pathognomonic then at least a cardinal one for the diagnosis of algodystrophy. The demineralization is particularly marked in the subchondral area, but it almost always spares the subchondral bone lamina, so that the bone contours persist and are visible as an opacity resembling a line drawn with a pencil.

There are also *two negative signs* which are of cardinal importance: absence of narrowing of the articular interspaces and absence of denser bone margins.

Biochemical Criteria

These consist only in the absence of biochemical signs of inflammation, particularly the absence of increased erythrocyte sedimentation rate.

Other biochemical anomalies may be found but they have no value for the diagnosis of algodystrophy.

Scintigraphic Criteria

Algodystrophy is one of the diseases in which bone scanning shows the most marked increased uptake of technetium ^{99m}, and this occurs very early and prior to the appearance of radiologic anomalies. Although increased uptake of tracer is not a specific feature, it is of great value for the diagnosis, as we recently pointed out in a study of 74 cases of algodystrophy.

Although bone scanning is not indispensable for diagnosing radioclinically typical forms, it affords a definite clue in atypical or misleading forms. It may also provide a valuable argument in forms which show no radiologic changes throughout the course of the disease or in very localized, partial and parcellar forms. Extension of the increased uptake to several articular areas is sometimes also a valuable clue for the diagnosis. It should also be kept in mind that there are also cases of algodystrophy which show no increased uptake throughout the course of the disease.

As we pointed out in Part 2, Chap. 3, there are also algodystrophies with evidence of hypoactivity at bone scanning. This finding should be confronted with the other clinical, radiological, and biochemical findings and should be taken as an argument in favor of algodystrophy.

Criteria Related to the Clinical Course and to the Treatment

Algodystrophy usually progresses toward recovery without sequels, and this has become the most important criterion for the diagnosis. Shortening of the clinical course due to the treatment may constitute a determining criteria in some instances.

Thus, in case of bone involvement suggesting metastasis or aseptic necrosis, the effectiveness of calcitonin treatment – total recovery in a few days in some instances – can permit the diagnosis of algodystrophy to be made, as in the case history already reported in Part 2, Chap. 3. This concerned a 63-year-old woman, suffering from pain in the root of the left lower limb with total functional disability, in contrast to preserved passive mobility. She had a history of uterine cancer. Bone scanning showed an isolated high uptake of the tracer. Treatment with calcitonin produced dramatic improvement of pain and functional disability and thus made it possible to diagnose algodystrophy of the left hip. This was confirmed subsequently by complete clinical recovery without sequel and by the return to normal of the scintigram within 3 months.

Recently Glick [312] proposed criteria for the *diagnosis of algoneurodystrophy,* namely pain, hyperalgesia, vascular changes, hyperhydrosis, and osteoporosis.

Glick states that when all five criteria are present, the diagnosis is definite; when there are four, the diagnosis is likely; when there are three, the diagnosis is possible.

Glick's five criteria do not include the scintigraphic findings, which, along with other workers, we recently showed to be important for the diagnosis of algodystrophy. Besides, the application of these criteria would lead to an excess of diagnoses of algodystrophy, particularly in pseudophlegmonous forms, since these too satisfy the first four criteria.

Therefore we propose the following five groups of criteria:

Group A:
1. Pain of locoregional or local, mechanical, inflammatory, or mixed type
2. Cutaneous hyperesthesia
3. Vasomotor disturbances, local or locoregional hyper- or hypothermia
4. Cutaneous changes: local or locoregional redness, pallor or cyanosis
5. Local or locoregional hyperhydrosis
6. Local or locoregional edema
7. Aponeurotic or tendinous retraction

Group B:
1. Local or locoregional bone demineralization of the homo- or heterogeneous type, without denser margins or changes in the joint spaces
2. Local or locoregional high or low uptake of tracer at bone scanning

Group C:
1. Absence of biochemical signs of inflammation

Group D:
1. Paucicellular joint fluid (mechanical type)
2. Synovial histology showing vascular congestion without significant cellular infiltration
3. Normal bone histology, or increased osteoclastic resorption

Group E:
1. Dramatic effectiveness of treatment with calcitonin or beta-blockers

The diagnosis of algodystrophy is *definite* or well-established when it satisfies at least one criterion in each of the groups A, B, and C, or A, C, and E. The diagnosis is *likely* when one criterion in each of the groups B, C, and D is satisfied, or two criteria in groups C and D, or also two criteria in group A and the criterion E. The diagnosis is *possible* when the case satisfies one of the criteria of the groups A and B, or A and C, or A and E, or B and C.

The way we propose these criteria be applied demonstrates the multiplicity of the radioclinical pictures which may be encountered.

Note that a definite diagnosis of algodystrophy requires criterion C to be satisfied. However, in cases of elevated erythrocyte sedimentation rate which can be correlated to an intercurrent or concomitant disease, it is admitted that the absence of criterion C is not an obstacle to establishing a definite diagnosis, although this can only be affirmed when criterion E is present.

Note also that the diagnosis of algodystrophy must always be confirmed by regression without sequels, or possibly with clinical sequels such as aponeurotic or tendinous retraction and/or radiological sequels such as thickened bone trabeculations.

It is mainly in cases of probable or possible algodystrophy that criterion E is important to confirm the diagnosis.

Use of diagnostic criteria is particularly important in atypical or misleading forms and even more in the early stages of the disease. Early diagnosis will then allow early application of treatment by calcitonin or beta-blockers, which seem to have more dramatic results the earlier they are given.

Part 6 Etiology

The polymorphism of the symptoms of algodystrophy has been stressed in Part 3. For a long time it has seemed justified to individualize numerous clinical pictures as constituting apparently distinct entities.

The same polymorphism is found in the etiology. Favoring factors or potential sources of algodystrophy are so numerous that they involve almost all fields of medicine and surgery.

The clinical and evolutive features of algodystrophy considered from the etiological point of view have led some workers to isolate more peculiar forms. It seems in fact that algodystrophy never has one single cause, but rather that certain factors can provoke algodystrophy under particular background circumstances.

A. General Etiologic Circumstances

I. Age

Algodystrophy may be encountered in all age groups. According to Bouvier et al. [97] it is most frequent in later adulthood, i.e., between 40 and 70 years. With reference to 140 cases, Louyot et al. [519] note that the range of ages is very wide, from 15 to 80 years, most of the cases occurring between 30 and 65 years. With reference to 45 cases of algodystrophy of the foot, Serre et al. [749] demonstrate that the disease predominantly affects subjects between 40 and 60 years, with extremes of 24 and 83 years. According to Lejeune et al. [464], three-quarters of the cases of algodystrophy occur after the age of 40 years. In our series of 250 cases of algodystrophy of the limbs, the average age was 52 years (range: 19 to 81 years). Algodystrophy can also occur in children, although there are few reports. In 1978 Bernstein et al. [54] observed 24 affected sites in 23 children between 9 and 16 years old; they emphasize that the frequency of algodystrophy in children is certainly underrated, the diagnosis of algodystrophy being frequently overlooked.

Some other isolated cases of algodystrophy in children have been published [120, 418, 421, 467]. Fermaglich [255] reported two cases affecting children aged 11 and 12 years, and Terlizzi et al. [807] reported 3 cases in children.

II. Sex

The classical predominance in males is not confirmed by all workers. According to Serre et al. [749] two third of the patients affected with algodystrophy are males. For Louyot et al. [519] the proportion is 67% males and 33% females, but the authors think this distribution is open to dispute, on the grounds that men are more exposed to injury. Moreover, in the idiopathic forms they did not find a sex-linked predominance (50% males to 50% females). In their series of 100 cases, Bouvier et al. [97] found only a slight predominance of male cases (55%). Among our 250 cases we recorded 59% in males and 41% in females.

B. Favoring Circumstances

Numerous favoring factors are recognized in algodystrophy. It is a matter either of releasing factors which play a determining part in the development of algodystrophy, or of favoring factors which may be single or multiple and constitute a peculiar background against which algodystrophy develops.

In some instances, finally, there is no evidence of a cause or favoring factor: these are the apparently primary or idiopathic algodystrophies.

It should also be pointed out that although some releasing or favoring factors frequently produce peculiar clinical pictures, there is no close or exclusive relationship between these factors and the clinical features and course of the disease, so that it is justifiable to group all these facts under the same heading, algodystrophy.

I. Traumatism

Traumatisms play an important part in algodystrophy, but this part is diversely estimated by the different workers. For some, e.g., Leriche [494], the role of the traumatism seems if not constant, at least essential. With knowledge of the various clinical features of algodystrophy, however the condition has in fact come to be recognized more and more often in the absence of a traumatism. Lejeune et al. [464] listed a traumatic origin in 42.5% of their cases, Harif [351] in 44%. For Serre et al. [754] traumatisms are the causal agent in 30% of algodystrophies of the upper limbs, and in 77% of those of the lower limbs. Schiano et al. [727] found a traumatism to be the origin of 47% of involvements of the upper limbs, and of 72% in the lower limbs. Bouvier et al. [97] consider algodystrophy of the lower limbs to be very often posttraumatic (77%). We elicited a traumatic etiology in 52% of our 250 cases; for the algodystrophies of the lower limbs, the rate was of 55%.

1. The Severity of the Causal Traumatism

The severity of the causal traumatism is very variable. It should be stressed that there is no correlation between the severity of the trauma and the occurrence or severity of algodystrophy. Very mild traumatisms may be followed by severe and extensive algodystrophy; this was noted by Serre et al. [754], for whom half of the responsible contusions are benign.

It should be added that the existence of the traumatisms supposed responsible is sometimes disputable. Not uncommonly the patient suffering from algodystrophy, especially of the foot, attributes this condition a priori to a sprain of the ankle, which can be ruled out on questioning the patient.

2. The Nature of the Traumatism

The nature of the traumatism is also very variable. It is usually a matter of a relatively minor, even minimal traumatism out of proportion with its consequences: contusions, direct blows, falls, abnormal or forced movements, or even wounds.

Reeducation or untimely mobilization frequently constitute favoring factors or even precipitating factors of posttraumatic algodystrophy of the limbs [716]. Very often also the causal agent is a benign sprain or an articular contusion. The symptomatology varies from one case to the other. The delay of occurrence with regard to the traumatism is very variable. We would like to stress once more a very frequent feature suggesting the diagnosis of algodystrophy, namely severe pain and functional disability, mainly of the feet, contrasting with the absence, or at least moderate degree, of anomalies revealed by clinical examination.

In more than one-half of cases algodystrophy is subsequent to a fracture, but Louyot et al. [519] stress one must keep in mind that bone attrition in not the only cause. Immobilization in a plaster cast plays an important part as well as the sometimes untimely reeducation [716].

Three to four weeks after a fracture, pain and swelling that resulted from the traumatism persist, worsen or even reappear if they had already regressed. Sometimes algodystrophy develops when the injured part resumes its function. Surgery upon the limbs, particularly the articulations, can also induce algodystrophy.

3. The Site of the Traumatism

As has been pointed out by Fontaine et al. [271] traumatisms involving the articular regions predispose more to algodystrophy than those affecting the diaphyseal bone parts. Classically the articulations of the feet and ankles are the most often involved. In the 61 cases of traumatic algodystrophy in the series of Schiano et al. [727], the traumatism was mild in 15 cases, severe in 46 cases, including 16 fractures of or surgery on the long bones of the limbs, 16 fractures of or surgery on the distal extremity of a limb, 7 sprains, 2 traumatisms to the spine with radiologically evident lesions, and 5 meniscectomies.

Of our series of 250 cases, 47% were posttraumatic, including 31% affecting the feet or ankles, 10% the knees, 5% the shoulders, and 4% the hands and wrists.

Burns and frostbite [607] may be complicated with algodystrophy.

Finally, one last point must be considered: although algodystrophies are frequently posttraumatic, traumatism being the most important favoring factor, the frequency of algodystrophies relative to the total number of traumatisms is very low (about 1%) and relative to fractures 5%–8%, according to Belenger [44]. This points to the role played by the involvement together of the etiologic factors, and thus the role of the predisposing background, as with the other etiologic factors.

In fact, as was noted by Belenger, fractures always provoke demineralization in the immediate neighborhood of the injured area, but there is usually no repercussion on the architecture of the bone structure. The bone only appears more translucent and regains normal appearance when normal function is resumed. Osteoporosis appears at the earliest 3 weeks after the trauma and may remain at the stage of trivial demineralization; on the other hand, it may also reach the stage of a heterogeneous spotty demineralization while remaining clinically entirely asymptomatic; even in this case there is subsequent complete remineralization. However, asymptomatic posttraumatic osteoporosis can be the first manifestation of "posttraumatic osteoporosis," i.e., of posttraumatic algodystrophy.

4. Algodystrophy of the Limbs and Immobilization

According to Fontaine et al. [271] inactivity alone does not suffice to provoke osteoporosis. He reports [272] that in a large number of rats after 57 days' immobilization of the posterior limb in a plaster, in the absence of the least traumatism, the bones had not undergone changes, namely as concerns the calcium and phosphorus rate. Fontaine adds moreover that a plaster applied smoothly and well does not provoke pain or swelling with subsequent demineralization. But he insists that this no longer holds true when the immobilization is of a previously injured limb which is the site of an infection or of a nervous lesion, or when an inadequate plaster itself constitutes a traumatism.

For other workers, namely Serre et al. [754], immobilization is the determining cause of algodystrophy (7 cases of Serre's 188) or the aggravating factor (37 cases of Serre's 188). In 1954 Weil and Gerard-Marchant [855] stressed the risk of unduly prolonged immobilization in plasters.

II. Nontraumatic Affections of the Locomotor Apparatus

Numerous diseases of the locomotor apparatus can be accompanied by algodystrophy or even precipitate it. These include the infections of the extremities: panaris, phlegmons, pasteurellosis. It may thus be very difficult sometimes to distinguish pseudophlegmonous algodystrophy of the hand from a true phlegmon of the synovial sheaths of tendons. Septic arthritis, microcrystalline arthritis, particularly gouty arthritis, or inflammatory arthritis may also be complicated by algodystrophy. Among the inflammatory articular affections during which we observed algodystrophy we would quote rheumatoid arthritis, ankylosing spondylarthritis, Reiter syndrome, and polymyalgia rheumatica [840]; connectivitis, periarteritis nodosa, Weber-Chistian disease, tendinitis, and acute bursitis of the shoulder [477] are also mentioned.

III. Diseases of the Nervous System

Already in 1901, Nonne [603] who worked in the same Hamburg hospital as Südeck, reports cases of "chronic or acute bone atrophy" occurring in neurologic affections.

1. Involvement of the Peripheral Nerves

Involvement of peripheral nerves may provoke algodystrophy. This is the case with algodystrophy, among which causalgia, reported about during the War of Secession by Mitchell et al. [575]. *Nerve contusions* or *nerve compressions* may provoke algodystrophy. Also *herpes zoster* may be followed by algodystrophy, as demonstrated by Südeck [793] and later by others [30, 57, 324, 387, 404, 455, 456, 536, 678, 809].

Cervicobrachial, sciatic, or crural *radiculalgiae* can also be responsible, as demonstrated by Serre et al. [754]. These authors identified lumbalgia, cruralgia, or lumbosciatica as a cause of algodystrophy of the lower limbs 12 times out of 188. In 1977, Carlson et al. [117] reported two cases of algodystrophy of the lower limbs following sciatica by *disk herniation,* subsequently confirmed by radiculosaccography. This examination was of course neither the cause nor an aggravating factor of the algodystrophy. Nevertheless, *radiculosaccography* may be the precipitating factor, as in the two cases reported by Morettin and Wilson [583]. In the second of these cases, in fact, the pseudoinflammatory signs of algodystrophy of the left lower limb appeared abruptly, immediately after introduction of the needle into the subarachnoid spaces, demonstrating that the mere traumatism of an injection can cause algodystrophy. There are also descriptions of cases following *polyneuritis* or *Guillain-Barré's polyradiculoneuritis* [740].

2. Diseases of the Central Nervous System
(8, 11, 111, 141, 348, 540, 596, 673)

A relatively large number of encephalic and meningeal diseases and some acute or chronic medullar involvements have been considered to be responsible for algodystrophic syndromes.

a) *Affections of the brain and of the meninges* [134, 814]. Among the *acute conditions,* let us first mention hemiplegia of vascular origin [137,245, 326, 579, 625, 799]. Davis et al. [178] carried out a retrospective study of 540 hemiplegic patients with a *thromboembolic middle cerebral artery vascular disease.* Some 68 (12.5%) were diagnosed as having shoulder-hand syndromes. Most patients developed symptoms and signs between the second and fourth months after onset of the hemiplegia. The full syndrome recurred in 6 patients.

Traumatisms to the skull [9], *intracranial hypertension. Cerebral tumors* [673, 825] and *neurosurgical interventions* [727] have also been implicated. Algodystrophies have also been reported to occur in *acute meningeal affections,* e.g., meningitis, meningoencephalitis, and meningeal hemorrhage, subsequently to various investigations such as *arteriography* of the carotid artery [97], *electroshocks*, and *gas encephalography.*

Among the *chronic affections* the following conditions are mainly mentioned: *epilepsy, Parkinson's disease* [307, 741, 762], *the thalamic syndromes, Wilson's disease, and para-osteoarthropathies* [111, 596, 673].

In all these diseases of the central nervous system it is in fact very difficult to distinguish what part is caused by the neurologic disease itself, what part by the complementary investigations, and what part by the medical (barbital) or surgical treatment. Moreover, it should be pointed out that the incidence of subsequent algodystrophy is very low relative to the total number of patients with these diseases.

b) *Medullar affections* are much more rarely incriminated. Cases of algodystrophy have been reported in *syringomyelia, amyotrophic lateral sclerosis, and medullar metastases* [742].

IV. Cardiovascular Disease

Disease of the coronary arteries is accompanied by algodystrophy in 4% of cases, according to Lenègre [468]. According to Froment [286], myocardial infarction results in algodystrophy in 10% of cases, whereas less than 1% of angina pectoris cases would be associated with algodystrophy. The occurrence of persistent painful disability of the shoulder as a complication of coronary heart disease has long been recognized. The conditions was noted even before the turn of the century, as is shown by Osler's [612] reference to "motor disability" at the shoulder as a sequel to "anginal attacks." Later, around 1930, Howard [374] reported cases with painful stiffness of the shoulders occurring at the same time as severe myocardial disease. Other publications [84, 459, 829] point out the frequency of this conditions, but none reports involvement of the hand. In 1940 Ernstene and Kinell [246] described 6 cases with involvement of shoulder and hand without correlating algodystrophy and coronaritis. Later came the publications of Askey [22], Johnson [393], and finally, in 1947, Steinbrocker. The most frequent clinical picture is painful disability of the shoulder (scapulohumeral periarthritis), the most rare is the shoulder-hand syndrome. In myocardial infarction [31, 138, 139, 148, 234, 235, 483, 619, 631, 718, 821, 853, 864], algodystrophy occurs 4 – 8 weeks after the onset of the cardiac involvement, it is bilateral in one-third of cases and affects the left upper limb or predominates on the left in more than 50% of cases. Algodystrophies have also been observed in *aortitis, aneurysms* of the aorta, *acute pericarditis* [581], and *infective endocarditis.* Kohler [413] describes a case of algodystrophy following *obliteration of the brachiocephalic trunk. Cardiac surgery* can also be responsible for algodystrophy [413]. Among the possible causes are also mentioned *thrombophlebitis, arteritis*, particularly diabetic arteritis [661, 754].

V. Pleuropulmonary Diseases

All pulmonary diseases and intrathoracic operations have been presumed to be the cause of algodystrophy, although this association is relatively rare [309].

Among the presumed causes we would mention: *pulmonary tuberculosis, bronchial cancer,* particularly of the apex, *pulmonary infarction,* spontaneous or therapeutic *pneumothorax, pleurisy, traumatisms to the chest, contusions, fractures of ribs, and hemothorax* [654].

VI. Hyperthyroidism

Quite a number of studies have been devoted to the rheumatismal manifestations observed in diseases of the thyroid gland. Some authors even speak of thyroid rheumatisms [454], whereas others describe algodystrophy occurring in hyperthyroidism [64, 80, 131, 150, 230, 231, 308, 412, 453, 470, 638, 770, 771, 826].

Algodystrophy occurs chiefly in hyperthyroidisms of the *Basedow disease* type. According to Ravault et al. [651], hyperthyroidism and algodystrophy would perhaps only be two different consequences of a single diencephalic disturbance. For Schiano et al. [727] hyperthyroidism itself is concerned, and uninfluenced by the treatment; out of 14 cases they note in fact 6 algodystrophies in untreated hyperthyroidism and 8 cases in hyperthyroidism treated either with antithyroid chemotherapy or with iodine 131. Among 720 patients suffering from hyperthyroidism and treated with radioactive iodine, Methlin et al. [563] found 20 algodystrophies subsequent to the treatment and only 4 which had occurred prior to any treatment. Clinically, half of the cases had evidence of capsulitis of the shoulder, the other half a shoulder-hand syndrome. These manifestations were bilateral in more than three-quarters of the cases. Pain was associated with vasomotor disturbances and restricted motion. Osteoporosis was more frequent in the wrist than in the hand. Methlin and one of us insist on the precipitating role of radioactive iodine resulting from an indirect action related to the sudden central hyperstimulation, following intense irradiation of the thyroid. In the last 5 years the frequency of algodystrophy secondary to treatment with iodine 131 seems to have clearly diminished. This is probably due to the fact that iodine 131 is no longer given without preparation with antithyroid and beta-blocking drugs.

VII. Diabetes Mellitus [476, 661]

Diabetes mellitus seems to be capable if not of provoking, at least of favoring algodystrophy, as reported by Lequesne et al. [481]. Schiano et al. [727] found this association in only 2 of their 103 cases. As for ourselves, we found 8 cases of patent or latent diabetes mellitus in a series of 108 algodystrophies. The frequency of diabetes in our series was certainly underrated, since we did not systematically carry out the oral glucose tolerance test. In fact, diabetes is often associated with other precipitating or favoring factors. In their series of 11 algodystrophies associated with diabetes, Lequesne et al. [482] point out the presence in 4 cases of another precipitating factor (angina pectoris, surgery, antituberculous treatment). According to Lequesne et al., the clinical manifestations are often mild, and algodystrophy more often affects the upper limb, with a tendency for capsulitis. Moreover the involvements are often plurifocal and recurrent. However, in our 8 cases of algodystrophy associated with diabetes we did not find these peculiarities. Indeed we noted involvement of the lower limbs 6 times out of 8 (2 times the knee and 4 times the foot). Our two remaining cases concerned a shoulder-hand syndrome. On the whole, diabetes does in fact seem to be more frequent in algodystrophy than in the general population, since in our series we found 7.4%, whereas the prevalence of diabetes in France is clearly lower, although diversely estimated (1.5 to 2 per thousand according to Derot [196], 20 per thousand according to Fromantin et al. [287]). Algodystrophy seems not to have peculiar characteristics in diabetics although Lequesne insists upon the fibrosis.

VIII. Hyperlipidemia

In 1970, Pinals and Jabbs [628] stressed the role of type IV hyperlipoproteinemia in algodystrophy. Recently Amor et al. [7] reported that patients with algodystrophy of the hip showed considerably increased alcohol-ingestion-induced hypertriglyceridemia with regard to the control group.

IX. Iatrogenic Algodystrophies

1. Phenobarbitals

Since the first description by Maillard and Renard in 1925 [529], barbiturate-induced algodystrophy has been the subject of numerous studies [17, 51, 75, 109, 111, 116, 466, 470, 530, 715, 755, 830]. In the literature on "barbituric rheumatisms" we found in fact two types of observation: the majority concern epileptic patients treated with barbiturates, the remainder concern other patients treated with barbiturates. The frequency of this condition is difficult to estimate, but taking into account the large number of patients who regularly take barbiturates, it is probably very low. It should also be remembered that algodystrophy is due to an association of factors and never to a single cause.

In our series of 250 algodystrophies we noted 6 patients treated with barbiturates, but only in two cases could this treatment be retained as the only causal factor. One of them concerns a 62-year-old man, suffering from hypertension, who had for several years been treated for severe insomnia with barbiturates (association of ballobarbital and secobarbital), when pain appeared in both shoulders, together with clinical inflammatory symptoms of both wrists and the metacarpophalangeal and proximal interphalangeal articulations, with morning stiffness lasting more than 12 h. After failure of numerous anti-inflammatory treatments, withdrawal of the barbiturates produced improvement within 1 month. In the other cases the treatment by barbiturates was only considered one of the possible etiologies. One of these cases concerns a 66-year-old woman who was also treated for a psychotic syndrome with diffuse arteriopathy, patent diabetes mellitus and hyperlipidemia with hypertriglyceridemia. Another case concerned a 60-year-old woman treated by barbiturates for epilepsy diagnosed 31 years earlier, who underwent angiography and gas encephalography subsequent to a new attack of epilepsy a few days before the occurrence of severe algodystrophy of both hands. Still another case concerned a 30-year-old man who had a traumatism to the skull. The last case is a 62-year-old woman who was operated upon for a frontal meningioma.

Nevertheless, whatever the nature of the treated disease, even in the absence of brain involvement, any treatment with barbiturates can cause algodystrophy, whichever sort of barbiturate is used. It seems however that relatively high doses administred over a prolonged period are necessary; there is a very wide range of delay between the onset of treatment and the time of occurrence of algodystrophy: from 19 days to 25 years, according to Arlet et al. [17]. Barbiturate-induced algodystrophy is more frequent in women and uncommon before the age of 30 years. From the clinical point of view it involves chiefly the upper limb, where it produces a shoulder-hand syndrome which develops in two phases: first a pseudoinflammatory appearance of the hands, and later, atrophy and retraction of the fingers and a sclerodactylic appearance with palmar aponeurotic nodules. Algodystrophy subsequent to barbiturates is often bilateral. Involvement of the hips is not uncommon. At the level of the lower limbs there may be plurifocal involvement, as in a case reported by Arlet et al.. The radiological signs vary: sometimes osteoporosis is very marked, sometimes it is lacking. The treatment of barbiturate-induced algodystrophy consists of withdrawal of the barbiturates, but continuation of treatment does not prevent spontaneous healing.

2. Tuberculostats

In 1961, Brouet et al. [105] reported cases with pseudorheumatismal signs in the upper limbs, particularly shoulder-hand syndromes, following chemotherapy of tuberculosis comprising the association of izoniazid and ethionamide.

In the same year McKusick and Hsu [556] reported the same facts in patients treated by isoniazid. Since then other studies have been done on "rheumatism and chemotherapy of tuberculosis" [169, 198, 304, 317, 318, 390, 470, 486, 534, 615, 675, 822]. At the same time, other authors [119, 239, 263, 281, 395] insist on the part played by the tuberculosis itself in the genesis of these conditions. The pseudorheumatismal manifestations of chemotherapy of tuberculosis concern electively the upper limbs and more particularly the shoulders. In half of the cases both shoulders are affected, producing the clinical picture of painful stiffening of the shoulders. The hands are affected in more than half of the cases, producing the typical but often bilateral shoulder-hand syndrome. Involvement of the elbow is much more rare. Involvement of the lower limbs may occur, but is rather uncommon (feet, ankles, knees, hips), sometimes associated with Ledderhose disease subsequently to treatment with isoniazid, ethionamide, cycloserine, or associations of these drugs. The evolution is usually favorable, especially when the chemotherapy of tuberculosis can be interrupted. Nevertheless, trophic disturbances of the extremities with contracture and even Dupuytren's disease may develop and constitute irreversible sequels.

As for other etiologic factors inducing algodystrophy, chemotherapy of tuberculosis is probably not the unique cause. Moreover, the frequency of the pseudorheumatismal signs is low relative to the number of tuberculoses treated. We would also stress the importance of the associated factors, i.e., diabetes, alcoholism, psychic conditions.

3. Pregnancy

Several studies have reported algodystrophies provoked by pregnancy. In 1953 Curtiss and Kincaid [168] described the first three observations of algodystrophy of the hip occurring during the third month of pregnancy. Others [42, 126, 458, 514, 841] have reported algodystrophic syndromes of the lower limb occurring during the last months of pregnancy. They are almost always involvements of the hip, although other sites were noted: in our series of 250 cases we found two cases: one concerns a 24-year-old woman who during the eighth month of pregnancy, developed an algodystrophic syndrome of the right foot with radiologic and scintigraphic signs of extension to the knee and to the right hip; the other concerns an algodystrophic syndrome affecting the hip of a woman in the seventh month of pregnancy. Algodystrophy can also occur after delivery, as pointed out by Guaquiere [333].

X. Other Etiologic Factors

Harada and Kozuma [348] report an algodystrophic syndrome subsequent to *carbon monoxide intoxication;* Horvath [373] reports a case occurring after a *dive in water.*

Electrocution has been incriminated in a certain number of cases. Thus Lièvre and Hubault [508] report the case of a 50-year-old man with intense and diffuse osteoporosis of the spine and multiple compressions of vertebrae subsequent to electrocution. The same authors report another case of electrocution of the upper limb with clinical and radiologic signs suggesting algodystrophy. Other causes, that may be considered as traumatizing, have been reported to be the origin of algodystrophies, namely *acupuncture, antitetanus* vaccinations [48], etc.

Dejour et al. [185] and Lequesne et al. [478] have reported cases of *osteoid osteoma,* one being of the acetabulum, the other of the femoral head, complicated by algodystrophy, which they termed capsulitis of the hip. Also under the term capsulitis of the hip, Lequesne et al. [478] described 4 cases of algodystrophy secondary to *chondromatosis* of the hip.

Algodystrophy has been said, by various authors, to occur in *Lobstein's disease* [149, 354, 382, 728]. Of our 250 cases, 2 were in Lobstein disease (1 involving the hip and 1 the foot).

XI. Apparently Primary Algodystrophies

In some cases of algodystrophy no precipitating or favoring factor can be elicited. These seem to be primary or idiopathic algodystrophies. In these cases as in the others, the problems of the algodystrophic "terrain" arises. Primary algodystrophies are frequent but diversely appreciated: for Ravault and Durant [648] one-third of the algodystrophies of the upper limbs are primary, for Lequesne et al. [474] 50% of the algodystrophies of the hip are primary, but only 25% of those of the feet; whereas Schiano et al. [727] found only 9 cases without known etiology among their 103 algodystrophies.

Among our material we have 36% of cases for which no precipitating or favoring cause could be elicited. Of our cases affecting the upper limb 27% only are primary conditions, whereas for the lower limb we found 43% to be primary, and for the hip, 75%.

But in fact it is always very difficult to establish the primary character of algodystrophy. There is indeed very often a peculiar "terrain": "neurovegetative dystonia," or even a frankly psychiatric condition is found in 17 of the 78 algodystrophies of the upper limb and in 5 of the 22 algodystrophies of the lower limb in Bouvier's paper [96]. Among our 250 cases we found a frankly anxious or anxiodepressive state in 30%.

It should be added that most of the time, several etiologic factors are mixed up together without it being possible to estimate the exact part played by each. Perhaps there is some determining factor which is still undetected, while all other factors would then be only favoring factors.

XII. Etiologic Factors in Our 250 Cases of Algodystrophy

We recorded the one etiologic factor which seemed to us to be predominant for each patient. As to the "terrain" (diabetes, hyperlipidemia, neurovegetative dystonia) this seems to be the most important factor in determining algodystrophy.

Traumatisms		120
Contusions, direct shocks	42	
Sprains	42	
Luxations	2	
Fractures	34	
Surgery on the limbs		11
Traumatism to the skull		1
Meningioma		1
Hemiplegia		1
Gas encephalography		1
Perfusion		1
Pregnancy		2
Myeloma		1
Polyglobulia		1
Myocardial infarction		1
Lobstein's disease		2
Cutaneous infection		1
Septic arthritis		2
Cancer		3
Rheumatoid arthritis		2
Ankylosing spondylarthritis		1
Reiter syndrome		1
Polymyalgia rheumatica		1
Phenobarbital		6
Radioactive iodine		1

Part 7 Physiopathology

The term algodystrophy covers a number of extremely varied pathological manifestations which seem to us to correspond to common mechanisms, all of which are not yet well known.

Numerous theories have been suggested in turn, incriminating traumatisms, infectious, inflammatory, or even tumoral processes, metabolic or endocrine disorders, chemical aggressions (diverse therapeutics), etc.

In fact, the small number of algodystrophies provoked by each of these different aggressions with regard to the large number of subjects who, in the same circumstances, did not experience algodystrophy, demonstrates that none of these factors is alone responsible for the occurrence of algodystrophy. But each of them, or several together, may be responsible for the excitation of sensitive fibers, which may provoke a pathologic reflex process on a particular background (terrain).

As concerns disturbances in the vegetative nervous system, Leriche [490, 494] was the first to put forward a satisfactory and coherent explanation of what we now call algodystrophy. He postulated that following any aggression, a reflex arc is formed which follows the routes of the sympathetic nervous system and provokes peripheral vascular disturbances.

The reflex arc consists of an efferent and an afferent route.

The afferent pathway is constituted by the sensitive fibers of the mixed nerves, for the locomotor apparatus, or by the sensitive fibers of the sympathetic nerves, for the viscera. The noci-influence reaches the spinal ganglion of the posterior spinal root, the medullar gray matter, and then through the internuncial neurones to the tractus intermediolateralis of the lateral gray column.

The internuncial pool [512, 516] consists of two main systems: a so-called multiple system, in which the stimulations successively reach the neurones of the second and then of the third order connected to each other and leading to the same center; and a closed system, placed in derivation on a synapse and forming there an autostimulation circuit. These internuncial neurones carry the influx not only to the lateral column of the same medullar level and to several over- or underlying medullar levels, but also to the tractus intermediolateralis on the contralateral side. This accounts for the extent of the reflexogenic area, and for the numerous topographic possibilities of the peripheral response for a given reflexogenic area.

As concerns the efferent pathway, it commences in the lateral column of gray matter and courses through the preganglionic fibers in the ventral roots via the white rami communicantes to join the corresponding ganglia on the sympathetic trunk. There a single preganglionic fiber may synapse with several postganglionic fibers. Through the gray rami communicantes these are distributed to the mixed nerves and, moreover, give off branches with a vasomotor function that accompany the blood vessels in their zone of supply.

The after-discharge phenomena are more marked the greater the number of internuncial neurones, this not being sufficient however to explain the long duration of this reflex arc and thus the prolonged persistence of the disturbances. According to Leriche [494] the peripheral "inflammatory" disorders would be perceived by the afferent fibers as a noci-influence. This is also the opinion of Ficat [257] who points out the importance of possible "irritative stimuli." A vicious circle would thus establish between central and peripheral processes.

The reflex arc is normally influenced by activities of higher levels in the brain stem and cerebral hemispheres. Algodystrophies secondary to central nervous system lesions could be explained by changes in the transmission pathways or by disinhibition in the upper control centers. Lequesne [471] explains thus the frequent occurrence of algodystrophy in neurotonic subjects who have a poor control of their impulsions and thus also of their corticosympathetic activity.

The sympathetic reflex arc may act on the periphery by two mechanisms. There may be a direct action of the sympathetic system on the cutaneous, subcutaneous, muscular, tendinous, capsular, and bony tissues. This direct action would explain capsular, aponeurotic, and tendinous retraction, by means of neurotissular chemical mediators.

The vasomotor action is certainly very complex: there seems to be a functional disturbance in the microcirculation, i.e., at the level of the thoroughfare channels which connect the terminal arteriole and the venule, including the metarterioles and the Sucquet's canals which connect the arteriole directly with the venule.

The precapillary sphincters situated on the metarteriole as well as the metarteriole itself, the arteriole, and the venule are sensitive to the mediators of the autonomic nervous system. The anatomic arrangement of this system explains why disturbances in the venous pole have a much more significant repercussion that those of the arterial pole.

Histamine and bradykinin, for instance, produce venous constriction and stasis in the capillaries situated upstream, and increased permeability of these capillaries.

On the other hand, adrenaline and noradrenaline produce vasoconstriction of the arteriole and of the precapillary sphincter with subsequent diminution in the blood flow and permeability of the capillaries, as well as venous vasoconstriction.

Finally, serotonin produces arteriolar and venular vasoconstriction, dilatation and stasis in the capillaries, increased capillary permeability, and, perhaps, dilatation in the arteriovenous anastomosis; there is moreover increased intracapillary pressure.

According to Belanger [44] the normal condition would comprise two phases, vasoconstriction and vasodilatation, but in algodystrophy there would be three phases. The first phase is short and consists of vasodilatation; during the second phase the metarterioles close and the blood passes electively through the Sucquet's canal. However, since the venules are spasmed, there is reflux of blood toward the metarteriole and the capillaries with increased blood pressure responsible for exsiccosis and edema. The third phase, finally, is inconstant and characterized by total vasomotor atony.

According to Ficat et al. [259], the reflex vicious circle is dominated by the capillary stasis, which is responsible for hyperpressure and hyperpermeability of the capillaries with plasmatic exsiccosis, microthrombosis, and sludged blood. These vascular phenomena cause stagnant anoxia with accumulation of protein metabolites and tissue acidosis, which also contribute to increase the permeability of the capillaries and to cause edema and increased pressure in all tissues, from skin to bone.

The bone shows vascular stasis and engorgement in the backflow. Ficat insists on the regional and segmental character of this disorder, which is particularly obvious when there are two affected sites separated by an unaffected area on the same limb. (In one of Ficat's cases the medullar pressure was 30 mm Hg in the diaphyseal area, and 1 cm from there, on the epiphysis, it was 50 mm Hg.) After the edema has regressed, fibrosis develops, diminishing the capillary permeability and hindering metabolic exchanges. At this stage definite sequels may set in. A chemical mediator, serotonin, provokes vasoconstriction in the arterioles and venules, dilatation and stasis in the capillaries, and increased permeability of the capillaries. It also has a sclerogenic action. According to Lequesne and Auquier [477] serotonin could be the natural chemical mediator between the sympathetic influx and the trophicity of the joint capsules and aponeuroses.

The role of serotonin would be particularly prominent in isoniazid- and barbiturate-induced iatrogenic algodystrophies. Zarafonetis and Kalas [871] have shown that isoniazid inhibits the degradation of serotonin. Feldberg and Fleischhauer showed that pentobarbital increased the liberation of serotonin and catecholamines in the central nervous system.

As concerns the peculiar "terrain," Ravault [649] pointed out that the neurovegetative terrain would be a favoring one, since algodystrophy often occurs in hyperemotive and anxious subjects. Besides, the dystonic state itself could be the consequence of the same disorder that causes algodystrophy. This disorder could be an anomaly in the chemical mediators, in particular serotonin.

Despite concerted efforts, at present we cannot provide more precise details about the causative physiopathologic mechanism.

Part 8 Treatment

Numerous methods have been advocated for the treatment of algodystrophy, since the condition was first described, about a hundred years ago.

The different methods answered to symptomatic or, sometimes, speculative pathogenic criteria. None of them has proved invariably effective. It was mainly on the basis of the physiopathology and the vasculosympathetic theory that the aim was established of suppressing or attenuating the vasomotor disturbances which are a fundamental feature of algodystrophy. Thus sympathetic blocks have been used, either by surgical sympathectomy or by injecting an anesthetic into the sympathetic chains, or also by means of the sympatholytic effect of different substances, from derivates of ergot to beta-blocking drugs. Numerous analgesic drugs and nonsteroid inflammatory products have been used with inconstant results to relieve the pain. The different modes of physiotherapy and kinesitherapy contribute to prevent vascular stasis and tissue contracture.

Calcitonin was first used because it had an inhibitory effect on osteoclastic activity, but it has in fact a much more complex mechanism.

The various metabolic disorders which are discovered in connection with algodystrophy and could have had a precipitating effect, should be overcome. Finally, the psychosomatic factors which we have seen to be quite frequent in patients suffering from algodystrophy, should also receive adequate therapy.

Chapter 1 Chemotherapy

A. Analgesics

Analgesics such as salicylates, glafenin, paracetamol, or clometacin are used as a complementary therapy for treating algodystrophies.

B. Nonsteroid Anti-inflammatory Drugs

These can also be useful but they expose the patient to complications, particularly digestive complications, and are therefore contraindicated in patients with gastroduodenal ulcers, whether these are active or not.

C. Systemic Corticosteroids

According to most authors, corticosteroids have no role in the management of algodystrophy [727, 749], although they are sometimes employed, with interesting results [83, 311, 313, 369, 588, 670, 706, 798]. It seems to us that there is no proof of the effectiveness of this therapy, and that it has more drawbacks than advantages in a disease which, at its onset, can be confused with aseptic osteonecrosis. This latter condition has a similar physiopathology, and is often related to corticotherapy.

D. Local Corticosteroids

[50, 306]

May [549] and Serre et al. [749] have obtained good results with this method. It is mainly used in retractile capsulitis of the shoulder.

E. Therapy Aimed at Vasodilatation

Numerous vasodilators have been advocated for the treatement of algodystrophy [332, 494, 645, 646].

I. Systemic Treatment

1. Alpha-blockers

The *derivates of ergotoxine,* especially dihydroergotoxine, obtained from ergot, raise the peripheral circulation rate [68, 147, 176, 358].

Nicergoline is a synthetic product recently used in therapy; it lowers the peripheral vascular resistance.

2. Ganglioplegics

These provoke increased vasodilatation.

Pentamethonium diminishes the vascular resistance but its use is somewhat delicate because of its adverse effects related to paralysis of the vegetative nervous system [452, 568].

3. Postganglionic Blockers [347]

Drugs producing blockade of the sympathetic postganglionic fibers, particularly guanethidine, have been advocated as producing local sympathetic blocks. According to McKay et al. [555] significant improvement has been obtained with intravenous perfusions of guanethidine. This sympathetic block is more complete than with surgical sympathectomy.

II. Local Treatment

In 1932, Leriche and Fontaine [499] reported their results on the effect of novocaine-induced anesthesia of the ligaments and periarticular tendinous insertions in sprains and "traumatic arthrites."

Whereas surgery of the sympathetic system had been introduced by the same author in 1924 [490, 491], it is from 1932 on [494] that catenoid, stellate, upper thoracic, and lumbar ganglion infiltrations were added to the therapeutic procedures and rapidly became known. These infiltrations are most helpful in the early phase of algodystrophy, where formerly sympathectomy was necessary. They were very much in fashion [19, 21, 85, 300, 389, 442, 633, 805] and their efficiency greatly reduced the application field of surgery to the sympathetic nerve, mainly periarterial sympathectomy. The technique of sympathetic blockade seems however to have been partly abandoned since the sixties, but it is regaining interest under the influence of anesthesists and physicians concerned with pain relief [140, 391].

The results are usually good. Steinbrocker et al. [779] studied a series of 69 patients and noted in 31.8% complete recovery, in 49.3% appreciable benefit, and failure in 18.9%. It is important to note that the results depend on the stage at which treatment is applied. When the disease is treated before the appearance of the trophic disturbances, recovery is almost complete, but once they are present, especially when they are severe, regression is much less frequent.

For the upper limb, stellate ganglion block is employed, preferably by anterolateral approach, and the effect is evaluated by the appearance of ocular signs and the feeling of warmth in the upper limb. For the lower limb, the lumbar sympathetic chain is infiltrated. The number of injections that is necessary depends on the patient's response to the therapy. The average is two injections per week with 5–10 ml of 2% procaine or lidocaine solution. In addition, periarterial sympathetic infiltrations or intra-arterial injections have also been used. The results are however poorer than with stellate or lumbar sympathetic ganglion block. It is advisable then to add a vasodilator to the novocaine derivative; Leriche [496] used acetylcholine.

F. Griseofulvin

Griseofulvin is a fungistatic antibiotic isolated from *Penicillium griseofulvium* and other penicilliums. Cohen et al. [142] and Serre et al. [746] obtained good results with it in patients with shoulder-hand syndrome. In 1974, Baudouin [37] obtained good results in 75% of 70 patients; also, in 1976, Laborie et al. [432] successfully treated shoulder-hand syndromes and posttraumatic algodystrophies. Beaufils [41] had 17 good results out of 26 treated cases.

The agent is administered orally at a dose of 3 g/day. Improvement occurs after 7–10 days. The drug is well tolerated; the only side effects are epigastralgiae.

The mode of action of griseofulvin seems to concern the microcirculation.

G. Beta-blockers

Beta-blocking drugs were first used in some isolated cases of algodystrophy and gave conflicting results [314, 526, 655, 656, 768]. In a more substantial series Schiano [726] obtained promising results, but it was mainly the studies of May et al. [550, 551, 552] and subsequently of Ziegler et al. [875] that demonstrated the usefulness of beta-blockers in algodystrophy.

Propranolol is the agent most often used, but pindolol, oxyprenolol, procinolol, or timolol are also employed. The posology must be progressive, and necessitates clinical and electrocardiographic control; the dose is increased every 3 days, until the effective dose is reached, which is indicated by a cardiac rhythm of about 60/min. Contraindications are asthma, peptic ulcers, diabetes, pregnancy, cardiac insufficiency, atrioventricular conduction disturbances, and concomitant intake of drugs such as barbiturate and antidepressants (monoamine oxidase inhibitors or tricyclics). The results vary with the authors; they appear sometimes to be excellent: 30 good or very good results out of 34 patients treated by May et al. [550]; 72% of excellent results and 13% of good results obtained by Ziegler et al. [875]. The best benefit is derived from treatment in the early phase. Improvement occurs promptly, as early as the 7th day according to May et al. [550]; it consists in decreased pain and swelling, and regression of the functional disability around the 15th day. The total duration of treatment was about 51 days for May et al. (from 15 to 150 days). Beta-blockers are usually well tolerated. These results merit confirmation in double-blind studies.

The mode of action of the beta-blockers is still poorly understood, insofar as the physiopathology of algodystrophy is itself much debated. The beta-blockers would intervene at different levels. First, they would have a central action of the anxiolytic type, a sympatholytic action on the cortical adrenergic circuits which regulate the preganglionic sympathetic tonicity. Finally, they would have a peripheral action on the reflex arc by slowing down the nerve conduction, and they would also react on the local vasomotricity by blocking the beta-receptors and inhibiting primarily the initial vasoconstriction and secondarily the vasodilatation.

H. Calcitonin

In 1974, Eisinger et al. [241] reported the results of treatment with calcitonin in 10 cases of algodystrophy, of which 7 showed a prompt favorable response. The authors confirmed their first results with a study bearing on 46 cases [241]. Other workers [171, 179, 212, 218, 276, 593, 725, 839, 876] have also confirmed the effectiveness of this treatment.

In these different studies the treatment has consisted in intramuscular injections of 160 units/day of porcine calcitonin for 10–20 days, and then every other day for several weeks, or of 50–100 units/day of salmon calcitonin with the same schedule of administration. The results are sometimes so dramatic that even in the absence of controlled studies, the remarkable efficiency of treatment by calcitonin can be affirmed. Eisinger et al. [242] obtained about 70% of good or very good results with total disappearance of pain, edema, and vasomotor disturbances, or an appreciable decrease, and persistence of only mild pain.

In our 60 cases of algodystrophy, including 28 posttraumatic conditions, we obtained good or very good results in 33 cases (55%), and healing within 1 month or less. In 16 cases (17%), total recovery was obtained within less than 8 days, improvement having occurred after the very first injections. Such an evolution is never seen in untreated algodystrophies or in cases given the classical vasodilator treatment [217].

As was already pointed out by Eisinger et al. [242], prompt response to treatment and the quality of this response depend on how early the treatment is started, although this is not a rule; as a matter of fact, we obtained a dramatic response to treatment within less than 1 month, in stage 2 algodystrophy with an 8-month history, and in 4 cases of stage 2 of several months' duration, whereas in 5 cases of stage 1 or 2, healing occurred within 3–6 months, the responsiveness to treatment being poor or nonexistent. Poor results are nevertheless usually observed in stage 3 conditions.

It seems that good results to treatment by calcitonin also depend on the daily dose. In 1978 Acquaviva et al. [2] reported the results of a study concerning 90 cases of algodystrophy (49 men and 41 women, aged 20–82 years) involving the upper limbs in 40 cases and the lower limbs in 50 cases. Of the 90 cases 66 were posttraumatic or postsurgical algodystrophies. Large doses of calcitonin (more than 100 units per day) were given to 79 patients; the others received low doses (1 unit per day). Of the

79 patients who had received large doses, 54 derived benefit from the treatment, whereas none of the 11 who had been given small doses improved. The authors also noted that the improvement was usually very prompt, occurring in the very first days of treatment.

Side effects were observed in 15 of the 79 patients who had received large doses of calcitonin (10 flushes, 4 dizziness, 3 nausea, 2 asthenia, 2 somnolence). The signs of intolerance appeared 1 h after the injection. They were very marked at the beginning of the treatment and were relieved by administration of antihistaminics. The signs of intolerance lasted usually 2 h, and their intensity decreased as treatment was continued.

A double-blind study has been carried out by two of us in collaboration with Meunier, Roy-Camille, Seguy, and Massias. This study was aimed at comparing the effect of 100 units of salmon calcitonin administered by intramuscular injection with the effect of a placebo, in 28 patients suffering from stage 1 algodystrophy of the lower limbs, taken at random. The results confirmed the action of calcitonin and demonstrated a significant difference with regard to the placebo, as concerns the early attenuation of pain. By the 28th day the patients who received a placebo had in fact improved, as well as those who were given calcitonin, but at the 14th day, the pain was significantly relieved in the patients receiving calcitonin, whereas the others reported no appreciable difference in the intensity of their pain. Thus by the 14th day, 64% of the patients were considered as having improved on calcitonin treatment, versus 25% with the placebo, and this difference is significant ($p<0.01$).

The various works, and especially this controlled study enable a schema to be recommended for the use of calcitonin in algodystrophy: the dose must be large – at least 100 units of salmon calcitonin and at least 160 units of porcine calcitonin – and it must be administered in the form of a daily intramuscular injection for 15 days. In case of failure, it is useless to prolong the treatment, since it has very little chance of becoming effective after a delay when it was not rightaway.

Tolerance toward calcitonin is not always excellent. We observed signs of intolerance in 20%–35% of the cases but they were seldom intense enough to necessitate interruption of the treatment. In Eisinger's series [242] interruption of treatment was never necessary, and in our 60 cases nausea and vomiting lasting 24 h after each injection caused us to interrupt the treatment in one case [217].

The side effects are usually only troublesome; they consist of vasomotor symptoms or flushes in 12 of our cases, nausea and vomiting in 20 cases, cephalagiae, somnolence, and asthenia. These manifestations appear from the first injections, within $^1/_2$–1 h, and last several hours, rarely 12–24 h. They may become attenuated in the course of the treatment, spontaneously or with the help of symptomatic therapy.

In our controlled study only the calcitonin-treated group showed signs of intolerance (flushes in 2 cases out of 15, nausea in 4, and somnolence in 1).

The mode of action of the calcitonin was first thought to be related to its antiosteolytic and antiosteoclastic properties with transient increase in osteoblasts. Eisinger [240] showed that calcitonin produces a decrease in the 24-h hydroxyprolinuria and, concomitantly, increased alkaline phosphatases, witnessing the osteoblast activity.

But the promptness of action of calcitonin not only on the pain but also on the vasomotor disturbances and the edema cannot be ascribed only to its inhibitory effect on the osteoclasts. Calcitonin has a properly vascular effect. Recently Vayssairat et al. [832] provided evidence of the vasoactive properties of calcitonin in Raynaud's phenomenon, in a controlled study of 20 cases: 50% of the patients treated with calcitonin improved, as against none of those who were given the placebo. The number of attacks fell by 35%, and the Doppler method showed the digital pulpar pulses reappearing subsequent to treatment by calcitonin.

The rapid improvement of the functional impairments could thus be ascribed to the vasculotropic effect of calcitonin; the inhibition of the activity of the osteoclasts would complement the reparation of the initial vasomotor disturbance.

Chapter 2 Physical Treatment

Physical modalities include all therapies which deliver energy in any form to the tissue. Thus the oldest physiotherapy is the mechanical energy afforded by massage, and the most sophisticated, in its mode of production as well as its effects, is roentgentherapy.

We shall consider successively massage, rehabilitation, hydrotherapy and its corrolaries, crenotherapy, thalassotherapy, vibrotherapy (mainly ultrasound), electrotherapy (continuous current, alternating low, medium and high frequency currents), roentgentherapy, and, finally, acupuncture.

There is great confusion concerning use of these physical modalities, depending on the stage of the disease, and concerning their results. This is due as much to the great variety of clinical pictures seen in algodystrophy as to the variable degree of pain or of atrophy, and to the stage of the disease at the time when therapy is administered.

After studying and discussing the reports which seemed to us the most significant and the most recent, we shall try to provide a scheme for the physiotherapic management of algodystrophy.

A. Massage

At the onset, massage should mainly help to overcome tendencies to contracture and should consist of kneading and vibrating to facilitate venous and lymphatic drainage; deep muscular massage should be avoided. Some authors [163] have proposed periosteal massage.

While trying to act upon vascular disorders, some authors thought of using the "Syncardon." This instrument produces a pressotherapy synchronous to the ventricular systole; it is widely used for treating chronic arteriopathies of the limbs. Of 42 patients with algodystrophy only 9 have received this treatment in the 3 months following the appearance of the syndrome. The main characteristic of this treatment is its antalgic effect, which is said to be constant and unrelated to the stage of the disease.

We were disappointed by the book of Dicke et al. [202] on massage of the reflex areas in the connective tissue (*Bindegewebsmassage*). We thought indeed that this technique could be utilized for the etiologic treatment by acting upon the reflex phenomena. The authors, however, employ their technique only at stage 2 and treat first the spine and only afterward the involved segment. Only when edema and pain have diminished do they apply their technique to the limb, and this very cautiously. Finally, as concerns the third or atrophic stage, the authors believe that improvement can only be obtained with the supplementary aid of excercises.

We think that the possibilities of this method have not been fully exploited [781] and that it should be most useful in the very early stages of the disease, provided the theoretical bases are what the authors believe them to be.

B. Hydrotherapy, Crenotherapy, Thalassotherapy [528]

Most of the authors avoid using hydrotherapy in the early inflammatory stages of the disease. Nevertheless, some patients derive benefit from warm hydrotherapy, others from cold hydrotherapy or even from the alternation of the two, which provides a true vasomotor gymnastic. Contrariwise, other patients are aggravated by one or both methods so that it has to be immediately abandoned. Merklen [562] is one of those who believe that simple crenotherapy can nevertheless be useful for the following two reasons: feebly mineralized saline hot springs would have an antifluxionary and disinfiltrative action on the skin. Moreover, Merklen noticed that in mild forms of mono- or oligoarticular algodystrophy very gentle mobilization under immersion never entails risks of reactivation, due to the hydrostatic pressure.

According to Rénier [669] thermal cures would be useful, from the end of the acute phase, to encourage healing, especially in sluggish forms.

From our observations of more than 80 patients sent to hot springs with saline water for 3–4 weeks as soon as the diagnosis of algodystrophy had been made, we think that this procedure appreciably shortens the duration of the disease. Merklen reviewed 60 case reports of patients who had been treated in Niederbronn-les-Bains (France) and he believes that medical treatment is not sufficient to avoid functional sequels in the articulations as well as the muscles and skin. Early kinebalneotherapy seems to accelerate return to function and minimize the sequels. Crenotherapy would still be useful in later stages, even in the atrophic stage in patients submitted for long months to treatments that have ceased to be effective. The impact of thermalism on the underlying "terrain" which is so important in algodystrophy, renders beneficial the neurovegetative changes brought about by the thermal cure.

Graber-Duvernay et al. [321, 322] believe that early crenotherapy may have a preventive effect in posttraumatic conditions. They refer to two statistics: the first concerns more than 1000 wounded persons in the First and (mainly) the Second World War; the second concerns about 1000 casualties treated in Aix-les-Bains (France) in 1951 and 1952. According to them treatment should be commenced as early as possible, and before irreversible lesions have developed, during the edematous phase in the 30 days following the traumatism. This treatment consists first in sedation. A few days later active and voluntary muscle contraction carried out under water can be undertaken, followed by active-assisted motor rehabilitation. By the combined action of the joints and muscles the first part of the excercise allows the muscles to regain their tonicity, the second part aims at accelerating return to function of the articulation. According to these authors crenotherapy would provide a 41% gain with regard to the transient incapacity to work, and also a 41% gain with regard to the partial permanent disablement. The authors believe mineral water to have a much more decisive action than plain water.

Levernieux and Kerzreho [505] report about treatment by thalassotherapy, including sea water baths, seaweed baths, and applications of sea-muds in patients with algodystrophy of the lower limbs.

C. Kinesitherapy and Rehabilitation

[45, 129, 302, 414, 504, 589, 642, 711, 752]

Kinesitherapy consists here in passive and active mobilization carried out during the period without weight-bearing on the affected limb. In the following phase, rehabilitation becomes necessary. These techniques are aimed at preventing aggravation of bone demineralization, and conservation or recuperation of the joint mobility.

We refer to the works of Minaire [573] concerning disuse osteoporosis. For this author the mechanical factor seems to be prominent, even at the level of the cell, where it certainly influences the bone resorption-formation sequence. The different dynamic methods seem to be insufficient to reestablish a bone with normal density. If we admit, along with Issekutz [388], that a minimum of 2 h walking per day is necessary to prevent osteoporosis, it would necessitate a much longer time to make it regress. Mobilization of the patient at rest helps only to maintain the joint mechanisms. Maximal use of muscle contracture is efficient by way of prevention. It allowed considerable reduction in the calcium loss in the cosmonauts of Gemini VII, by comparison with their predecessors in Gemini IV and V, in spite of a longer flight duration. According to Covalt et al. [160] and to Nordin et al. [604] the reestablishment of the longitudinal pressure forces would be of capital importance. Two hours per day of walking and upright position would suffice to avoid immobilization osteoporosis.

All methods based on these principles could be useful in algodystrophy. We have already pointed out the interest of hydrokinesitherapy. As to "dry" kinesitherapy, this consists of passive and active mobilization. It must be done "cautiously, progressively and perseveringly" [646] by means of "short and repeated sessions." It must not be painful or brisk, so as to avoid reactivation of the algodystrophic process. Methods which are forbearing to the articulation should be proscribed.

Although it should be done as early as possible, active mobilization can only be undertaken when at least partial sedation of pain has been obtained. Serre et al. [752] provided an accurate description of the rehabilitation procedures in algodystrophy of the lower limb. Passive mobilization is performed with the patient supine, his lower limb being raised by 30°. It consists in passive mobilization, joint by joint, from the ankle to the interphalangeal articulations. The active mobilization is also performed with the patient supine. He is told to perform movements of the foot and toes at maximal range, while taking care to neutralize the ankle. Then the same movements are carried out against a resistance. Combined movements of foot and toes are also associated. Postural maneuvers are employed when muscular contracture or retraction tend to appear. This helps to prevent a faulty walking posture establishing itself.

The techniques and principles which are described here for the foot, are also valuable for the other joints of the lower limb and for the upper limb.

D. Electrotherapy

The term electrotherapy designates treatment by the following physical agents: electricity, electromagnetic radiation, and mechanical vibration.

All these electrotherapic methods have been used for more than 50 years for the treatment of algodystrophy [32, 204, 227, 232, 328, 330, 335, 423]. From our experience it seems that short waves (30–300 MHz), diathermy (3–30 MHz), and other applications of heat are contraindicated. Böhler [86], on the contrary, currently uses warm air, short waves, and diathermy.

Ertem et al. [247], to obtain a sympathetic block, used a fixed modulation of a sinusoidal current which produces a sympatholytic effect. They took advantage of the anti-inflammatory action of low frequency and of the analgesic effect of high frequency current.

Commandre et al. [145] advocate pulsated high frequencies with nonthermic effect, applied to the stellate ganglion, the lumbar chain, or periarterial sympathetic system. The effects seem remarkable, since, out of 50 patients so treated they obtained 39 cures within 3–5 weeks, improvement starting only 3–6 days after the onset of treatment. Only stage IV conditions (our irreversible stage III) seem to be poorly influenced by this treatment.

Guillemin et al. [335] provide the following indications concerning the application of electrotherapy. "Galvanic currents with their analgesic action, microwaves with their anti-edematous action, interferential currents used as vasodilators, and slow-frequency excitomotor currents are to be used for stage I conditions. For stage II, short waves and, moderately, ultrasound are used for their relaxant and hyperemic effect. Diadynamic currents with analgesic action and modulated or interferential low frequency currents will create a real 'electrokinesitherapy'. Dielectrolysis of relaxant, anti-inflammatory, anabolizing, analgesic and muscular eutrophic agents will be associated to the above listed methods and improve the course of functional rehabilitation. At stage III, finally, short waves, simple or pulsated microwaves influence the neurovegetative disorders and favor the dielectrolysis of the group B vitamins, of vasodilators, anabolics, of phosphorus and calcium. Ultrasound is associated because of its sedative and hyperemic effect and also of its local mechanical action."

As the authors point out, electrotherapy cannot of course be considered a major therapeutic procedure, but should always be used in addition to the medical and physical treatments.

Bargy [32] associates calcic ionizations and roentgentherapy.

E. Roentgentherapy

A certain number of good results have been reported to be due to treatment of algodystrophy by roentgentherapy [101, 592]; thanks to the works of Vieten [838] the method has been standardized. Patients receive the X-radiation in the cervical and upper thoracic or the lumbosacral sympathetic chains. In very advanced or severe cases, it is also possible to irradiate the axilla, Scarpa's triangle or the popliteal space. In principle doses of 50–100 roentgen are employed, six sessions for each field, the sessions being spaced 3–6 days apart.

According to this author the results are better the sooner treatment is done. In stage I conditions, the analgesic effect appears after two to three sessions, but the trophic disturbances take 3–4 months to disappear completely. In stage

II, the effect is less prompt. The author often performs a second series of radiotherapy, and sometimes even a third. In the atrophic stage III, no significant result should be hoped for.

In their report on the indications and interpretation of the mode of action of roentgentherapy Böni and Faidherbe [88] studied more particularly the treatment of scapulohumeral periarthritis. Unfortunately they do not distinguish the different anatomoclinical types, i.e., simple or calcifying tendinitis, rupture of the rotator cuff, and retractile capsulitis. They do not give their view concerning the technique which consists of isolated irradiation of the scapulohumeral articulation alone or of associated irradiation of the shoulder and cervical spine. They note that posttraumatic periarthritis is cured in 18% of cases, and improved in 58%, whereas those which appeared spontaneously are cured in 29% of cases, and improved in 52%.

As for ourselves, we use roentgentherapy mainly in algodystrophies of the shoulder, i.e., frozen shoulder. We never give X-radiation to the cervical spine and we content ourselves with an irradiation of the scapulohumeral articulation. Our aim is mainly to relieve the pain, so as to permit the application of a rehabilitation program. It should however be noted that we obtain by this method a gain of about 10° in the range of motion, this being probably due to the analgesic action. The improvement becomes evident after 4–6 weeks and the maximal effect is obtained after 2 months.

In some severe forms of algodystrophy of the hand or foot, after the medical treatment had failed and with the severity of pain preventing any modality of physiotherapy, roentgentherapy on the cervical or lumbar sympathetic chains provided a definite improvement after a few sessions.

F. Acupuncture

We owe to Schrodi [733] the main part of the data concerning the treatment of algodystrophy by acupuncture. Details of the different techniques of treatment are beyond the scope of this chapter, but a few basic principles will be given. It seems to us that acupuncture could have a therapic utility in a reflex sympathetic dystrophy.

As concerns acupuncture, algodystrophy would be a lack of balance between the energetic circulation from the depth of an organ to the periphery. In the normal condition the yin energy is in the depth. Under the action of a certain number of factors, causing algodystrophy, the yin energy would suddenly accumulate at the periphery, an area usually occupied by yang energy. In the superficial tissues it will thus be necessary to mobilize the yin by supplying yang (heat, movement) and this via all points available for acupuncture. Thus, the yin will be released and will circulate again and join the depth to play its normal nutritional role there.

Experience and practice showed that sessions should be performed every 2 or 3 days and that a therapic response occurs only around the tenth or twelfth session, i.e., after about 3–4 weeks. No controlled study has ever been made, as far as we know.

Chapter 3 Surgery

Heymann [364] of Mount Sinai Hospital published in 1924 the first case report of *sympathectomy*. "A man aged 21 years, complained of pain in the left foot ... Five months had elapsed since his injury ... Roentgen-ray examination showed a very marked osteoporosis of all bones in the foot.

Arterial sympathectomy was advised in the hope of breaking up the vicious circle ... The externa was stripped from the femoral artery in Hunter's canal ... Three hours later it was observed that there was a full bounding pulse, and the foot was warm .. Two months after operation he returned to his shop work ... A roentgenogram taken that day (seven and a half months after sympathectomy) showed a normal appearance of the bones in the foot."

In 1926 Leriche [491], being anxious to know the action of periarterial sympathectomy on tuberculous arthritis, carried out this intervention in a man suffering from what he believed to be a white swelling of the wrist. The effect was so dramatic that Leriche had doubts about the diagnosis.

Thus, periarterial sympathectomy became in Strasbourg the method of choice for the treatment of osteoporotic syndromes.

From 1932 on, analgesic infiltrations were widely used. Surgery was only considered for a relatively small number of cases, those for which all therapic procedures had failed and also those which came with already longstanding functional disturbances.

As concerns algodystrophy, periarterial sympathectomy or catenoid sympathectomy (including for the upper limb stellectomies and upper thoracic sympathectomies, and for the lower limb, upper or lower lumbar sympathectomies) can be taken into account. Periarterial sympathectomies do not seem to be effective enough in advanced syndromes; as soon as particularly powerful vasodilating action is desired, catenoid operations are preferred.

After Leriche, numerous authors [249, 266, 310, 448, 515, 699] reported isolated cases of sympathectomy, but only in 1955 did Fontaine et al.'s statistics [275] permit a judgement to be made on this surgical technique. Their series comprised 59 cases.

In longstanding osteoporosis of the upper limb upper thoracic sympathectomy provided, out of 12 cases, 7 excellent or very good results; out of 30 cases stellectomy provided 10 excellent or very good results; out of 10 cases perihumeral sympathectomy obtained only 1 very good result.

If the results are similar in the case of upper thoracic sympathectomy and stellectomy, they are clearly insufficient in perihumeral sympathectomy. The results of lumbar sympathectomy for osteoporosis of the lower limb were very good 7 times out of 7.

The symptom which usually regresses most rapidly is the pain. It disappears sometimes almost instantaneously, as soon as the postoperative vasodilatation takes effect. In the good cases, the vasomotor and cutaneous disturbances, the edema, and the contractures are also quickly attenuated. Osteoporosis however needs several months to regress.

Sympathectomy should be considered in obstinate forms, but it would seem that nobody has recourse to it. Does that mean that there are no more obstinate forms or that the medical and physical modalities are sufficient to content the patient?

It was mainly Ficat and Arlet [257] who used *drill biopsy* for diagnostic and therapeutic purposes in reflex algodystrophies of the hip, and mainly in aseptic necroses of the femoral head.

Surgical treatment of tendinous and aponeurotic retractions is most often disappointing since the retractions have a regrettable tendency to recur.

In two cases of algodystrophy with hypercalciuria, Leriche and Jung [501] decided to attempt *parathyroidectomy*. In both cases they found the parathyroid glands to have an increased volume. They obtained considerable improvement but not healing.

Finally, *amputation* of the painful limb constitutes the ultimate failure. Leriche [494] had to take this decision in two cases, as did other workers [680]. These amputations allowed a certain number of pathologic findings to be reported (Part 2, Chap. 8).

Chapter 4 Management of Algodystrophies

Respect of the fundamental rule of avoiding and eliminating pain must be the major concern of the therapist in any case. Thus each case of algodystrophy should benefit from all means aimed at suppressing the pain: avoidance of weight-bearing in involvements of the lower limbs, rest positions for involvements of the upper limbs, postural drainage, the upper limb placed in an elevated position.

But it is at least as important to ensure passive and above all active mobilization, as soon as possible, even if only small-range movements can be carried out, without ever going so far as to provoke the pain.

Return to activity should be done very progressively but as early as possible, i.e., as soon as pain is sedated.

At the onset the treatment consists of analgesics, nonsteroid anti-inflammatory agents, anxiolytics, and correction of any metabolic disorders; psychotherapy is desirable and should be aimed at explaining to the patient the nature of his disease, and telling him that it usually ends in healing although this may be only obtained after a variable and perhaps very long delay, without underlining the risks of recurrence and of possible extension of the process.

The different drugs which we have reviewed could be administered successively since it is not possible to indicate definitely which would be the most effective and best tolerated.

Nevertheless, three of these drugs seem to have a definite value, namely griseofulvin, beta-blockers, and above all calcitonin; all three have been successful in a significant number of cases.

If these treatments fail, we have recourse successively to the different modalities of physiotherapy, kinesitherapy, hydrotherapy, crenotherapy, etc.

For all these methods the same rule is applied, that of avoiding and eliminating pain.

Chapter 5 Prevention

We have seen the causes of algodystrophy to be multiple, often intertwined, sometimes difficult to demonstrate; we have also seen that the physiopathology of this condition is not yet entirely understood.

It is nevertheless perhaps possible to limit the incidence of algodystrophy by treating the etiologic factors which we have already pointed out.

The metabolic disorders, namely hyperglycemia and hyperlipidemia should be diagnosed and overcome.

An anxious "terrain" justifies the use of anxiolytics.

As we saw, traumatisms play an important part in algodystrophy. In traumatisms without fracture (contusions, sprains, etc.) plaster casts should be applied only when absolutely necessary; and when a cast is necessary care should be taken to place the patient in a declive position so that the weight does not increase the edema, but rather help to diminish it.

In traumatisms with fracture a certain number of rules should be observed. The repair of damage caused by the traumatism should be done as soon as possible; the injured area should be rigorously immobilized to favor rapid cicatrization of the tissues.

Immediate mobilization is undertaken without compromising the immobility of the injured area. This mobilization must be absolutely painless.

The traumatized limb must moreover be placed on an abduction splint, for the upper limb, or on a declive splint for the lower limb. A cast for the lower limb permitting walking can be used provided there appears no edema, cyanosis, or pain, in which case walking is prohibited and the lower limb is placed in a declive position and submitted to active mobilization several times per day.

Chemotherapy, especially treatment with phenobarbital, tuberculostats, in particular isoniazid, and radioactive iodine may be responsible for algodystrophy. It is of course not a question of abstaining from such treatment, when the patient's state requires it. Nevertheless, excessive use of hypnotic medications containing phenobarbital should be avoided. Hypnotics such as the products of the benzodiazepine series should be preferred.

In order to prevent posttraumatic or postoperative comitiality, it is preferable to use in the first place, anticonvulsive agents of the hydantoin or primidone group, and to reserve phenobarbital in case they fail.

In hyperthyroidism, for the preparation of patients for treatment with radioactive iodine or surgery, beta-blockers are to be used; we have already pointed out the usefulness of these drugs for the treatment of algodystrophy.

Part 9 Clinical Course and Prognosis

Chapter 1 Clinical Course

The clinical course of algodystrophy is extremely variable depending on the site which is affected, and for a given localization it varies also from one case to another.

We have seen (Part 1, Chap. 2) however, that the evolution of this condition is most often favorable and ends with healing without sequels. Regression occurs more or less rapidly, however, depending partly on whether treatment is given. When the disease is treated, the evolution depends on the nature and modality of treatment and on when it is commenced.

A. Clinical Course of Untreated Algodystrophy

When it is not treated, algodystrophy usually progresses very slowly toward recovery without sequels. This spontaneous course is however very variable and lasts several months to several years, depending on the site that is affected.

The course of algodystrophy of the upper limbs, whether it consists of isolated involvement of the shoulder, of the hand, or of a shoulder-hand syndrome, is frequently very long with the possibility of sequels, such as fibroaponerotic retraction of the hand causing an irreducible claw, with vasomotor and trophic disturbances.

In involvements of the feet, the evolution is usually also very long, but recovery without sequels usually occurs after from 6 months to 1–2 years, or even later.

In the knee, recovery occurs within a relatively shorter period, rarely more than 1 year, and without sequels.

It is however mainly in the hip that evolution of algodystrophy is relatively rapidly favorable, even in the absence of a treatment. Healing may occur within a few weeks, but the average duration is 4–6 months. Forms which have a duration of more than 8 months to 1 year are quite uncommon. There are never sequels in this localization.

When one episode of algodystrophy, whatever the site affected, is healed, the patient is not secure from other involvements, which may occur shortly after the first, sometimes even before it is healed, or also several years later and, in some rare instances, more than 10 years later. Note however that only exceptionally does the second episode involve the same site as the first.

B. Clinical Course of Treated Algodystrophy

We have seen in Part 8 that the evolution of this condition can be influenced by treatment.

Only a few controlled studies have been made concerning the different modalities of treatment applied to algodystrophy. Moreover, the great variability in the spontaneous evolution makes it difficult to evaluate objectively the efficiency of the different treatments which have been proposed.

The classical treatment combines diverse medications, e.g., vasodilators, antalgics, or even nonsteroid anti-inflammatory drugs, associated with cautious and very forbearing reeducation; it has the advantage of preventing trophic sequels. But it cannot be affirmed that the duration of the disease is really shortened by this treatment.

Follow-up studies over a period of 3 months to 10 years (average duration of follow-up: 3 years) were made by Serre et al. [754] on 122 cases of algodystrophy of the foot. The mean duration of the disease was 12 months, with extremes of 4 and 28 months. According to the authors, early treatment diminished the duration of the course, and the only sequels consisted in pain provoked by fatigue and weather changes.

In recent years three drugs seem to have proven their effectiveness in reducing the duration of the disease: griseofulvin, which has proved very effective, within a few days sometimes; beta-blocking drugs are also quite effective, within a few days in some instances; and finally, calcitonin, results with which have been particularly striking from the first injections, sometimes even the first day after onset of treatment;

complete healing occurs within a few days even in severe forms.

But response to treatment is inconstant and, in about half of the cases the clinical course is about the same with and without treatment, in spite of these new therapeutics; the classical treatments which are successively given concomitantly with very cautions and persevering kinesitherapy, only permit avoidance or limitation of the sequels, especially in the upper limbs.

It should also be pointed out that all these treatments are more active when they are administered during the so-called warm or hyperemic phase, i.e., at the onset of the course or, at least, during the first few weeks; this is not however an absolute rule.

Finally, the sometimes very dramatic effectiveness of these three drugs does not prevent the unforeseeable occurrence of algodystrophic involvements of other sites; but these too may respond to the same treatment.

Chapter 2 Prognosis

The prognosis of algodystrophy is unpredictable. The apparent severity of the affection, the importance of the inflammatory signs, the intensity of pain, and the importance of functional disability are not constantly correlated with the response to treatment, the total duration of the episode, and the eventual existence of sequels.

Thus, a pseudophlegmonous form may heal within a few days to several months. On the contrary, algodystrophy of the foot, for instance, which is characterized by pain on weight-bearing, almost invisible heterogeneous demineralization and moderately increased uptake at bone scanning, may have a desperately prolonged course of 1 year and more, in spite of the different treatments administered early and successively.

All the same, the severity of the radiologic signs, the extent of the algodystrophic process, the intensity of the increased uptake at bone scanning are no clues for the prognosis. Thus the only one of our observations which had, from the onset very clear hypofixation at bone scanning, had a sluggish course of about 1 year.

The degree of hydroxyprolinuria has no value for the prognosis, and in particular does not allow one to foresee the response to calcitonin treatment.

On the other hand, the site of algodystrophy can have an undeniable prognostic value. Thus certain areas are usually the site of relatively benign and short involvements; this is the case with the hips, knees, and elbows, even in the absence of treatment.

The rapidity of the response to treatment, namely pain relieved within a few hours or several days following treatment with griseofulvin, beta-blockers, and especially calcitonin, is a good prognosis.

Fournié et al. [276] showed the interest of calcitonin-induced acute hypocalcemia. A decrease of 6 mg or more in the calcium rate 4–10 h after the injection of 160 units of porcine calcitonin, or of 80 units of salmon calcitonin was consistent, in 5 patients suffering from algodystrophy, with a good response to treatment with calcitonin, whereas 5 other patients, in whom the calcitonin test had been negative, failed to derive benefit from treatment with calcitonin. The authors believe that the calcitonin-induced hypocalcemia indicates the degree of osteclastosis, since the calcitonin-induced decrease in the calcium rate is above 10 mg in Paget's disease, whereas it is less than 3 mg in controls.

This test could thus be really valuable for the prognosis of algodystrophy, namely for predicting the effectiveness of calcitonin treatment. But these results should be confirmed by further studies.

Finally, early treatment, particularly by beta-blockers and by calcitonin, is for most of the authors a ground for a good prognosis. This is however not always the case; indeed, one of our best results was obtained in 4 days by calcitonin in a stage II affection which had already lasted 8 months when we started the treatment.

Part 10 Medicolegal Considerations

Posttraumatic algodystrophies raise delicate medicolegal problems concerning compensation for bodily damage subsequent to a professional accident, to a common law injury or to a casualty covered by an individual insurance policy [136, 236, 346, 500, 701, 823].

We shall consider successively the causality, the eventual part played by an anterior status, the duration of total transient disability, the date of consolidation, and finally, the pretium doloris.

Causality

Assessment of the causality requires proof that a traumatism has existed, definite diagnosis of algodystrophy, and temporospatial concordance between the traumatism and the algodystrophy.

Past Status

We have several times pointed out that algodystrophy occurs preferentially in patients with neurovegetative instability and precarious neurosympathetic balance.

As concerns professional accidents, the past status is not taken into account since responsibility for it is assumed. In common law injuries, only the damage resulting from the traumatism is taken into account, so that only a possible aggravation of an anterior status can be considered for estimating reparation. Finally, as concerns individual insurances the compensation is estimated on the direct sequels of the traumatism, after elimination of all pathological antecedents.

Duration of Total Transient Disability

This is very variable and depends on the duration of the course of the algodystrophic syndrome.

Date of Consolidation

It is often very difficult to fix this date, which does not necessarily coincide with the date when the patient returns to work. It corresponds to the moment when the status has become sequellar and no longer susceptible to improvement by any treatment whatsoever.

Now, algodystrophy has an unpredictable course. One must therefore be very prudent and wait as long as is necessary, but without prolonging unduly the interruption of work which always has a prejudicial effect on the course of the disease. It is however possible to fix a date for resuming professional activities with a rate of transient disability and prolongation of medical care for 6–12 months, after which another examination permits one to appreciate the evolution and to make a statement as to the consolidation.

If the initial plurifocal forms do not raise problems since the relation between the traumatism and the lesion seems obvious, secondarily extensive forms, whether, these are forms with multiple episodes or plurifocal recurrent forms, still instigate discussion among medical experts. One may indeed discuss the relation between the initial episode and the subsequent localizations.

Is it possible to fix a date after which a relation between the traumatism, the initial episode of algodystrophy, and later algodystrophic manifestations will no longer be admitted?

Also, should a new localization of algodystrophy appearing after a variable delay, sometimes after several years, and affecting a segment of the limb which had not been injured or involved in the first algodystrophic episode, be taken into account for compensation?

The task of the expert will be very delicate since he should avoid denying any link between the different episodes as well as correlating anything to the traumatism.

Fixation of Permanent and Partial Disability

This will be done at the same time as consolidation, i.e., when the lesions are stabilized. As concerns professional accidents, the rate of permanent and partial disability is always revisable, and an estimation which the later course of the disease proves to be erroneous – improvement or aggravation having occurred in the meantime – can always be reviewed. On the other hand, in common law, the judgment can only exceptionally be reviewed.

As concerns the rate of permanent and partial disability, this is very difficult to assess, since each case is peculiar.

The Pretium Doloris

This takes into account the pain endured by the patient during the period preceding consolidation. It also depends mainly on the severity of the initial traumatism, on the duration of hospitalization, on the distressing character of medical treatments, and also on the painful element of the syndrome in so far as this pain is not a part of the definitive sequels.

In the great majority of cases the evolution of algodystrophy is favorable and tends toward recovery without sequels within unpredictable delays.

But in contradiction to this optimistic view, there also exist, fortunately rather rare cases with irreversible sequels of major functional severity. This is the case for instance with the hand where tendinous retraction in the flexed position and fibrous ankylosis involving the metacarpo-phalangeal and proximal and distal interphalangeal articulations of the 3 or 4 last fingers cause the classical neurotrophic claw with definitive functional disablement.

Such fibrotic sequels have been described in detail by Ravault et al. [649] and by Steinbrocker et al. [778]. More recently, Rubens Duval et al. [702] reported their follow-up studies in 7 patients after 1 year's intensive treatment: 4 still have a major functional disablement preventing the use of the hand in professional life, the 3 others could return to work but still experience marked discomfort due mainly to the fibrotic ankylosis of the 4th and 5th fingers.

Analogous sequels due to fibrotic ankylosis have been reported in the shoulder and the feet.

Return to professional life depends mainly on the duration of the course of the algodystrophic process, which is very variable from patient to patient and is also related to the site affected. Thus, Serre et al. [749] report, in a series of 45 algodystrophies of the foot followed up for about 3 years, an average duration of interruption of work of 11 months, with extremes of 1 month and 2 years.

References

1. Abergel S (1978) Algodystrophies et hyperlipidémies. Mémoire CES Rhumatologie, University of Paris
2. Acquaviva P, Eisinger JB, Schiano A, Recordier AM (1976) Traitement des algodystrophies par la Calcitonine. Mediterr Med 4:33–44
3. Acquaviva P, Schiano A (1976) Les algodystrophies. Vie Med 34:2761–2766
4. Algodystrophy (1978). Br Med J 6111:462–463 (Editorial)
5. Allison N, Brooks B (1921) Bone atrophy. An experimental and clinical study of the changes in bone which result from non-use. Surg Gynecol Obstet 33:250–260
6. Amick LD, Gilmer WJ, Sutton FD (1966) The holistic approach to the shoulder-hand syndrom. South Med J 59:161–167
7. Amor B, Gery A de, Saporta L, Abergel S, Delbarre F (1980) Algodystrophies et hyperlipidémies. Rev Rhum Mal Osteoartic 47:353–358
8. Andrews CG, Armitage KJ (1971) Sudeck's atrophy in traumatic quadriplegia. Paraplegia 9:159–165
9. Arendt J (1945) Bone rarefaction after skull injuries. Radiology 45:608–613
10. Arens W (1967) Sudecksche Dystrophie des Fußes nach leichter Distorsion. Monatschr Unfallheilkd Versicherung Versorg Verkehrsmed 70:187–190
11. Arieff AJ, Bell JL (1956) Epilepsy and Dupuytren's contracture. Neurology (Minneap) 6:115–117
12. Arieff AJ, Bell JL, Tigay EL (1964) Reflex physiopathic disturbances. Surg Gynecol Obstet 118:1029–1034
13. Aristoff H, May V, Guillon C (1979) A case of partial sympathetic reflex dystrophy of the knee. (Abstr. 432) IX European Congress of Rheumatology Wiesbaden
14. Arlet J (1979) Histopathologie comparée de la nécrose de la tête fémorale et de l'algodystrophie sympathique réflexe de la hanche. Rhumatologie (Aix les Bains) 31:377–378
15. Arlet J, Durroux R, Girou DE, Gercourt G (to be published) Histopathologie de l'algodystrophie sympathique du genou. A propos de 15 observations. Rev Rhum Mal Osteoartic
16. Arlet J, Ficat P, Durroux R, Theallier JP, Mazieres B, Bouteiller G (1978) Histopathologie des lésions osseuses dans 9 cas d'algodystrophie de la hanche. Rev Rhum Mal Osteoartic 45:691–698
17. Arlet J, Rascol A, Mole J, Roger JM (1967) Observations de "rhumatisme gardénalique". Rev Rhum Mal Osteoartic 34:193–198
18. Arnstein A (1972) Regional osteoporosis. Orthop Clin North Am 3:585–600
19. Arnulf G (1944) Traitement par les infiltrations sympathiques des troubles réflexes post-traumatiques, dits physiopathiques. Rev Chir Orthop 30:161–168
20. Arnulf G (1954) A propos des troubles réflexes post-traumatiques. Rhumatologie (Aix les Bains) 3:130–133
21. Arnulf G (1957) A propos de la thérapeutique sympathique des osteoporoses posttraumatiques. Acta Chir Belg [Suppl] 1:282–283
22. Askey M (1941) The syndrome of painful disability of the shoulder and hand complicating coronary occlusion. Am Heart J 22:1–12
23. Avouac B (1979) L'étiologie de la périarthrite scapulo-humérale. Rhumatologie (Aix les Bains) 31:125–126
24. Ayrolles C, Fournié A, Ruffié R (1970) La hanche neurotrophique isolée et primitive. Rev Med Toulouse 6:663–674
25. Babinski J, Froment J (1915) Contribution à l'étude des troubles nerveux d'ordre réflexe. Examen pendant l'anesthésie chloroformique. Rev Neurol (Paris) 28:925–933
26. Babinski J, Froment J (1916) Des troubles vasomoteurs et thermiques d'ordre réflexe. Rev Neurol (Paris) 29:410–414
27. Babinski J, Froment J (1917) Hystérie-pithiatisme et troubles nerveux d'origine réflexe. Masson, Paris
28. Babinski J, Froment J, Heitz J (1916) Des troubles vasomoteurs et thermiques dans les paralysies et les contractures d'origine réflexe. Ann Med (Paris) 3:461–497
29. Bacri J, Mutin S (1951) Les manifestations osseuses du zona (à propos d'une observation). Rev Rhum Mal Osteoartic 18:618–620
30. Baer RD (1966) Shoulder-hand syndrome: its recognition and management. South Med J 59:790–794

31. Barcelo P, Juncadella-Ferrer E (1948) El llamado sindrome de hombro y mano en el infarto de miocardio. Rev Espan Reum Enferm Osteoartic 2:480–487
32. Bargy P (1972) Electrothérapie des algodystrophies réflexes. In: EMC Appareil loco-moteur 26205 A-10. Editions techniques, Paris
33. Barnett E, Nordin BEC (1960) The radiological diagnosis of osteoporosis. A new approach. Clin Radiol 11:166–174
34. Barraud F, Gerster JC, Saudan Y (1979) Polyarthrite rhumatoïde et algodystrophie post-traumatique. Rev Med Suisse Romande 99:57–61
35. Batisse R, Doury P, Pattin S, Garreta L (1976) L'algodystrophie coxo-fémorale unifocale. Ann Radiol (Paris) 19:519–524
36. Baud CA, Pouëzat JA (1973) Données microradiographiques quantitatives sur le minéral osseux dans l'ostéoporose posttraumatique. Rhumatologie (Aix les Bains) 22:75–77
37. Baudoin P (1974) Algodystrophies et Griséofulvine (Griséfuline). Concours Med 35:5277–5279
38. Baum F (1954) Schulter-Arm Syndrom und vegetatives Nervensystem. Aerztl Wochenschr 9:774–777
39. Bauss A (1957) Über Beziehungen von Sudeck-Syndromen nach Traumen. Aerztl Wochenschr 12:213–216
40. Bayles TB, Judson WE, Potter TA (1950) Reflex sympathetic dystrophy of the upper extremity (Hand-shoulder syndrome). JAMA 144:537–542
41. Beaufils C (1965) Traitement des algodystrophies réflexes par la Griséofulvine. MD dissertation, University of Paris
42. Beaulieu JG, Razzano CD, Levine RB (1976) Transient osteoporosis of the hip in pregnancy. Clin Orthop 115:165–168
43. Beckmann KH (1955) Vitaminotherapie beim Sudeckschen Syndrom. Chirurg 26:57–62
44. Belenger M (1956) Aspect clinique et méthodes thérapeutiques des ostéoporoses post-traumatiques. Acta Chir Belg [Suppl] 1:219–440
45. Benezis C (1973) Place de la réadaptation dans le traitement des algodystrophies réflexes du membre inférieur (à propos de 188 observations). MD dissertation, University of Montpellier
46. Benichou M (1966) Maladie de Dupuytren et traitement antituberculeux par l'isoniazide et l'éthionamide. MD dissertation, University of Paris
47. Benkwitz I (1906) Ueber akute Knochenatrophie (Sudeck). Strassburger Med Zeitung 3:129–131
48. Bensasson M, Lanoe R, Assan R (1977) Un cas de syndrome algodystrophique du membre supérieur survenu après vaccination antitétanique. Sem Hop Paris 53:1965–1966
49. Berard L, Dargent M, Trillat A (1936) A propos des troubles physiopathiques. Lyon Chir 33:433–439
50. Berger H (1954) The treatment of post-myocardial infarction shoulder-hand syndrome with local hydrocortisone. Postgrad Med 15:508–511
51. Beriel L, Barbier J (1934) Le rhumatisme gardénalique. Lyon Med 153:77–83
52. Bernard J (1954) Contribution à l'étude des algodystrophies réflexes sympathiques. MD dissertation, University of Paris
53. Bernard J, Mauvoisin F (1955) L'ostéoporose vasculaire et sympathique. In: Le rhumatisme. Etudes cliniques, biologiques et thérapeutiques. Expansion Scientifique Française, Paris
54. Bernstein BH, Singsen BH, Kent JJ, Kornreich H, King K, Hicks R, Hanson U (1978) Reflex neurovascular dystrophy in childhood. J Pediatr 93:211–215
55. Berthel M, Kuntzmann F, Moyses B, Méthlin G (1980) Evaluation de la minéralisation osseuse mesurée par radiodensitomètrie directe en fonction de l'âge: étude par méthode transversale et longitudinale. In: Rapport de la VI Conférence Internationale des Maladies Rhumatismales, Aix les Bains
56. Berthelen MC (1976) Contribution à l'étude de l'algodystrophie de la hanche. MD dissertation, University of Strasbourg
57. Berthier L (1949) Zona et périarthrite scapulohumérale. Rev Rhum Mal Osteartic 16:28
58. Bertrix GP (1959) Contribution à l'étude des algodystrophies réflexes des membres (à propos de 5 observations). MD dissertation, University of Clermont-Ferrand
59. Betcher AM, Casten DF (1955) Reflex sympathetic dystrophy: criteria for diagnosis and treatment. Anesthesiology 16:994–1003
60. Bianchetti CF (1925) Edema duro post-traumatico della mano; simpatectomia periarteriosa; guarigione. Giorn Acad Med Torino 31:39–47
61. Bianchi M (1966) La sindrome di Sudeck posttraumatica. Immagini radiografiche. Minerva Orthop 17:110–113
62. Bibergeil E (1911) Traumatische Neurose und Sudecksche Knochenatrophie. Med Klin 7:921–923
63. Bienfait A (1907) Un cas d'atrophie osseuse de Sudeck. J Neurol 12:149–151
64. Bion P (1963) Les périarthrites et rhumatismes neurotrophiques du membre supérieur consécutifs au traitement des hyperthyroïdies par l'iode radioactif. MD dissertation, University of Paris
65. Bircher JL (1970) Sudecksche Dystrophie. Handchirurgie 2:193–199
66. Bircher JL (1973) Algodystrophie réflexe et fractures de la main. Acta Orthop Belg 39:1024–1032
67. Bircher JL (1973) Le syndrome de Sudeck-Leriche. Rhumatologie (Aix les Bains) 25:21–24
68. Bircher JL (1974) Klinische Sudeckprophylaxie und Therapie. Tierexperimentelle Grundlagen. Springer, Berlin Heidelberg New York
69. Bircher JL, Arnim D von (1972) Behandlung des

Sudeck Syndroms. Muench Med Wochenschr 114:1951–1952
70. Bircher JL, Schieweck C, Schenk R (1967) 77 Versuche zur experimentellen Erzeugung einer Sudeckschen Dystrophie und deren Prophylaxie. Arch Klin Chir 319:454–457
71. Blanc D (1976) Le test aïgu à la Calcitonine synthétique de saumon. Son intérêt en pathologie osseuse. MD dissertation, University of Grenoble
72. Blanc D, Chapuy MC, Meunier P (1977) Evaluation de l'activité ostéoclastique par le test d'hypocalcémie provoquée par la calcitonine de saumon. Nouv Presse Med 6:2489–2494
73. Blanchet CM (1932) De l'ostéoporose infectieuse et de l'ostéoporose algique post-traumatique. MD dissertation, University of Paris
74. Blankoff MB (1956) Tuberculose et ostéoporose de Sudeck. Acta Chir Belg [Suppl] 1:497–508
75. Blanquart F, Moudent G, Deshayes P (1974) L'algodystrophie iatrogène gardénalique. Sem Hop Paris 50:499–503
76. Blauth W (1962) Die Sudecksche Dystrophie des Kniegelenks. Arch Orthop Unfall Chir 53:231–249
77. Blini J (1957) Le distrofie post-traumatiche della mano. Minerva Orthop 8:429–432
78. Bloch-Michel H, Salomon A (1964) Traitement des algodystrophies réflexes par la Griséofulvine. Rhumatologie (Aix les Bains) 16:345–347
79. Bloch-Michel H, Salomon A, Revuz J (1968) Affections "médicales" post-traumatiques de la main. Rev Prat 18:2037–2044
80. Bloch-Michel H, Vallee G, Bion P (1964) Manifestations rhumatismales consécutives au traitement des hyperthyroïdies. Ann Endocrinol (Paris) 25:319–322
81. Blumensaat C (1952) Zur Phasen-Deutung des Sudeckschen Syndroms. Chirurg 23:449–457
82. Blumensaat C (1955) Durchblutungstörungen bei Sudeck-Syndrom. Z Rheumaforsch 14:94–101
83. Blumensaat C (1956) Der heutige Stand der Lehre von Sudeck-Syndrom. 51. Beiheft z. Unfallheilkunde. Springer, Berlin Heidelberg New York
84. Boas EP, Levy H (1937) Extracardiac determinants of site and radiation of pain in angina pectoris, with special references to shoulder pain. Am Heart J 14:540–554
85. Boely C (1958) Traitement de l'ostéoporose algique post-traumatique par les injections intraartérielles de procaïne. Lyon Chir 51:84–85
86. Böhler L (1956) Ist das Sudeck-Syndrom nach geschlossenen Verletzungen eine unabwendbare Unfallfolge oder eine vermeidbare Behandlungsfolge? Arch Klin Chir 284:43–53
87. Bollinger A (1954) Gefässereaktion und ihre Rolle bei der Entstehung des Sudeckschen Syndroms. Helv Chir Acta 21:61–86
88. Böni A, Faidherbe P (1964) Indications et interprétation du mode d'action de la roentgentherapie des affections rhumatismales. In: Rapports de la IV Conférence Internationale des Maladies Rhumatismales, Aix les Bains
89. Bonica JJ (1973) Causalgia and other reflex sympathetic dystrophies. Postgr Med 53:143–148
90. Bordier P, Hioco D, Tunchot S (1970) Calcitonin acute effects upon serum calcium, urinary hydroxyproline excretion and osteoclasts in man. In: Calcitonin 1969, Heinemann, London
91. Boucher M (1948–1949) Le pied décalcifié douloureux. MD dissertation, University of Lyon
92. Boulet-Gercourt J (1955) Le syndrome épaule-main d'origine aorto-coronarienne. Clinique 50:129–134
93. Bourjat P, Dirheimer Y, Singer S (1969) L'exploration thermographique dans les affections rhumatismales. J Radiol Electrol Med Nucl 50:185–187
94. Bouvier M (1969) Le rhumatisme neurotrophique du membre supérieur (syndrome "épaule-main"). Algo-dystrophie réflexe du membre supérieur. Cah Coll Med Hop Paris 10:321–326
95. Bouvier M (1970) Le pied décalcifié douloureux ou algo-dystrophie réflexe du pied. Rev Med Lyon 19:275–280
96. Bouvier M (1976) Le pied algodystrophique. Rev Mediter Sci Med Fr 1:491–496
97. Bouvier M, Lejeune E, Bocquet B, Richard D (1973) Circonstances d'apparition des algo-neurodystrophies (A propos d'une série personnelle de 100 observations). Rhumatologie (Aix les Bains) 25:27–32
98. Bouvrain Y, Bidoux L (1954) Le syndrome épaule-main associé à la coronarite et son traitement par la cortisone. Rev Prat 4:2845–2847
99. Brandt G (1954) Betrachtungen zur Pathophysiologie des Sudeckschen Syndroms; reaktiver Gewebeumbau Dystrophie. Med Klin 49:600–602
100. Braun S (1975) Une algodystrophie du membre inférieur. Gaz Med Fr 82:4737–4740
101. Breitländer K (1947) Beitrag zur Röntgenbehandlung der Extremitäten-Dystrophie (Sudecksches Syndrom). Dtsch Gesundheitswes 2:321–327
102. Bressot E (1930) Osteoporose douloureuse posttraumatique de Leriche (à propos d'une observation). Bull Mem Soc Chir Paris 22:461–465
103. Brito M, Barcelo P (1972) Algodistrofias. Problemas conceptuales y etiopatogenicos. Revision casuistica. Rev Esp Reum Enferm Osteoartic 15:175–213
104. Brouet G, Marche J (1964) Les complications d'ordre métabolique et endocrinien produites par la chimiothérapie antibacillaire. Rev Tuberc Pneumol 28:5–76
105. Brouet G, Marche J, Chevallier J, Nicolle MH, Nevot T (1961) Traitement d'attaque de la tuberculose commune par l'association d'izoniazide et d'éthionamide. Rev Tuberc Pneumol 25:145–190
106. Bruskewitz HW, Ewell GH (1949) Osteoporosis

of pelvic bones (acute bone atrophy of Sudeck). Am J Surg 77:705–712
107. Buchmann J (1928) Traumatic osteoporosis of carpal bones. Ann Surg 87:892–910
108. Buchmann J (1943) Post-operative, post-traumatic osteoporosis or Sudeck's atrophy. Bull Hosp Joint Dis 4:55–61
109. Bulgheroni EM, Puricelli R, Ferrerio A (1977) Un'algodistrofia iatrogena: il reumatismo de barbiturici, in rapporto all'osservazione di alcuni casi. Minerva Med 68:369–374
110. Burdeaus BD, Hutchinson WJ (1953) Etiology of post-traumatic osteoporosis. J Bone Joint Surg 35A:479–489
111. Cabanel G, Butel J, Berthon MP (1971) Association algodystrophie-paraostéoarthropathies après coma barbiturique. Rhumatologie (Aix les Bains) 23:23–27
112. Cabanel G, Phelip X, Verdier JM, Butel J, Bally M (1973) Les circonstances de diagnostic des algoneuro-dystrophies post-traumatiques. Rhumatologie (Aix les Bains) 25:33–34
113. Caillens JP (1974) L'arthrographie de l'épaule. Masson, Paris
114. Cameron JR, Sorenson JA (1963) Measurement of bone mineral in vivo: an improved method. Science 142:230–232
115. Camus JP, Crouzet J (1973) Les syndromes algoneurodystrophiques. Rev Prat 23:4805–4812
116. Camus JP, Paul D (1972) Rhumatisme gardénalique. Rev Prat 22:1963–1967
117. Carlson DH, Simon H, Wegner W (1977) Bone scanning and diagnosis of reflex sympathetic dystrophy secondary to herniated lumbar disc. Neurology 27:791–793
118. Caroit M, Djian A, Hubault A, Normandin C, Sèze de S (1963) Deux cas de capsulite rétractile de la hanche. Rev Rhum Mal Osteoartic 30:784–789
119. Carriere J, Kerambrun G (1967) Périarthrite scapulo-humérale et syndrome épaule-main en millieu sanatorial. Rev Tuberc Pneumol 31:267–276
120. Carron H, Mc Cue F (1972) Reflex sympathetic dystrophy in a 10 year old. South Med J 65:631–632
121. Casten DF (1955) Reflex sympathetic dystrophy. Anesthesiology 16:994–1003
122. Castex M (1955) L'atrophie osseuse de Sudeck. Presse Med 35:79–81
123. Catchpole BN (1964) Erythromelalgia. Lancet 7339:909–911
124. Causalgia (1972) Lancet 7761:1170–1171 (Editorial)
125. Cayla J, Chaouat Y, Labrousse C, Coste F (1965) La forme décalcifiante de la chondromatose de la hanche. A propos de 3 observations. Rev Rhum Mal Osteoartic 32:646–653
126. Cayla J, Chaouat Y, Rondier J, Guerin K, Frugier JC (1978) Les algodystrophies réflexes des membres inférieurs au cours de la grossesse. Rev Rhum Mal Osteoartic 45:89–94
127. Cayla J, Rondier J (1973) Algodystrophies réflexes des membres inférieurs d'origine vertébro-pelvienne. Rhumatologie (Aix les Bains) 25:67–68
128. Cayla J, Rondier J (1974) Algodystrophies réflexes des membres inférieurs d'origine vertébro-pelvienne (23 cas). Sem Hop Paris 50:275–286
129. Cervetti R, Soave G (1965) L'osteoporosi posttraumatica di Sudeck; profilassi e trattamento farmacologico e fisiocinetico. Minerva Radiol 10:453–460
130. Cervini C (1953) In terma di rapporti fra periartrite della spalla e sindrome spalla mono. Minerva Med 44:1235–1239
131. Chabot J (1961) Périarthrite scapulo-humérale et hyperthyroïdie (A propos de 11 cas). Sem Hop Paris 37:2247–2249
132. Chamberlain MJ, Fremlin JH, Peters D, Philip H (1968) Total body calcium by whole body neutron activation: new technique for study of bone disease. Br Med J 2:581–583
133. Chappel R, Mortier G, De Cuyper H, De Neve M (1976) De Behandeling van het algodystrofisch syndroom naar de bevindingen van JL Bircher bij dieren. J Belge Rhumatol Med Phys 31:80–86
134. Charcot JM (1868) Sur quelques arthropathies qui paraissent dépendre d'une lésion du cerveau ou de la moëlle. Arch Phys Norm Path 1:379
135. Charcot JM (1883) Leçons sur les maladies du système nerveux faites à la Salpétrière. Vol III. Progrès médical, Paris
136. Chavigny P, Fontaine R (1932) Les ostéoporoses en médecine légale. Ann Med Leg Criminol 14:42–43
137. Chevallier PE (1867) De la paralysie des nerfs vasomoteurs dans l'hémipléglie. MD dissertation, University of Paris
138. Chierici F, Cussini G (1957) Sulla sindroma spella-mano in corso di infarto miocardio. G Clin Med (Bologna) 38:1180–1200
139. Chitwood WR (1951) Importance of recognizing post-infarction shoulder-hand syndrome. N Engl J Med 243:813–814
140. Churcher MD (1977) Local blocks in the treatment of pain. Sympathetic blocks. In: Boerhaave Course (Anaesthetists and pain relief): Faculteit der Geneeskunde Rijksuniversiteit Leiden, 14–16
141. Cluzet J (1915) Paralysie du plexus brachial avec troubles de la main, sans blessure ni contusion apparente provoquée par l'explosion d'un obus. Lyon Med 125:20
142. Cohen A, Goldman J, Daniels R, Kanenson W (1960) Treatment of shoulder-hand syndrome with Griseofulvin (preliminary communication). JAMA 173:542–543
143. Cohn SH, Dombrowski CS, Fairchild RG (1970) In vivo activation analysis of calcium in man. Int J Appl Radiat Isot 21:127–137

144. Cohn SH, Ellis KJ, Wallach S, Zanzi I, Atkins HL, Aloia JF (1974) Absolute and relative deficit in total skeletal calcium and radial bone mineral content in osteoporosis. J Nucl Med 15:428–435
145. Commandre F, Kalaschnikoff P, Auzias J, Guillemin R, Viani JL, Lengrand J, Mercati E (1976) Algoneurodystrophies réflexes et hautes fréquences pulsées. Lyon Mediterr Med 12:3205–3215
146. Corbett M, Colston JR, Tucker AK (1977) Pain in the knee associated with osteoporosis of the patella. Ann Rheum Dis 36:188–191
147. Cormier F (1955) Traitement de l'ostéoporose algique post-traumatique par l'Hydergine. MD dissertation, University of Bordeaux
148. Cosby RS, Giddings JA, See JR, Mayo M (1976) Late complications of myocardial infarction. JAMA 236:1717–1720
149. Coste F (1969) Décalcifications idiopathiques de la hanche. Rev Rhum Mal Osteoartic 36:517–521
150. Coste F, Delbarre F, Braun S, Forette B, Panahi F (1967) Algodystrophie réflexe et sclérodermie chez une hyperthyroïdienne après administration de radio-iode. Bull Mem Soc Med Hop Paris 118:451–458
151. Coste F, Delbarre F, Massias P (1956) Remarque sur une algodystrophie de la main. Rev Rhum Mal Osteoartic 23:42–44
152. Coste F, Illouz G (1962) Syndrome épaule-main et canal carpien. Rev Rhum Mal Osteortic 29:29–30
153. Coste F, Laurent F, Manigand G, Chouraki (1961) Sur un cas familial de polyfibrose. Rev Rhum Mal Osteoartic 28:322–325
154. Coste F, Piguet B (1956) Dystrophie réflexe indolente des membres inférieurs. Rev Rhum Mal Osteoartic 23:153–155
155. Coste F, Piguet B, Bernard J, Antoine B (1954) Un cas de dystrophie réflexe du membre supérieur au cours d'une polyarthrite chronique évolutive. Rev Rhum Mal Osteoartic 21:46–47
156. Coste F, Piguet B, Cayla G (1956) Nouveau cas de dystrophie réflexe indolente d'un membre inférieur. Rev Rhum Mal Osteoartic 23:581–584
157. Costen JB (1936) Neuralgias and ear symptoms associated with disturbed function of temporomandibular joint. JAMA 107:252–255
158. Cotta H (1969) Therapie des Sudeck-Syndroms. Dtsch Med Wochenschr 94:1505
159. Coudouy G (1980) A propos du traitement d'un syndrome algodystrophique du membre supérieur. Sem Hop Paris 56:487
160. Covalt DA, Cooper LS, Roen TL, Rusk HA (1953) Early management of patients with spinal cord injury. JAMA 151:89–94
161. Cravener EK (1936) Acute "reflex" bone atrophy (Sudeck's disease); short summary of literature and 2 typical cases. NY State J Med 36:815–820
162. Crémieux G (1974) Les algodystrophies, pathologie de confins. Marseille Med 111:193–204
163. Crémieux G (1975) Traitement des algodystrophies. Rev Med Ther 16:1786–1792
164. Crespo LA, Gerster JC, Boussina I, Gabay R, Fallet GH (1973) Algodystrophie décalcifiante post-traumatique du pied. Rev Med Suisse Romande 93:581–593
165. Creyssel J (1955) Syndrome d'ostéoporose spontanée à bascule et à évolution cyclique des deux pieds. Lyon Chir 50:576–578
166. Crinetz S (1934) Contribution à l'étude médicolégale de l'ostéoporose algique post-traumatique. MD dissertation, Strasbourg
167. Crutchlow WP (1970) Sr 85 scintimetry of the hip in osteoarthritis and osteonecrosis. Am J Roentgenol 109:803–812
168. Curtiss PH, Kincaid WE (1959) Transitory demineralization of the hip in pregnancy. A report of three cases. J Bone Joint Surg 41 A:1327–1332
169. Cury M, Rénier J, Bregeon CH, Tuchais E (1969) Les syndromes algo-dystrophiques au cours de la chimiothérapie. Arch Med Ouest 1:121–136
170. Dammann F (1972) Isoliertes Sudeck-Syndrom nur an drei Fingern. Beitrag zur Entstehung eines peripher-neurogenen Sudeck-Syndroms. Monatsschr Unfallheilkd Versicherung Versorgung Verkehrsmed 75:13–22
171. Darriulat M (1979) Algodystrophie de la hanche. Intérêt de la scintigraphie et du traitement par la thyrocalcitonine. A propos de six cas. MD-dissertation, University of Paris
172. Dausset J (1976) Le complexe HLA. Immunogénétique du système HLA. Nouv Presse Med 5:1301–1304
173. Dauw W (1957) Fracture fémorale avec ostéoporose, qui a mené à la déformation osseuse du genou et du pied. Acta Chir Belg [Suppl] 1:518–520
174. David-Chaussé J (1962) Le rhumatisme neurotrophique du membre supérieur. J Med Bordeaux 139:1256–1259
175. David-Chaussé J (1976) Syndromes dystrophiques chez les traumatisés des membres inférieurs. Bordeaux Med 9:605–618
176. David-Chaussé J, Cormier F (1957) Le traitement de l'ostéoporose algique post-traumatique par l'Hydergine. J Med Bordeaux 134:837–847
177. David-Chaussé J, Pimouguet CL, Dehais J (1973) Algodystrophies extensives des membres. Rhumatologie (Aix les Bains) 25:69–73
178. Davis SW, Petrillo CR, Eichberg RD, Chu DS (1977) Shoulder-hand syndrome in a hemiplegic population: a 5 year retrospective study. Arch Phys Med Rehabil 58:353–356
179. De Bastiani G, Nogarin L, Perusi M (1978) Trattamento della sindromi algodistrofiche con la calcitonina. Minerva Med 69:1485–1495
180. Dechaume M, Descrozailles C, Carlopeau F,

Robert J (1955) Nécrose mandibulaire localisée au décours d'un zona du trijumeau. Rev Stomatol Chir Maxillofac 56:516–521

181. Decoulx P, Lemerle (1957) Utilisation de la fluorescéine dans les ostéoporoses traumatiques. Acta Chir Belg [Suppl] 1:272–273
182. Decoulx P, Rieunau G (1958) Les fractures du rachis dorso-lombaire sans troubles nerveux. Rev Chir Orthop 44:254–322
183. Decourt J, Gregoire J (1932) Rôle des troubles sympathiques dans les arthropathies des hémiplégiques. Ann Med (Paris) 21:375–387
184. Dehm A (1964) Ca47 in clinical studies of bone physiopathology. In: International Atomic Energy Agency, Vienna, 32:50–55
185. Dejour H, Leclerc P, Nourissat C (1975) Ostéome ostéoïde du fond du cotyle. Rev Chir Orthop 61:755–758
186. Delaye R, Migayron A, Lieux A (1931) Ostéoporose post-traumatique du poignet avec début de dislocation spontanée du carpe. Bull Soc Med Milit Franç 25:165–171
187. Delbart P, Bernard MH, Rousseaux P, Scherpereel B, Freneaux B (1978) Les algodystrophies rachidiennes existent peut-être. A propos d'une observation. Rhumatologie (Aix les Bains) 30:303–305
188. Delcroix M (1957) Ostéoporose post-traumatique. Acta Chir Belg [Suppl] 1:287
189. Delorme E (1916–1917) De la décalcification consécutive aux traumatismes de guerre. Arch Med Pharm Milit 66:1–54
190. Delorme E (1917) Chirurgie de guerre. Les fractures; déplacements, séquelles, décalcifications, raideurs articulaires consécutives. Fournier, Paris
191. De Marchi E, Santacroce A, Solarino GB (1966) Su di una peculiare artropatia rarefacente dell'anca. Arch Putti Chir Organi Mov 21:62–75
192. Demilly J (1958) Le syndrome de Kümmell-Verneuil n'existe pas. MD dissertation, University of Lille
193. Denis A (1967) Contribution à l'étude de l'algodystrophie décalcifiante du pied (Maladie de Sudeck-Leriche). J Med Paris 87:9–18
194. De Palma AP (1950) Surgery of the shoulder. Lippincott, London
195. Deplante JP, Michel CR, Courpron P, Queneau P, Laurent J (1975) Algodystrophie de la hanche. Cahiers Med 1:329–353
196. Derot M (1962) Diabète et maladies de la nutrition. Flammarion, Paris
197. Desaive P (1957) Considérations à propos de l'ostéoporose radiologique. Acta Chir Belg [Supp] 1:491–496
198. Deshayes P, Houdent G, Morere P, Lemercier JP, Desseauve P, Simonin JL (1969) Algodystrophie de la chimiothérapie anti-tuberculeuse: à propos de 22 observations. Rev Rhum Mal Osteoartic 33:316–322
199. Desplats R (1934) Radiothérapie fonctionnelle sympathique et glandulaire dans les séquelles de traumatismes. J Radiol Electrol Med Nucl 18:575–579
200. Destot C (1904) Ostéotrophies traumatiques. Lyon Med 103:236–238
201. Destot C, Mouisset (1898) Décalcification des os. Radiographie. Echo Med Lyon 3:23
202. Dicke E, Schliack H, Wolff A (1968) Bindegewebsmassage. Hippokrates, Stuttgart
203. Dietrich J (1974) Les algodystrophie réflexes. J Med Strasbourg 5:475–491
204. Dilsen G (1979) The therapeutic effect of diadynamic current applied over stellate ganglion in 65 cases of shoulder-hand syndrome. (Abstr. 439) IX European Congress of Rheumatology, Wiesbaden
205. Dini P, Faussone F (1971) L'algodystrophia decalcifiante primitiva dell'anca. Arch Putti Chir Organi Mor 26:101–110
206. Dirheimer Y, Roethinger J (1971) Algodystrophie isolée et primitive de la hanche. France Med 34:19–21
207. Dolle PM (1975) Composantes psychologiques du syndrome algodystrophique du type Sudeck. Rev Med Psychosom 17:167–170
208. Douillet C (1868) Contribution à l'histoire des fractures et luxation du rachis. MD dissertation, University of Paris
209. Doury P (1979) L'épaule bloquée. Rhumatologie (Aix les Bains) 31:121–122
210. Doury P, Delahaye RP, Granier R, Pattin S, Metges PJ (1978) Highly localized transient osteoporosis of the knee. Arthritis Rheum 21:992–993
211. Doury P, Delahaye RP, Granier R, Pattin S, Metges PJ, Fabresse F (1979) L'algodystrophie parcellaire. Rev Rhum Mal Osteoartic 46:37–44
212. Doury P, Delahaye RP, Pattin S, Batisse R, Metges PJ, Roue R, Darriulat M, Pouchat JM, Larroque P, Duriez R (1977) L'algodystrophie de la hanche; intérêt de la scintigraphie aux polyphosphates de technetium pour le diagnostic et de la Calcitonine pour le traitement. Med Armees 5:697–704
213. Doury P, Dirheimer Y, Pattin S (1980) Abstract 26, IV Congrés Latin de Rhumatologie, Liège. Critères pour le diagnostic de l'algodystrophie
214. Doury P, Granier R, Pattin S (1980) Algodystrophie du pied avec hypofixation à la scintigraphie osseuse par les pyrophosphates de technetium 99m. Nouv Presse Med 42–3189
215. Doury P, Granier R, Pattin S (1979) La place de la scintigraphie osseuse aux pyrophosphates de technetium 99m dans le diagnostic des algodystrophies. A propos de 74 observations. Ann Med Int 130:553–557
216. Doury P, Louyot P, Pattin S, Pourel J, Hannequin JR (1973) L'algodystrophie récidivante plurifocale. Rev Rhum Mal Osteoartic 40:399–406

217. Doury P, Pattin S (1980) Le traitement de l'algodystrophie par la thyrocalcitonine: à propos de soixante observations. Rhumatologie (Aix les Bains) 32:111–113
218. Doury P, Pattin S, Delahaye RP, Metges PJ, Batisse R (1975) La thyrocalcitonine dans le traitement des algodystrophies. Nouv Presse Med 4:2527–2528
219. Doury P, Pattin S, Delahaye RP, Metges PJ, Granier R (1978) L'algodystrophie parcellaire du genou. Nouv Presse Med 7:3156
220. Doury P, Pattin S, Granier R (1979) La place de la scintigraphie osseuse aux pyrophosphates de technetium 99m dans les algodystrophies. (Abstr 434) IX European Congress of Rheumatology Wiesbaden
221. Doury P, Pattin S, Granier P, Metges PJ, Delahaye RP (1980) Le diagnostic précoce des algodystrophies. Entretiens de Bichat. Medecine 311–315.
222. Drai M (1957) Manifestations consécutives à un déséquilibre de l'articulé dentaire. Syndrome de Costen-Hennebert-Dechaume. MD dissertation, University of Paris
223. Dreux C (1970) L'hydroxyproline. In: Problèmes actuels de biochimie appliquée. n° 43 (3ème série). Masson, Paris
224. Dubrulle P, Claeys C, Amoudru C, Constant A (1956) Traitement endocrinien des ostéoporoses post-traumatiques. Therapie 11:1199–1207
225. Dulap R, Ivins J (1952) Unusual lesions of sternum associated with shoulder pain. JAMA 149:552–553
226. Dumoulin J (1974) Etude électrologique des modifications musculaires au cours de l'ostéoporose post-traumatique. Bull Acad Nat Med Paris 158:328–333
227. Dumoulin J, De Bisschop G, Clauses I (1974) L'éléctrothérapie des algodystrophies. Electrodiagn Ther 11:128–131
228. Duncan H, Frame B, Frost HM, Arnstein AR (1967) Migratory osteolysis of the lower extremities. Ann Intern Med 66:1165–1173
229. Duncan H, Frame B, Frost H, Arnstein AR (1967) Regional migratory osteoporosis of the lower limbs. Arthritis Rheum 10:276
230. Duncan WS (1928) Relationship of hyperthyroïdism to joint conditions JAMA 91:1779–1782
231. Duncan WS (1932) Relationship of thyroïd disease to chronic non specific arthritis. JAMA 99:1239–1243
232. Ebbetts J (1971) Autonomic pain in the upper limb. Physiotherapy 57:270–279
233. Ecoiffier J, Geerts A (1957) Aspect radiologique des ostéoporoses posttraumatiques. Acta Chir Belg [Supp] 1:203–216
234. Edeiken J (1957) Shoulder-hand syndrome following myocardial infarction with special reference to prognosis. Circulation 16:14–19
235. Edeiken J, Wolferth CC (1936) Persistent pain in shoulder region following myocardial infarction. Am J Med Sci 191:201–210
236. Egyed B, Kazar G (1967) Die Bedeutung des Sudeck-Syndroms in der Rehabilitation Unfallverletzter. Z Gesamte Hyg 13:795–798
237. Ehlert H (1974) Neue Gesichtspunkte zur Genese des Sudeck-Syndroms. Monatschr Unfallheilkd Versicherung Versorgung Verkehrsmed 77:417–421
238. Ehlert J (1956) Beitrag zur Genese des Sudeckschen Syndroms. Arch Klin Chir 284:55–57
239. Einaudi G (1956) La periartrite della spalla e la sindrome spallamano in corso di tuberculosi pulmonare. Reumatismo 8:71–81
240. Eisinger J (1967) L'hydroxyprolinurie. MD dissertation, University of Marseille
241. Eisinger J, Acquaviva P, d'Omezon Y, Recordier AM (1973) Traitement des algodystrophies par la Calcitonine, Résultats préliminaires. Marseille Med 110:373–376
242. Eisinger J, Acquaviva P, d'Omezon Y, Schiano A, Recordier AM (1974) L'hydroxyprolinurie au cours des algodystrophies. Déductions thérapeutiques. Rev Rhum Mal Osteoartic 41:455–458
243. Eisinger J, d'Omezon Y, Schiano A, Recordier AM (1973) L'hydroxyprolinurie au cours des algodystrophies. Rhumatologie (Aix les Bains) 25:79–80
244. Eisinger J, Serratrice G, Recordier AM (1966) A propos des effects des interventions sympathiques sur le métabolisme phospho-calcique. Rhumatologie (Aix les Bains) 18:357–359
245. Ellis LB, Weiss S (1936) Vasomotor disturbance and edema associated with cerebral hemiplegia. Arch Neurol Psychiatry 36:362–372
246. Ernstene AC, Kinell J (1940) Pain in the shoulder as a sequel of myocardial infarction. Arch Intern Med 66:800–806
247. Ertem O, Erturk M, Yamanel G (1979) Les courants diadynamiques dans le traitement de l'atrophie de Sudeck. "R" 8:465–467
248. Eufinger H (1957) Das Sudeck Syndrom. Med Klin 52:805–807
249. Evans JA (1946) Sympathectomy for reflex sympathetic dystrophy. JAMA 132:620–623
250. Evans JA (1947) Reflex sympathetic dystrophy. Report on 57 cases. Ann Intern Med 26:417–426
251. Exner A (1902) Beiträge zur Kenntnis der akuten Knochenatrophie. Fortschr Geb Roentgenstr 6:1–12
252. Farkas TA, Nemes GA (1975) Beitrag zur Morphologie des Sudeck-Syndroms. Z Orthop 113:421–424
253. Faulong L (1952) Dystrophie reflexe du membre supérieur (syndrôme épaule-main). Rev Rhum Mal Osteoartic 19:554–563
254. Faulong L (1959) Les ostéoses raréfiantes posttraumatiques. Rev Prat 9:1107–1112

255. Fermaglich DR (1977) Reflex sympathetic dystrophy in children. Pediatrics 60:881–883
256. Ficat P (1973) Les déséquilibres rotuliens. De l'hyperpression à l'arthrose. Masson, Paris
257. Ficat P, Arlet J (1977) Ischémie et nécrose osseuse. L'exploration fonctionnelle de la circulation intra-osseuse et ses applications. Masson, Paris New York Barcelone Milan
258. Ficat P, Arlet J, Lartigue G, Pujol M, Tran MA (1973) Algodystrophies reflexes post-traumatiques. Etude hémodynamique et anatomopathologique. Rev Chir Orthop 59:401–414
259. Ficat P, Arlet J, Pujol M, Vidal R (1971) Traumatisme, dystrophie réflexe et ostéonécrose de la tête fémorale. Ann Chir 25:911–917
260. Ficat P, Mansat Ch, Roudil J (1967) Epaules bloquées et dystrophies réflexes. Rev Med Toulouse 3:295–304
261. Figar S, Eis E, Gregar M (1974) The value of plethysmography in Sudeck's dystrophy (in Czech). Acta Chir Orthop Traumatol Cech 41:289–291
262. Fischer F, Key JA (1934) Local atrophy of bone; effects of vitamine D and of calcium on local atrophy and union. Arch Surg 29:312–315
263. Fisher H, Mankin H, Mooney V (1963) The painful shoulder in patients with pulmonary tuberculosis. Am Rev Respir Dis 87:88–92
264. Fleming A, Dodman S, Beer TC, Crown S (1976) Personality in frozen shoulder. Ann Rheum Dis 35:456–457
265. Florescu A (1928) Quelques considérations sur les ostéoporoses algiques post-traumatiques. Presse Med 36:1661–1664
266. Fokin AA, Orekhova LA (1978) Treatment of Sudeck's atrophy by means of thoracic sympathectomy through the thoracoscope (in Russian). Orthop Travmatol Protez 8:61–62
267. Fontaine R (1958) Posttraumatische Osteoporose und Sudecksche Krankheit. Wien Med Wochenschr 108:679–683
268. Fontaine R, Herrmann L (1931) Les ostéoporoses douloureuses dans le cadre des troubles vasomoteurs post-traumatiques des membres. Questions médicales d'actualité 1:7–60
269. Fontaine R, Herrmann L (1933) Post-traumatic painful osteoporosis. Ann Surg 97:26–61
270. Fontaine R, Mandel P, Muller JN, Sibilly A (1953) Le rôle du système nerveux végétatif dans les dystrophies post-traumatiques. Rev Acc Travail 2:67–100
271. Fontaine R, Mandel P, Muller JN, Sibilly A, Bollack C, Wagner R (1957) L'ostéoporose post-traumatique. Acta Chir Belg [Suppl] 1:19–74
272. Fontaine R, Mandel P, Muller JN, Sibilly A, Bollack C, Wagner R, Ebel A, Burckard J, Viaud J (1957) Contribution à la physiopathologie de l'ostéoporose post-traumatique. Acta Chir Belg [Suppl] 1:173–201
273. Fontaine R, Mandel P, Muller JN, Sibilly A, Burckard J (1954) Les répercussions pondérales et biochimiques de l'inactivité simple ou combinée à un traumatisme sur l'os de rat normal et castré. Contribution à l'étude de l'ostéoporose post-traumatique. J Chir (Paris) 70:797–809
274. Fontaine R, Miloyevitch D (1927) Contribution à l'étude expérimentale des troubles vasomoteurs post-traumatiques des membres. Rev Chir 46:385–395
275. Fontaine R, Muller JN, Sibilly A (1956) Résultats de la chirurgie du sympathique dans l'ostéoporose post-traumatique des membres. Acta Chir Belg [Suppl] 1:457–489
276. Fournié A, Ayrolles C, Guyard C (1979) Résultats de l'épreuve d'hypocalcémie aiguë à la Calcitonine dans les algodystrophies décalcifiantes. Rev Rhum Mal Osteoartic 46:55–56
277. Fournié A, Valverde C, Tap G, Bazerque JJ, Ayrolles C (1977) Test d'hypocalcémie aiguë à la calcitonine de porc et de saumon. Rev Rhum Mal Osteoartic 44:91–98
278. Frank E (1969) Über das "Sudeck-Syndrom". Muench Med Wochenschr 111:600–603
279. Frank R, Kern R, Fontaine R (1957) Etude histopathologique de l'ostéoporose post-traumatique au microscope électronicque. Pathol Biol (Paris) 5:2203–2208
280. Frank R, Kern R, Fontaine R (1957) Microscopie et diffraction électronique dans l'étude de l'ostéoporose post-traumatique. Ann Anat Path (Paris) 2:5–23
281. Franklin EC, Nemcick FJ (1959) Shoulder dysfunction in pulmonary tuberculosis. Ann J Med Sci 227:601–608
282. Freudiger A (1950) Die pathologische mechanische Konstellation als ätiologischer Faktor der Sudeckschen Atrophie nach Frakturen. Helv Chir Acta 17:426–448
283. Freund E, Hüttner JH, Schröder H (1970) Morbus Sudeck als Komplikation der Radiusfraktur. Monatsschr Unfallheilkd Versicherung Versorgung Verkehrsmed 73:569
284. Fried K (1970) Beitrag zum Verlauf und zur Pathogenese der neurotrophischen Osteoarthropathien. Fortschr Geb Röntgenstr 113:560–575
285. Froelich R, Mouchet A (1930) Spondylite traumatique (Maladie de Kümmell-Verneuil). J Chir 36:601–606
286. Froment D, Perrin A, Gonin A, Jandet R (1956) Périarthrites scapulo-humérales et autres manifestations neurotrophiques d'origine corona rienne. III Conférence du Rhumatisme. Aix les Bains
287. Fromantin M, Freyria J, Bressac F, Bon R (1975) Dépistage du diabète chez le jeune adulte. Enquête portant sur 161500 sujets de sexe masculin. Nouv Presse Med 4:1272–1274
288. Frost HM (1972) Bone remodeling and metabolic

bone diseases. Orthopaedic lecture series III. Thomas, Springfield
289. Frost HM (1973) Bone remodeling and its relationship to metabolic bone diseases. Orthopaedic lecture series V. Thomas, Springfield
290. Frost HM (1979) Treatment of osteoporoses by manipulation of coherent bone cell populations. Clin Orthop 129:227–244
291. Galley AM (1952) Caudal analgesia. Clinical applications in vaso-spastic diseases of the legs and in diabetic neuropathy. Proc Roy Soc Med 45:748–752
292. Garnett ES, Bowen BM, Coates G, Nahmias C (1975) An analysis of factors influencing the local accumulation of bone seeking radiopharmaceuticals. Invest Radiol 10:564–568
293. Garot H (1955) Introduction à une étude thermométrique et oscillographique dans les syndromes douloureux dystrophiques des membres supérieurs. Acta Physioth Rheum Belg 10:236–242
294. Gaucher A (1979) La scintigraphie osseuse. Documenta Geigy, Laboratoires Ciba-Geigy
295. Gaucher A, Colomb JN, Naoun A, Netter P, Faure G, Pourel J, Robert J (1978) Caractéristiques scintigraphiques des coxopathies. Leur valeur étiologique. Rev Rhum Mal Osteoartic 45:641–648
296. Gaucher A, Colomb JN, Naoun A, Pourel J, Netter P, Robert J (1979) L'exploration scintigraphique du genou. Ann Med Nancy 18:1295–1299
297. Gaucher A, Naoun A, Pourel J, Faure G, Netter P, Colomb JN, Robert J (1976) Valeur diagnostique des hypofixations localisées en scintigraphie osseuse. Rev Rhum Mal Osteoartic 43:715–721
298. Gaucher A, Robert J, Naoun A (1975) Quelques indications de la scintigraphie osseuse en rhumatologie. J Med Strasbourg 6:695–697
299. Gaud M (1968) Etude critique de la notion d'algodystrophie. MD dissertation, University of Marseille
300. Gautier P (1960) Traitement des algodystrophies sympathiques de l'extrémité distale du membre supérieur par les injections intra-artérielles de xylocaïne. Rev Rhum Mal Osteoartic 27:31–33
301. Gburek Z (1979) Reflex algodystrophies of extremities: therapeutic values of Griseofulvin Forte (Abstr. 433). IX European Congress of Rheumatology: Wiesbaden
302. Geiser M (1957) The role of muscular fonction in post-traumatic osteoporosis. Arch Orthop Unfall Chir 49:268–281
303. Geiser M, Trueta J (1958) Muscle action, bone rarefaction, and bone formation. J Bone Joint Surg 40-B:282–311
304. Gemperli R (1969) Beitrag zur isoniazidinduzierten fibrosierenden Arthropathie ("Algodystrophie"). Helv Med Acta [Suppl] 46:151
305. Genant HK, Kozin F, Bekerman C, McCarty DJ, Sims J (1975) The reflex sympathetic dystrophy syndrome. A comprehensive analysis and using fine detail radiography, photon absorptiometry and bone and joint scintigraphy. Radiology 117:21–32
306. Gerhardt A (1956) Erfahrungen mit lokaler Hydrocortisonbehandlung beim Sudeckschen Syndrom. Arch Klin Chir 284:75–78
307. Gilbert-Dreyfus, Faulong (1936) L'acro-rhumatisme parkinsonien. Rev Rhum Mal Osteoartic 3:2–79
308. Gineste J (1946) Le rhumatisme thyroïdien. Rev Rhum Mal Osteoartic 23:173–176
309. Girard PF, Allegre, Lanternier (1951) Troubles neurovégétatifs de l'épaule et de la main apparus après une thoracoplastie. Rev Neurol (Paris) 84:55–57
310. Girardier J de (1933) Ostéoporose douloureuse post-traumatique du pied avec troubles vasomoteurs traitée par sympathectomie périartérielle. Lyon Chir 30:357–362
311. Glick EN (1973) Reflex dystrophy (algoneurodystrophy) results of treatment by corticosteroids. Rheumatol Rehabil 12:84–88
312. Glick EN (1979) Algodystrophy: proposal of diagnostic criteria. (Abstr. 431) IX European Congress of Rheumatology, Wiesbaden
313. Glick EN, Helal B (1976) Post-traumatic neurodystrophy. Treatment by corticosteroids. Hand 8:45–47
314. Godde JL, Schiano A (1978) Les bêta-bloquants en rhumatologie. Mediterr Med 974:39–47
315. Goldsmith NF, Johnston JO, Picetti G, Garcia C (1973) Bone mineral in radius and vertebral osteoporosis in an insured population. J Bone Joint Surg 55A:1276–1293
316. Goldsmith NF, Johnston JO, Ury H, Vose G, Colbert C (1971) Bone mineral estimation in normal and osteoporotic women. J Bone Joint Surg 53A:83–100
317. Good AE (1970) Rheumatism and chemotherapy of tuberculosis. Ann Intern Med 72:752–753
318. Good AE, Green RA, Zarafonetis CJ (1965) Rheumatic symptoms during tuberculosis therapy. A manifestation of isoniazid toxicity? Ann Intern Med 63:800–807
319. Gougeon J (1973) Les algodystrophies des membres inférieurs. Concours Med 95:3415–3433
320. Gougeon J, Moreau-Huttin J (1966) Les formes récidivantes des algodystrophies des membres inférieurs. Rhumatologie (Aix les Bains) 18:395–399
321. Graber-Duvernay J (1954) La maladie post-traumatique: sa prévention, son traitement. Rhumatologie (Aix les Bains) 6:110–126
322. Graber-Duvernay J, Trepsat P, Rozier M, Deslous-Paoli P (1973) Intérêt de la crénothérapie précoce dans la prévention de la maladie post-traumatique. Rhumatologie (Aix les Bains) 25:89–91

323. Graille R (1961) Le pied décalcifié douloureux idiopathique ou ostéoporose algique essentielle du pied. Lyon Med 10:533–534
324. Graudal H (1959) Shoulder-hand syndrome and herpes zoster. Report of a case with signs of vasodilatation and vasoconstriction in the same hand. Acta Rheum Scand 5:157–163
325. Gray RG, Gottlieb NL (1976) Rheumatic disorders associated with diabetes mellitus: literature review. Semin Arthritis Rheum 6:19–34
326. Gregoire JJ (1931) Arthropathie des hémiplégiques. MD dissertation University of Paris
327. Griessmann, Damman F (1956) Osteitis pubis-Sudecksche Krankheit? Z Urol 49:321–329
328. Gromo G, Ceroni P, Sosso A (1974) La ioniforesi con enzime diffusore (Thiomucase) associata alle correnti diadinamiche nel trattamento fisio kinesiterapico delle sindromi edematose algodistrofiche post-traumatiche degli arti. Minerva Med 656:4015–4025
329. Gros C, Butz JM, Daladouire P, Dirheimer Y, Gilliot M, Singer S, Weille Y, Bourjat P (1968) Thermographie des affections rhumatismales de la main et du poignet. Rhumatologie (Aix les Bains) 20:51–64
330. Grosbois B, Brissot R, Allas T, Bouffant T, Louvigne Y (1978) Quelle est la place de l'électrothérapie dans le traitement des algodystrophies réflexes? Electrodiagn Ther 15:61–65
331. Grosclaude-Cugnardey S (1976) L'algodystrophie de hanche: à propos de 5 observations. MD dissertation, University of Grenoble
332. Gross D (1971) Therapie des Sudeck-Syndroms. Dtsch Med Wochenschr 96:345–346
333. Guaquiere A (1969) Les algodystrophies du membre inférieur à localisation coxo-fémorale prédominante. MD dissertation, University of Nancy
334. Guerin C (1974) Les algodystrophie réflexes secondaires à la grossesse. MD dissertation Paris
335. Guillemin R, Bonelli AJ, Commandre F (1973) Place de l'électrothérapie dans le traitement des algodystrophies post-traumatiques. Rhumatologie (Aix les Bains) 25:85–86
336. Guillermet J (1952) Le rhumatisme neurotrophique du membre supérieur (Syndrome épaule-main). MD dissertation, University of Lyon
337. Guntheroth WG, Chakmakjian S, Brena SC, Ricketts HJ, Wiederhielm CA (1971) Posttraumatic sympathetic dystrophy. Am J Dis Child 121:511–514
338. Gupta RC, Popovtzer MM, Huffer WE, Smyth CJ (1973) Regional migratory osteoporosis. Arthritis Rheum 16:363–368
339. Gurd FB (1934) Post-traumatic acute bone atrophy (Sudeck's atrophy). Ann Surg 99:449–469
340. Gurd FB (1936) Post-traumatic acute bone atrophy – clinical entity. Arch Surg 32:273–291
341. Guyon C (1965) Les algodystrophies des membres inférieurs principalement sous la forme d'apparence idiopathique. MD dissertation, University of Nancy
342. Gyorgyi G, Bozoky L (1961) Der lineare Schwächungskoeffizient als ein Masstab des Mineralgehaltes der Knochen. Die roentgendensitometrische Bestimmung des Mineralgehalts der Knochen. Fortschr Geb Röntgenstr 94:667–672
343. Hackethal KH (1958) Das Sudeck-Syndrom; Medizin, Theorie und Klinik in Einzeldarstellungen. Hüthig, Heidelberg
344. Hackethal KH (1956) Moderne Sudeck-Behandlung – eine Kausal-Therapie? Arch Klin Chir 284:64–67
345. Halipre A (1914) Décalcifications osseuses posttraumatiques; évolution des lésions; intérêt de la question dans les accidents du travail. Rev Med Normandie 6:209–215
346. Hannequin JR (1972) Algodystrophie plurifocale et traumatisme. Diplôme d'études médicales réparation dommage corporel, University of Paris
347. Hannington-Kiff JG (1977) Relief of Sudeck's atrophy by regional intravenous guanethidine. Lancet 8022:1132–1133
348. Harada M, Kozuma Z (1968) A case of carbon monoxid poisoning with so-called Sudeck's syndrome and various neurologic symptoms (in Japanese). Brain Nerve 20:1095–1099
349. Harff J (1956) Das Zusammentreffen des Sudeckschen Syndroms mit Krankheiten anderer Genese. Arch Klin Chir 284:61–64
350. Harff J, Stuth HW (1954) Zum Problem des Sudeckschen Syndroms. Z Orthop 84:359–369
351. Harif V (1962) Les algodystrophies sympathiques du membre inférieur. MD dissertation, University of Paris
352. Harif V (1974) Les algodystrophies des membres inférieurs. Phlébologie 27:47–60
353. Hartenbach W (1956) Erfahrungen über posttraumatische Knochenumbaustörungen und ihre Behandlung. Arch Klin Chir 284:67–69
354. Hasche HH, Meyer W (1974) Idiopatische Algodystrophie der Hüfte. Z Rheumatol 33: 206–213
355. Hector A (1956) Ostéoporose algique du tarse, complication tardive des fractures du membre inférieur. Presse Med 64:2211–2213
356. Hector A (1957) A propos de l'étiologie des ostéoporoses postfracturaires algiques du tarse. Acta Chir Belg [Supp] 1:218
357. Heikinheimo R, Sallas O (1957) Capillary resistance in the shoulder-hand syndrom, and the effect of anesthesic therapy. Arch Rheum Scand 3:289–296
358. Heinzel J (1956) Behandlungsergebnisse des Sudeckschen Syndroms in den Jahren 1945–1955 an der Heidelberger Klinik. Arch Klin Chir 284:74–75
359. Hennebert P (1939) Syndrôme douloureux et

fonctionnel par mauvais articulé dentaire. Ann Otolaryngol 58:371–377

360. Hermann LG (1934) Diagnosis and treatment of post-traumatic painful osteoporosis. Intern J Med Surg 47:510–513
361. Hermann LG, Reineke HG, Caldwell JA (1942) Post-traumatic painful osteoporosis: clinical and roentgenological entity. Am J Roentgenol 47:353–361
362. Heuck F, Schmitt E (1961) Die praktische Anwendung einer Methode zur quantitativen Bestimmung des Kalksalzgehalts gesunder und kranker Knochen. Fortschr Geb Roentgenstr 93:761–783
363. Heyate D (1953) Hypothèse sur la pathogénie de l'ostéoporose douloureuse post-traumatique. Sem Hop Paris 29:561–562
364. Heymann CH (1924) Osteoporosis relieved by sympathectomy. JAMA 32:1333
365. Hildebrand O (1921) Über neuropathische Gelenkerkrankungen. Arch Klin Chir 115:443–493
366. Hilgenreiner H (1923) Gibt es eine Sudeck'sche Knochenatrophie? Beitr Klin Chir 129:683–699
367. Hilker AW (1949) Shoulder-hand syndrome: complication of coronary artery disease. Ann Intern Med 31:303–311
368. Hirschmann J (1948) Die neurogene Form des Sudeckschen Syndroms. Arch Psych Neurol 180:681–686
369. Hochheuser W, Souvatzoglou A (1970) Kortikoid-Therapie mit Fluocortolon (Ultralan). Muench Med Wochenschr 112:892–896
370. Homans J (1940) Minor causalgia: a hyperesthetic neurovascular syndrome. New Eng J Med 222:870–874
371. Hoppe W (1969) Das Zentrogen Sudeck-Syndrom. Psychiatr Neurol Med Psychol (Leipz) 21:389–394
372. Hoppe W, Geidel H (1977) Das nichttraumatische Sudeck-Syndrom. Z Aerztl Fortbild (Jena) 71:1102–1106
373. Horvath G (1966) Algodystrophic syndrome following a dive into the water (in Czech). Acta Chir Orthop Traumatol Cech 33:64–66
374. Howard T (1930) Cardiac pain and periarthritis of the shoulder, angina pectoris, aortitis or cardiac infarct complicated by stiff and painful shoulder. Med J Rec 131:364–365
375. Hoyt WH (1966) The shoulder-hand syndrome: observations and review of the literature. J Am Osteopath Ass 65:943–953
376. Huaux JP, Nagant de Deuxchaisnes C (1973) Le syndrome épaulemain. Louvain Med 92:173–203
377. Huaux JP, Nagant De Deuxchaisnes C (1977) L'algodystrophie sympathique réflexe. Acta Rhum Belg 1:223–256
378. Hubault A (1970) Algoneurodystrophies reflexes des membres. J Kinesitherapie 180:3–8
379. Hubault A, Dry J (1968) Algoneurodystrophies réflexes des membres. In: EMC Appareil locomoteur 14285 A 10. Editions Techniques, Paris
380. Hueston JT (1963) Dupuytren's contracture. Livingstone, London
381. Huet P, Huguier J (1946) Le rôle probable de la stase capillaire réflexe en pathologie générale (hypothèse pathogénique à propos des réactions post-traumatiques). J Chir (Paris) 62:184–195
382. Hunder GG, Kelly PJ (1968) Roentgenologic transient osteoporosis of the hip. A clinical syndrome? Ann Intern Med 68:539–552
383. Hunder GG, Kelly PJ (1971) Bone scans in transient osteoporosis. Ann Intern Med 75:134
384. Hunter J (1843) Oeuvres complètes. Vol I: Tortin-Masson, Paris
385. Imbert A, Gagniere J (1903) Les atrophies osseuses calcaires consécutives à un traumatisme. Rev Chir 23:689–703
386. Iselin M (1957) Ostéoporose-ostéarthrite dystrophique et reflexes conditionnés. Acta Chir Belg [Suppl] 1:469–471
387. Isemein L, Fournier AM (1956) Complications osseuses du zona. Rhumatologie (Aix les Bains) 8:211–213
388. Issekutz B, Blizzard JJ, Birkhaed N, Rodahl K (1966) Effect of prolonged bed rest on urinary calcium output. J App Physiol 21:2013
389. Jacob A (1934) Ostéoporose post-traumatique de l'épaule avec pseudo-ankylose, guérie par infiltrations périarticularies de novocaïne. Strasbourg Med 94:580
390. Jacquot, Morel, Peltier, Delgove (1968) Manifestations algodystrophiques de la chimiothérapie antituberculeuse (à propos de 8 observations). Rhumatologie (Aix les Bains) 20:282–284
391. Jespersen K (1949) Cervical sympathetic block in periarthrosis of the shoulder joint with secondary reflex dystrophy. Ann Rheum Dis 8:220–222
392. Jochheim KA (1970) Die Sudecksche Atrophie. Med Welt 17:759–763
393. Johnson AW (1943) Disabling changes in the hand resembling sclerodactylia following myocardial infarction. Arch Intern Med 19:433–456
394. Johnson AW, Pannozzo AN (1966) Management of shoulder-hand syndrome. JAMA 195:108–110
395. Johnson JTH (1959) Frozen shoulder syndrom in patients with pulmonary tuberculosis. J Bone Joint Surg 41-A:877–882
396. Jung A (1937) Les mécanismes de la résorption osseuse. Rev Chir 75:473–511
397. Kahlmeter G (1930) A form of omarthritis accompanied by vasomotor disturbances in corresponding hand and anxiety neurosis. Rheumatologica (Amsterdam) 6:20–22
398. Kaiser H (1976) Medikamentöse ausgelöste Algodystrophien. Z Rheumatol [Suppl 4] 35:358–361
399. Kallabis M (1968) Zur Symptomatologie und Therapie des Sudecksyndroms. Med Klin 63:1227–1229

400. Kammerling E, Lewis GN, Ehrlich L (1950) Recurrent postinfarctional shoulder-hand syndrom: report of a case with unusual clinical evolution. New Eng J Med 242:701–702
401. Keane BE, Spiegler G, Davis R (1959) Quantitative evaluation of bone mineral by a radiographic method. Br J Radiol 32:162
402. Keller E (1939) Sudeckscher fleckförmiger Knochenbau nach Blitzschlagverletzung. Zentralblatt Chir 66:24–29
403. Kelly M (1953) Chronic rheumatic diarthritis and shoulder-hand syndrom. Med J Aust 1:330–334
404. Ketz E, Schliack M (1968) Zoster in C5–C6 mit Sudeckscher Krankheit. Nervenarzt 39:180–181
405. Key JA, Elzinga E, Fischer F (1934) Local atrophy of bone; effect of local heat, massage and therapeutic exercise. Arch Surg 28:943–947
406. Key JA, Fischer F, Elzinga E (1934) Local atrophy of bone: effect of immobilization and of operative procedures. Arch Surg 28:936–942
407. Kienböck R (1901) Über akute Knochenatrophie bei Entzündungsprocessen an den Extremitäten (fälschlich sogenante Inactivitätsatrophie des Knochens) und ihre Diagnose nach dem Röntgenbild. Wien Med Wochenschr 51:1346–1347, 1390–1392, 1427–1430, 1462–1466, 1507–1511, 1591–1596
408. Kienböck R (1904) Ein Fall von eigentümlicher wahrscheinlich trophoneurotischer Erkrankung der Hand nach Trauma. Wien Klin Wochenschr 17:262
409. Kim HJ, Kozin F, Johnson RP, Hines R (1979) Reflex sympathetic dystrophy syndrome of the knee following meniscectomy. Report of three cases. Arthritis Rheum 22:177–181
410. Kirsch K (1955) Das Sudecksche Syndrom als Fernwirkung gestörter Organ-funktion durch vermittlung des vegetativen Nervensystems. Z Orthop 86:95–112
411. Kirsch K (1978) Das Sudeck-Syndrom als Fernstörung (Klinik und Histologie). Z Orthop 116:199–203
412. Kissel P, Hartemann P, Royer R, Leclerc J (1965) Syndromes rhumatismaux après traitement de l'hyperthyroïdie. A propos d'une étude portant sur 76 hyperthyroïdiens. Ann Med Nancy 4:695–702
413. Kohler R (1968) A propos de l'étiologie de l'algoneurodystrophie du membre supérieur: deux observations d'algoneurodystrophie de cause exceptionnelle. Rev Rhum Mal Osteoartic 35:670–672
414. Kohlrausch W (1953) Sudecksches Syndrom und Bewegungstherapie. Arch Phys Ther (Leipzig) 7:16–22
415. Konings L (1951) Remarques sur la thérapeutique par les agents physiques de l'ostéoporose post-traumatique. Acta Chir Belg [Suppl] 1:478–482
416. Koschitz-Kosic H (1967) Zur Therapie der Sudeckschen Atrophie im akuten Stadium. Klin Med (Vienna) 22:79–81
417. Köstlin H (1956) Beziehung des Sudeck-Syndroms zu Unfall und Berufskrankheit. Arch Klin Chir 284:29–32
418. Koszla MM, Niemirska-Rebalska M (1967) Sudeck's syndrome in children (in Polish) Chir Narzadow Ruchu Orthop Pol 32:605–607
419. Kouka-Bemba D, Bouchot M, Froment J, Brichard JM, Pluvinage C (1977) Forme compliquée d'algodystrophie bilatérale de hanche au cours de la grossesse. Ann Med Nancy 16:173–177
420. Kozin F, Genant HK, Bekerman C, Mc Carty DJ (1976) The reflex sympathetic dystrophy syndrome. Roentgenographic and scintigraphic evidence of bilaterality and of periarticular accentuation. Am J Med 60:332–338
421. Kozin F, Haughton V, Ryan L (1971) The reflex sympathetic dystrophy in a child. J Pediatrics 90:417–419
422. Kozin F, Mc Carty DJ, Sims J, Genant HK (1976) The reflex sympathetic dystrophy syndrome. Clinical and histologic studies: evidence for bilaterality, response to corticosteroids and articular involvement. Am J Med 60:321–331
423. Kübler E (1952) Der Einfluss des Ultraschalls auf das Sudecksche Syndrom. Strahlentherapie 87:575–584
424. Kümmell H (1895) Ueber die traumatischen Erkrankungen der Wirbelsäule. Dtsch Med Wochenschr 21:180–181
425. Kümmell H (1921) Die posttraumatische Wirbelerkrankung (Kümmellsche Krankheit). Arch Klin Chir 118:878–901
426. Kümmell H (1928) Die posttraumatische Wirbelerkrankung, sogenante Kümmelsche. Monatschr Unfallheilkd Versicherung Versorg Verkehrsmed 35:67–76
427. Kunlin J, Bitry-Boely G (1957) Remarques sur l'ostéoporose douloureuse post-traumatique et son traitement. Acta Chir Belg [Suppl] 1:513–517
428. Kuntz D, Rain JD, Lemaire V, Sainte-Croix A, Ryckewaert A (1975) Intérêt diagnostic de la scintigraphie osseuse au pyrophosphate de technetium. Etude de 250 malades. Rev Rhum Mal Osteoartic 42:19–24
429. Kutzner J, Hahn K, Grimm W, Brod KH (1974) Skelettszintigraphische Untersuchungen bei der Sudeckschen Knochendystrophie. Fortschr Geb Roentgenstr 121:361–369
430. Kutzner J, Hahn K, Hulse (1975) Knochenszintigraphie mit 87m Strontium bei der Sudeckschen Knochendystrophie. Strahlentherapie 74:357–360
431. Kux P (1968) Beitrag zur Chirurgie des Schulter-Arm-Syndroms. Wien Med Wochenschr 118:809–811
432. Laborie G, Arramon JY (1976) La Griseofulvine en rhumatologie. Etude d'une nouvelle présentation. Bordeaux Med 9:897–906

433. Laborit H (1969) Neurophysiologie. Aspects métaboliques et pharmacologiques. Masson, Paris
434. Lachmann E (1955) Osteoporosis: potentialities and limitations of its roentgenologic diagnosis. Am J Roentgenol 74:712–715
435. Lacoste P, Roucoules B, Loiseau P (1975) Algoneurodystrophies post-traumatiques des membres supérieurs et syndrome de Babinski-Froment. Approche psychosomatique. Bordeaux Med 8:2365–2373
436. Lacroix P, Ponlot R (1956) Remarques sur l'histopathologie de l'ostéoporose post-traumatique. Acta Chir Belg [Suppl] 1:149–164
437. Lagier R (1972) L'approche anatomo-pathologique du concept d'arthrose. Rev Rhum Mal Osteoartic 39:545–557
438. Lagier R (1975) Anatomo-pathologie des arthroses post-traumatiques des membres inférieurs. Z Unfall med Bernfskr 1:3–21
439. Lagier R, Van Linthoudt D (1978) Dystrophie de Sudeck de l'arrière pied. Confrontation anatomo-radiologique. Ann Radiol (Paris) 21:539–544
440. Lagier R, Van Linthoudt D (1979) Articular changes due to disuse in Sudeck's atrophy. Int Orthop 3:1–8
441. Laine VA (1953) Incidence of reflex sympathetic dystrophy of the upper extremity, shoulder-hand syndrome. Ann Rheum Dis 12:315–316
442. Lance P (1944) Un cas d'ostéoporose post-traumatique guéri par les infiltrations stellaires. Rev Orthop 30:44–47
443. Landoff GA (1942) Experimentelle Untersuchungen über die „Knochenatrophie" infolge einer Immobilisation und einer akuten Arthritis. Acta Chir Scand [Suppl] 71:1–198
444. Landoff GA (1948) On the influence of the bone salts on the radiography of so-called acute atrophy of bone. Roentgen-experimental and histological examinations as well as a new alizarin staining technique. Acta Orthop Scand 17:270–300
445. Langeron P, Bayart M (1969) Algodystrophie reflexe et problèmes circulatoires distaux après section tendineuse. A propos de deux cas. J Sc Med Lille 87:449–454
446. Langloh ND, Hunder GG, Riggs BL, Kelly PJ (1973) Transient painful osteoporosis of the lower extremities. J Bone Joint Surg 55 A:1188–1196
447. Lantier R, Fortin J (1964) Atrophie de Sudeck. Union Med Canada 93:745–747
448. Larget M, Lamare JP, Gourdon R (1932) Ostéoporose post-traumatique. Sympathectomie périartérielle. Amélioration considérable. Bull Mem Soc Chir Paris 58:155–157
449. Latorzeff S, Arlet J, Gayrard M, Pujol M (1977) Pied douloureux décalcifié et ostéopathie raréfiante. In: Le pied inflammatoire. Les atteintes du pied au cours des rhumatismes inflammatoires. Maloine, Paris
450. Laurent C (1949) Les troubles reflexes consécutifs aux traumatismes des membres. Le syndrome physiopathologique de Babinski-Froment. Conception pathognomonique. MD dissertation, University of Lyon
451. Laval-Jeantet M, Tristant H, Chaumont P, Katz M (1972) Causes d'erreur en densitométrie osseuse. Possibilités et limites d'une méthode simplifiée. J Radiol Electrol Med Nucl 53:457–464
452. Laviec G (1974) Traitement des algodystrophies des membres. J Med Strasbourg 5:45–52
453. Layani F (1946) Les rhumatismes endocriniens. Rev Rhum Mal Osteoartic 13:300–312
454. Layani F (1948) Réflexions sur les rhumatismes endocriniens. Sem Hop Paris 24:608–612
455. Layani F, Durupt L, Paquet J (1959) L'ostéoporose zostérienne. Sem Hop Paris 35:1273–1281
456. Layani F, Poinsard G (1948) Ostéoporose zostérienne. Les troubles trophiques et les arthropathies du zona cervico-brachial. Rev Rhum Mal Osteoartic 2:56–59
457. Le Chevalier PL (1969) Le syndrôme épaule-main. Rev Med Tours 3:831–835
458. Lee DR (1973) A quasi-Sudeck's atrophy of the hip and knee in pregnancy. S Afr Med J 47:2191
459. Leech CB (1938) Painful shoulder in association with coronary artery disease. Rhode Is Med J 21:104–106
460. Leffman R (1947) Zur Problematik der traumatischen Reflexdystrophie der Extremitäten. Schweiz Med Wochenschr 77:451–455
461. Lefur S (1960) Les bilans calciques dans les décalcifications post-traumatiques. Presse Med 68: 1931–1932
462. Le Gallou Y (1978) Les algodystrophies. A propos de 86 observations Intérêt de la scintigraphie. MD dissertation, University of Lyon
463. Lejeune E (1966) Le traitement du rhumatisme neurotrophique du membre supérieur. Sem Hop Paris 42:1862–1864
464. Lejeune E, Bouvier M, Maitrepierre J, Siradj El Dine A (1966) Le pied décalcifié douloureux ou algodystrophie du pied; à propos d'une statistique personnelle de 40 observations. Rhumatologie (Aix les Bains) 18:377–393
465. Lelièvre J (1971) Pathologie du pied. Masson, Paris
466. Le Mouroux P (1977) Le rhumatisme gardénalique. Ouest Med 30:963–964
467. Lenart G (1975) Seltene posttraumatische Zustände des kindlichen Fußes. Beitr Orthop Traumatol 22:106–109
468. Lenègre J, Flament J (1946) Angine de poitrine et épaules douloureuses et raides. Paris Med 1:1–7
469. Lenggenhagger K (1971) Sudeck's osteodystrophy. It's pathogenosis, prophylaxis and therapy. Minn Med 54:967–972
470. Lequesne M (1967) L'algodystrophie d'origine

chimiothérapique. Pseudo-rhumatisme de l'isoniazide, de l'ethionamide, du phéno-barbital et de l'iode radio-actif. Sem Hop Paris 43:2581–2595

471. Lequesne M (1968) Etiologie et pathogénie des algodystrophies. Presse Med 76:953–954
472. Lequesne M (1968) L'algodystrophie décalcifiante de la hanche. Une série de dix cas. Rev Rhum Mal Osteoartic 35:183–195
473. Lequesne M (1968) L'algodystrophie de la hanche. Presse Med 76:973–976
474. Lequesne M (1968) Transient osteoporosis of the hip. A non-traumatic variety of Sudeck's atrophy. Ann Rheum Dis 27:463–471
475. Lequesne M (1969) L'algodystrophie iatrogène. Gazette Med Fr 76:5051–5064
476. Lequesne M (1970) Algodystrophie et diabète sucré. 12 observations personnelles. Rev Rhum Mal Osteoartic 37:237–244
477. Lequesne M, Auquier L (1968) Etiologie et pathogénie de la rétraction capsulaire de l'épaule (Rôle du système neuro-végétatif). Rev Prat 18:189–196
478. Lequesne M, Bard M, Becker JC (1979) La rétraction capsulaire de la hanche. In: L'actualité rhumatologique 1978. Expansion Scientifique, Paris
479. Lequesne M, Bensasson M (1976) Les algodystrophies décalcifiantes partielles. In: L'actualité rhumatologique 1975, Expansion Scientifique, Paris
480. Lequesne M, Cassan P (1976) La coxarthrose par contusion. Rev Rhum Mal Osteoartic 43:61–68
481. Lequesne M, Dang N, Bensasson M, Chimenes H, Mery C (1974) Le diabète, «nouvelle» cause prédisposante de capsulite de l'épaule et de syndrome épaule-main. In: Journées de diabétologie de l'Hôtel-Dieu. Flammarion, Paris
482. Lequesne M, Dang N, Bensasson M, Mery C (1977) Increased association of diabetes mellitus with capsulitis of the shoulder and shoulder-hand syndrome. Scand J Rheumatol 6:53–56
483. Lequesne M, Dreiser R (1976) Polycapsulite chez les cardiaques. A propos de 2 observations. Rev Rhum Mal Osteoartic 43:81–84
484. Lequesne M, Kerboull M, Bensasson M, Perez C, Dreiser R, Forest A (1977) Partial transient osteoporosis. Skeletal Radiology 2:1–9
485. Lequesne M, Mauger B (1979) L'algodystrophie décalcifiante de la hanche. Rhumatologie (Aix les Bains) 31:369–376
486. Lequesne M, Moghtader R (1966) L'algodystrophie de l'isoniazide et de l'éthionamide. Rev Rhum Mal Osteoartic 33:727–734
487. Lequesne M, Spartien O (to be published) L'algodystrophie dite décalcifiante infraradiographique. Rev Rhum Mal Osteoartic
488. Leriche R (1923) Déséquilibres vaso-moteurs post-traumatiques primitifs des extrémités. Lyon Chir 20:746–753
489. Leriche R (1923) Oedème dur aigu post-traumatique de la main avec impotence fonctionnelle complète. Transformation soudaine cinq heures après sympathectomie humérale. Lyon Chir 20:814–818
490. Leriche R (1924) Les réflexes d'axone et les traumatismes périphériques. Importance de leur connaissance et la chirurgie d'accident. Rev Chir 62:579–589
491. Leriche R (1926) Traitement par la sympathectomie périartérielle des ostéoporoses traumatiques. Bull Mem Soc Chir Paris 52:247–251
492. Leriche R (1927) Sur quelques maladies osseuses et articulaires d'origine vasomotrice et sur leur traitement. Bull Mem Soc Chir Paris 53: 1022
493. Leriche R (1928) De l'importance en pathologie et en thérapeutique des réactions vasomotrices post-traumatiques. Médecine (Paris) 9:341–342
494. Leriche R (1939) Physiologie et pathologie du tissu osseux. Masson, Paris
495. Leriche R (1939) The surgery of pain. Williams and Wilkins, Baltimore
496. Leriche R (1941) Traitement de l'ostéoporose algique post-traumatique. Presse Med 49:609
497. Leriche R (1952) De la nature des troubles trophiques. Importance vraisemblable de ces troubles dans la physiologie pathologique tissulaire. Presse Med 60:1375–1377
498. Leriche R, Fontaine R (1930) Des ostéoporoses douloureuses post-traumatiques. Presse Med 30:617–621
499. Leriche R, Fontaine R (1932) De la valeur thérapeutique des infiltrations périarticulaires à la novocaïne dans les entorses et arthrites traumatiques. Presse Med 32:280–282
500. Leriche R, Fontaine R (1935) Les séquelles trophiques et douloureuses des traumatismes de la main et des doigts. Rapport au VII Congrès International des Accidents et des Maladies du Travail, Bruxelles, vol II. pp 645–689
501. Leriche R, Jung A (1937) Retentissement de certains traumatismes ostéolysants sur les parathyroïdes. De l'existence d'un facteur parathyroïdien secondaire dans l'évolution de certaines ostéoporoses algiques post-traumatiques. Rev Chir 56:649–653
502. Leriche R, Policard J (1926) Les problèmes de la physiologie normale et pathologique de l'os. Masson, Paris
503. Les algoneurodystrophies décalcifiantes post-traumatiques (1973) I – Historique, nosographie, circonstances d'apparition, clinique. II – Anatomie et physiologie pathologiques des AND. Traitement préventif et curatif. Rhumatologie (Aix les Bains) 25:3–19
504. Levame JH (1967) Aspects pratiques du traitement et de la rééducation des algodystrophies de la main. Cahiers Reeduc Readapt Fonct 2:357–359
505. Levernieux J, Kerzreho F (1973) Les résultats obtenus en cure marine dans l'algodystrophie du

membre inférieur. Rhumatologie (Aix les Bains) 25:87–88

506. Levy P, Hinterbruckner C (1976) Transient or migratory osteoporosis of lower extremity. NY State J Med 76:739–742
507. Lichwitz A (1946) Les ostéoporoses aiguës; ostéoporose d'immobilisation ou ostéoporose d'alarme. Presse Med 54:654–655
508. Lièvre JA, Hubault A (1951) Ostéoporose rachidienne et pelvienne par électrocution. Rev Rhum Mal Osteoartic 18:609–611
509. Lin SR, Lee KF (1971) Relative value of some radiographic measurements of the hand in the diagnosis of acromegaly. Invest Radiol 6:126–131
510. Lippitt AG (1976) Post-traumatic patellitis. A case report. Bull Hosp Joint Dis 37:54–58
511. Little N (1939) Sudeck's atrophy. Med J Aust 26:263–265
512. Livingston WK (1938) Post-traumatic pain syndromes, interpretation of underlying pathological physiology. West J Surg Obstet Gynecol 46:341–426
513. Longstreth PL, Malinak LR (1972) Hydroxyproline and transient osteoporosis. Ann Intern Med 76:833
514. Longstreth PL, Malinak LR, Hill CS (1973) Transient osteoporosis of the hip in pregnancy. Surg Gynecol Obstet 41:563–569
515. Lord Jr JW (1970) Post-traumatic vascular disorders and upper extremity sympathectomy. Orthop Clin North Am 1:393–398
516. Lorente De No R (1938) Analysis of the activity of the chain of internuncial neurons. J Neurophysiology 1:207–244
517. Losada M, Zanartu J (1953) Sindrome hombromano. Rev Chir Esp 50:298–304
518. Louyot P, Gaucher A, Guyon G, Benoit P (1966) Les algodystrophies idiopathiques du genou. J Radiol Electrol Med Nucl 47:450–455
519. Louyot P, Gaucher A, Montet Y, Combebias JF (1967) Algodystrophie du membre inférieur. Rev Rhum Mal Osteoartic 34:733–737
520. Louyot P, Montet Y, Demonte S (1971) Importance de la localisation coxo-fémorale dans l'algodystrophie du membre inférieur. Ann Med Nancy 10:85–104
521. Louyot P, Montet Y, Pourel J, Demonte S (1970) La place de la hanche dans le syndrome d'algodystrophie du membre inférieur. J Agreges 3:249–259
522. Louyot P, Pourel J, Netter P, Duc ML, Schmidt C (1973) Etude hémodynamique et électrographique de l'algodystrophie. J Agreges 6:389–394
523. Louyot P, Rauber G, Baumgartner JC, Pourel J, Hannequin JR (1972) Les capsuloligamentites iatrogènes. Ann Med Nancy 11:13–37
524. Luccherini T (1956) Sindrome neurodistrofica del piede. Reumatismo 8:235–265
525. Lund M (1941) Dupuytren's contracture and epilepsy. The clinical connection between Dupuytren's contracture, fibroma plantae, periarthrosis humeri, sclerodermia, induration penis plastica and epilepsy with an attempt at a pathogenic valuation. Act Psychiatr Scand 16:465–492
526. Magee CP, Grosc JH (1974) Propanalon for causalgia. JAMA 228:826–827
527. Magiera J (1965) Das Sudeck-Syndrom. Arch Orthop Unfall Chir 58:88–97
528. Maignien L (1980) Les algodystrophies d'origine traumatique et la cure de Bourbonne les Bains. Personal communication
529. Maillard G, Renard G (1925) Un nouveau traitement de l'épilepsie la phénylmalonylurée (Rutonal). Presse Med 33:315–317
530. Maillard G, Thomazi P (1931) Douleurs provoquées par certains dérivés barbituriques au cours du traitement de l'épilepsie. Presse Med 39:851–852
531. Majd M (1979) Bone scintigraphy in children with obscure skeletal pain. Ann Radiol 22:85–95
532. Majello G (1970) Contributo clinico alla conoscenza della sindrome spalla-mano. Riforma Med 84:986–992
533. Mansat MM (1976) Algodystrophie réflexe (ADR) post-traumatique et syndromes canalaires du membre supérieur. Etude d'une artérioleptique: le Benfurodil. Bordeaux Med 9:1083–1094
534. Marche J, Chatard P (1967) Le pseudo-rhumatisme de la chimiothérapie antituberculeuse. Contribution à l'étude étiopathogénique du rhumatisme neurotrophique. Rev Rhum Mal Osteoartic 34: 11–33
535. Marchin P de (1955) Syndrôme épaule-main. Rev Med Liège 10:357–358
536. Margarot J, Rimbaud P, Izarn P, Bertrand A (1952) Séquelles trophiques avec ostéoporose d'un zona du membre supérieur. Montpellier Med 42:414–416
537. Marino A, Morosini C (1969) Aspetti etiopatogenetici, clinici e terapeutici della sindrome dolorosa spalla mano. Europa Mediocophys 5:51–53
538. Marti T (1954) Wesen und Behandlung des Sudeckschen Syndroms. Praxis 43:742–745
539. Martin JL, Sachs M, Corre X (1977–1978) Algodystrophie décalcifiante partielle de la hanche associée à un kyste intra-sacré. «R» 38:329–338
540. Mascher WL (1950) Über die Rolle des zentralen Nervensystems für die Entstehung des Sudeck-Syndroms. Nervenarzt 21:67–74
541. Matles AL (1971) Reflex sympathetic dystrophy, in a child. A case report. Bull Hosp Joint Dis 32:193–197
542. Mauger B (1979) L'algodystrophie décalcifiante de la hanche. Forme classique. Aspects nouveaux. A propos de 40 cas. Mémoire CES Rhumatologie, University of Paris
543. Maurer C (1978) Analyse minérale osseuse par densitométrie directe. Application de la méthode

à l'étude du vieillisement. MD dissertation, University of Strasbourg

544. Mauvoisin F, Bernard J (1954) Le syndrome épaule-main. Toulouse Med 55:597–604
545. Mauvoisin F, Bernard J (1955) A propos des algodystrophies reflexes. Rhumatologie (Aix les Bains) 7:19–24
546. Mauvoisin F, Bernard J (1961) Algodystrophies reflexes. In: EMC Appareil loco-moteur 14380 A 10. Editions Techniques, Paris
547. Mauvoisin F, Bernard J, Arnaudet M (1959) Les algodystrophies reflexes. Presse Therm Clin 96:175–179
548. May E (1931) Le rhumatisme chronique vasomoteur. Bull Mem Soc Med Hop Paris 47:646–649
549. May V, Aristoff H, Glowinski J (1973) Algodystrophie post-traumatique du membre supérieur. Rhumatologie (Aix les Bains) 25:35–39
550. May V, Aristoff H, Glowinski J, Geraro A, Dupaquier Y (1977) Les béta-bloquants dans le traitement des algo-neurodystrophies (à propos de 34 cas). Rev Rhum Mal Osteoartic 44:249–252
551. May V, Aristoff H, Glowinski J, Guillon G (1979) Treatment of the sympathetic reflex dystrophy (Abstr 437). IX European Congress of Rheumatology Wiesbaden
552. May V, Glowinski J (1979) Algoneurodystrophie: traitement par les bétabloquants. Nouv Presse Med 13:1095
553. Mazière B, Kuntz D, Coma D (1976) Variation de la concentration calcique de l'os en fonction de l'âge et du sexe étudiée par activation neutronique localisée «in vivo». Proceedings of the 1976 International Conference: Modern trends in activation analysis. Munich 1:229
554. McCord WC, Nies KM, Campion DS, Louie JS (1978) Regional migratory osteoporosis. A denervation disease. Arthritis Rheum 21:834–838
555. McKay NN, Woodhouse NJ, Clarke AK (1976) Post-traumatic reflex sympathetic dystrophy syndrome (Sudeck's atrophy): effects of regional guanethidine infusion and salmon calcitonin. Br Med J 6076:1575–1576
556. McKusick AB, Hsu JM (1961) Clinical and metabolic studies of the shoulder-hand syndrome in tuberculosis patients. Arthritis Rheum 4:426
557. McLean K, Stranks G (1950) Reflex dystrophy in upper extremity. Canad Med Assoc J 63:568–570
558. Meema HE, Schatz DL (1970) Simple radiologic demonstration of cortical bone loss in thyrotoxicosis. Radiology 97:9–15
559. Meissner F, Sieber E (1954) Stoffwechsel und pathologischanatomische Untersuchungen der Muskulatur beim Sudeckschen Syndrom. Arch Klin Chir 278:123–133
560. Melzack R (1975) Prolonged relief of pain by brief, intense transcutaneous somatic stimulation. Pain 1:357–373
561. Menke HE (1973) Reflex sympathetic dystrophy. Dermatologica 147:186–190
562. Merklen YG (1976) Concept du traitement physique et rééducatif en milieu thermal de l'algodystrophie des membres à l'établissement thermal de Niederbronn-les-Bains en fonction des données cliniques et étiopathogéniques. Interprétation statistique sur soixante cas. MD dissertation, University of Strasbourg
563. Methlin G, Moyses B, Grob JC, Dirheimer Y (1971) Algodystrophie du membre supérieur au cours des hyperthyroïdies et de leur traitement par l'iode radioactif. A propos de 24 cas. Rhumatologie (Aix les Bains) 23:185–188
564. Meunier P (1980) Personnal communication.
565. Meunier PJ, Courpron P, Edouard C, Alexandre C, Bressot C, Lips P, Boyce BF (1979) Bone histomorphometry in osteoporotic states. Osteoporosis 2:27–47
566. Meyer A (1960) Recherches sur l'infrastructure du tissu osseux à l'état normal et au cours de l'ostéoporose post-traumatique. MD dissertation, University of Strasbourg
567. Meyer-Laack H (1950) Über das Sudecksche Syndrom und seine Röntgentherapeutische Heilung. Strahlentherapie 82:231–246
568. Mikes K (1966) The treatment of Sudeck's dystrophy with neuroplegics (in Czech). Acta Chir Orthop Traumatol Cech 33:124–135
569. Miller D, Blaesel KF (1956) Cervical nerve root compression and shoulder-hand syndrome. Med J Aust 43:448–450
570. Miller DS, Takats de G (1941) Post-traumatic dystrophy of the extremities; Sudeck's atrophy. Surg Gynecol Obstet 75:558–581
571. Miller HI, Miller GF (1950) Posttraumatic reflex dystrophy. Am J Surg 79:814–818
572. Miller R (1965) Tanderil zur Behandlung des Sudeck-Syndroms. Med Welt 52:2931–2932
573. Minaire P (1973) L'ostéoporose d'immobilisation. Données biologiques et histologiques quantitatives. MD dissertation, University of Lyon
574. Minaire P, Meunier P, Edouard C, Bernard J, Coupron P (1974) Quantitative histological data on disuse osteoporosis: comparison with biological data. Calcif Tissue Res 17:57–73
575. Mitchell SW, Morehouse GR, Keen WW (1864) Gunshot wounds and other injuries of nerves. Lippincott, Philadelphia
576. Moberg E (1955) The shoulder-hand-finger syndrome as a whole. Acta Chir Scand 109:284–292
577. Monastero G (1951) Considerazioni sulla patogenesi e cura della cosidetta atrofia ossea di Sudeck. Minerva Orthop 2:242–248
578. Monnerot-Dumaine M (1951) Le syndrome épaule-main, clef de voûte des syndromes sympathi-

ques du membre supérieur. Rev Rhum Mal Osteoartic 18:581–588

579. Montgomery BM, King WW (1962) Hemiplegic migraine. A case with paroxysmal shoulder-hand syndrome. Ann Intern Med 57:450–455
580. Moojer D (1956) Diagnostik und Therapie des Schulter-Arm-Syndroms. Zentralblatt Chir 81: 2525–2528
581. Moreau R, Coste F, Lequesne M (1955) Syndrome épaule-main et péricardite aiguë primitive. Rev Rhum Mal Osteoartic 22:688–690
582. Moreau R, Rénier JC, Minier JF, Jallet P, Bernat M (1978) Explorations dynamiques à l'aide d'hématies marquées au 99m Tc dans les algodystrophies. Résultats préliminaires. J Fr Biophys Med Nucl 2:121–122
583. Morettin LB, Wilson M (1970) Severe reflex algodystrophy (Sudeck's atrophy) as a complication of myelography. Report of two cases. Am J Roentgenol 110:156–158
584. Morgensen EF (1953) Reflex vasodilatation-test in patients with periarthrosis humeroscapularis and the shoulder-hand syndrom. Acta Med Scand 145:1–14
585. Moriame G, Thiel A, Bast C de, Kugler I (1971) Algodystrophie sympathique symétrique des mains. Arch Belg Dermatol Syphiligr 27:309–312
586. Morsier G (1971) Les dystrophies réflexes et les lésions des nerfs consécutives aux traumatismes des membres. Arch Suisses Neurol Neurochir Psych 108:223–238
587. Moser H (1953) Über Pathophysiologie, Klinik und Therapie der Sudeckschen Krankheit. Arch Klin Chir 275:124–137
588. Mowat AG (1974) Treatment of the shoulder-hand syndrome with corticosteroids. Ann Rheum Dis 33:120–123
589. Muller AG (1955) Physiothérapie de la maladie traumatique. Rhumatologie (Aix les Bains) 7: 1–9
590. Müller P (1979) Neue Therapiemöglichkeiten bei Sudeckscher Dystrophie (Abstr. 438). IX European Congress of Rheumatology Wiesbaden 1979
591. Müller U (1952) Posttraumatische Dystrophie bei Kindern. Z Unfallmed Berufskr 45:252–255
592. Munford EB (1938) Roentgenotherapy in acute osteoporosis. New type of treatment. J Bone Joint Surg 20:949–959
593. Munzenberg KJ (1978) Therapie des Sudeck Syndroms mit Calcitonin. Dtsch Med Wochenschr 103:26–29
594. Navarro A (1952) El sindrome hombro-mano en las afecciones coronaris. Prensa Med Argent 39:421–428
595. Navratil J (1969) Reflex algodystrophic syndrome after tuberculostatic agents (in Czech). Fysiatr Reumatol Vestn 47:73–81
596. Navratil J (1972) Paraostéoarthropathies de la schizophrénie et rhumatisme neurotrophique des membres inférieurs. Rev Rhum Mal Osteoartic 39:469–471
597. Neviaser JS (1945) Adhesive capsulitis of the shoulder. J Bone Joint Surg 27:211–222
598. Nicole R (1944) Über die Ursache der Sudeckschen Atrophie bei Frakturen. Helv Med Acta 11:533–538
599. Nilsson BE (1966) Post-traumatic osteopenia: a quantitative study of bone mineral masse in the femur following fracture of the tibia in man using americium 241 as a photon source. Acta Orthop Scand 37 [Suppl 91]: 1–55
600. Nilsson BE, Westlin NE (1969) Osteoporosis following injury to the semilunar cartilage. Calcif Tissue Res 4:185–187
601. Noble TP, Hauser EDW (1926) Acute bone atrophy. Arch Surg 12:75–94
602. Noel G (1959) Les manifestations articulaires au cours des hyperthyroïdies. Entretiens de Bichat. Médecine:449–452
603. Nonne M (1901–1902) Über radiographisch nachweisbare akute und kronische „Knochenatrophie" (Sudeck) bei Nerven-Erkrankungen. Fortschr Geb Roentgenstr 5:293–297
604. Nordin BEC, Hodgkinson A, Peacock M (1967) The measurement and the meaning of urinary calcium. Clin Orthop 52:293–322
605. Nuraa A, Franz A (1952) La malattia di Sudeck. Minerva Orthop 3:217–226
606. O'Connor FM (1958) Reflex sympathetic dystrophy. Arch Dermatol 8:314–317
607. Oehlecker F (1942) Die Sudecksche Krankheit insbesondere nach Erfrierungen. Chirurg 14:422–428, 459–472
608. Oehlecker F (1948) Zu der Bezeichnung „Sudecksches Syndrom" oder kurz „Sudeck". Chirurg 19:398–403
609. Oehlecker F (1953) Beitrag zur Entstehung des Sudeckschen Syndroms durch versehentliche Strophantininjektion in die Arteria cubitalis. Med Klin 52:1673–1677
610. O'Mara RE, Pinal RS (1970) Bone scanning in regional migratory osteoporosis. Case report. Radiology 97:579–581
611. Ordonneau P (1961) Formes rhumatologiques des pasteurelloses. In: Aux Confins de la rhumatologie. Expansion, Paris
612. Osler W (1901) The principles and practice of medicine. 4th edit. Pentland, Edinburgh London
613. Ostapowicz G, Schulze HA (1952) Das Sudecksche Syndrom als Komplication einer Fremdkörperverletzung. Beit Klin Chir 194:300–309
614. Otte P (1964) Verkalkungs- und Entkalkungsprozesse im Schulterbereich. Z Orthop 98:405–419
615. Oury M, Rénier JC, Bregeon C (1969) Syndromes algodystrophiques au cours de la chimiothérapie antituberculeuse (à propos de 25 observations). Arch Med Ouest 1:121–135
616. Pak JJ, Martin GM, Magness JL, Kavanaugh

GJ (1970) Reflex sympathetic dystrophy. Review of 140 cases. Minn Med 53:507–512
617. Pantazopoulos T, Exarchou E, Hartofilakidis-Garafalidis G (1973) Idiopathic transient osteoporosis of the hip. J Bone Joint Surg 55A:315–321
618. Papier MJ, Papier MJ (1976) Sudeck's atrophy. A case report. J Am Podiatry Assoc 66:327–331
619. Parade GW, Bockel P (1955) Zur Pathogenese und Differentialdiagnose des Schulter-Hand Syndroms; das kardiale und zervikovertebrale Irritationssyndrom. Dtsch Med Wochenschr 80:1417–1420
620. Pasquali F, San Martino A (1957) La photopléthysmographie dans l'ostéoporose post-traumatique. Acta Chir Belg [Suppl] 1:283–287
621. Patel M (1943) Ostéoporose post-traumatique du carpe. Lyon Chir 38:472–473
622. Patman RD, Thompson JE, Perrson AV (1973) Management of post-traumatic pain syndromes. Report of 113 cases. Ann Surg 177:780–787
623. Pena Arrebola A (1977) Las algiodistrofias simpatico reflejas de los miembros inferiores. Rev Esp Reumat Enferm Osteoartic 20:247–276
624. Pender JW (1959) Basic concepts about shoulder-arm syndrome. JAMA 169:795–797
625. Perisson (1925) Troubles sympathiques dans l'hémiplégie. MD dissertation, University of Paris
626. Perrigot M, Veaux V (1978) Les algodystrophies: aspects, cliniques physiologiques et traitement. Rev Med (Paris) 19:2459–2464
627. Piguet B (1964) Diathèse fibroplastique de Jansen (polyfibromatose de Touraine et Ruel) et épilepsie essentielle. Rev Rhum Mal Osteoartic 31:290–296
628. Pinals RS, Jabbs M (1972) Type IV hyperlipoproteinemia and transient osteoporosis. Lancet 2 783:929
629. Plewes LW (1956) Sudeck's atrophy in the hand. J Bone Joint Surg 38B:195–203
630. Pohl W, Hinz G (1976) Reflexdystrophische Pseudoarthritis oder Sudeck-Syndrom. Kritische Betrachtungen zur Differentialdiagnose, Ätiologie und Pathogenese. Z Orthop 114:38–44
631. Pojer J, Ninger E (1954) On atypical cases of the shoulder-hand syndrome following myocardial infarction. Cardiologia 24:215–224
632. Polakova Z (1965) Prevention of reflex bone dystrophy in Colles' fracture (in Czech). Acta Chir Orthop Traumatol Cech 32:356–358
633. Pollosson, Arnulf (1936) Syndrome physiopathique post-traumatique de l'épaule. Guérison par anesthésie à la novocaïne du ganglion stellaire. Lyon Chir 33:357–359
634. Portias LH (1975) Les algoneurodystrophies réflexes des membres supérieurs. Etude basée sur l'observation de 106 cas. Sem Hop Paris 51:2687–2695
635. Portias LH (1977) Les algo-neuro-dystrophies réflexes des membres inférieurs. Résultats d'une étude basée sur l'observation de 78 cas (de 1969 à 1975). Sem Hop Paris 53:133–138
636. Poznanski AK (1974) The hand in radiologic diagnosis. Saunders Philadelphia London Toronto
637. Prats-Estève M, Vidal-Lopez F, Puigdomenec M, Arisa L, Puigtoro EM (1976) La télé-thermographie dans le contrôle du blocage sympathique du membre supérieur. Mediterr Med 4:17–18
638. Prévôt R, Horst W (1952) Über arthritische und rheumatoide Erscheinungen bei radiojodid behandelten (I 131) Thyreotoxicosen. Strahlentherapie 88:253–260
639. Prewitt G (1955) Symposium on pain in the neck, shoulder, and arm. The role of sympathetic influence. Portland Clin Bull 8:111–120
640. Prinzmetal M, Massuni RA (1955) The anterior chestwall syndrom. JAMA 159:177–184
641. Queloz J, Papayannopoulos E, Candardjis F (1970) Ostéodystrophie (de Sudeck) de l'astragale après fracture du tubercule externe. J Radiol Electrol Med Nucl 51:763–766
642. Queneau P, Maitrepierre J, Bocquet B, Lami M (1956) La massokinésitherapie en rhumatologie: les algodystrophies réflexes. Cah Med Lyon 8:260–264
643. Rain JD, Kuntz D, Najean Y (1973) Importants progrès en scintigraphie osseuse grâce à l'emploi du pyrophosphate de technetium. Nouv Presse Med 2:186
644. Rampon S, Bussiere SL, Prin P, Sauvezie B, Leroy V, Missioux D, Docy J, Suss P, Jourde H, Lapalus F (1974) A propos de 250 observations de scintigraphie osseuse par le pyrophosphate d'étain marqué au technetium 99m. Rev Rhum Mal Osteoartic 41:745–751
645. Ravault PP (1951) Le rhumatisme neurotrophique du membre supérieur. Rev Rhum Mal Osteoartic 18:74–82
646. Ravault PP, Bouvier M (1966) Les algodystrophies. Rev Prat 16:2529–2545
647. Ravault PP, Durant J (1956) Atteinte des hanches au cours des rhumatismes neurotrophiques des membres supérieurs. Rhumatologie (Aix les Bains) 8:260–264
648. Ravault PP, Durant J (1961) Le rhumatisme neurotrophique du membre supérieur. Rev Lyon Med 10:3–32
649. Ravault PP, Guinet P, Berthier L, Emery J, Carrier F (1974) Rhumatismes chroniques de la main et rhumatisme neurotrophique du membre supérieur. J Med Lyon 28:363–374
650. Ravault PP, Guinet P, Carrier P (1945–1946) Une cause d'erreur dans le diagnostic des polyarthrites: le rhumatisme neurotrophique du membre supérieur. Arch Rhum 6:129–134
651. Ravault PP, Lejeune E, Noel G, Franchet G (1963) Périarthrites scapulo-humérales et rhumatismes neurotrophiques du membre supérieur au

cours de l'hyperthyroïdie. Rev Rhum Mal Osteoartic 30:257–262
652. Ravault PP, Maitrepierre J, Riffat G (1959) Le pied décalcifié douloureux idiopathique (ou ostéoporose algique essentielle du pied) Rev Rhum Mal Osteoartic 26:393–407
653. Ravault PP, Thiers H, Berthier L (1949) Rhumatismes chroniques et arthropathies pseudorhumatismales au cours de maladies du système nerveux. Rev Rhum Mal Osteoartic 16:1–13
654. Ravault PP, Vignon G, Ponsonnet G (1955) La périarthrite scapulo-humérale d'origine thoracique et pleuro-pulmonaire. Rev Rhum Mal Osteoartic 22:421–428
655. Reboul M, Faye C, Reboul D, Firouzabadi R (1975) Deux observations de la sympathectomie chimique par les béta-bloquants dans les algodystrophies reflexes des membres. Phlébologie 28:317–322
656. Reboul M, Faye CL, Reboul P, Firouzabadi H (1975) Les algodystrophies réflexes des membres. Sympathectomie chimique par les béta-bloquants. Nouv Presse Med 4:1049
657. Reboul H, Vergoz L (1971) Les lésions et contractures artérielles dans les retards de consolidation, les pseudarthroses et les ostéoporoses post-traumatiques. Phlebologie 1:65–67
658. Recordier AM, Mouren P, Serratrice G (1961) Les ostéo-arthropathies nerveuses. Expansion, Paris
659. Recordier AM, Serratrice G, Eisinger JB, Valente P, Ragnoni R (1967) Modifications de l'hydroxyprolinurie après thérapeutique à effet vasculaire (à propos de 25 observations). Rhumatologie (Aix les Bains) 19:223–225
660. Reichle R (1956) Das Sudeck-Syndrom. Arch Klin Chir 284:18–29
661. Reinhardt K (1974) Die diabetische Arthropathie. Saarland Aertztebl 27:302–306
662. Reinstein H (1956) Das hypersensitive Halbseitensyndrom als Grundlage der Angina Pectoris und des Schulterarmsyndroms. Arch Phys Ther (Leipzig) 8:375–382
663. Remé H (1940) Über das Wesen des akuten Knochenumbaus (Sudecksche Knochenatrophie) und seine Beziehung zu den trophischen Störungen der Gliedmassen. Med Klin 36:827–829
664. Remé H (1940) Verlaufsformen des akuten Knochenumbaues. Dtsch Z Chir 253:76–89
665. Remé H (1943) Experimentelle Studien über den Knochenumbau aus verschiedenen Ursachen. Dtsch Z Chir 257:115–183
666. Remé H (1956) Das Sudeck Syndrome. Arch Klin Chir 284:32–39
667. Remé H (1965) Therapie der Sudeckschen Dystrophie. Intern Praxis 5:459–464
668. Remé H (1978) Sudeck Syndrom. Med Klin 73:1527–1533
669. Rénier JC (1958) Les algodystrophies du membre inférieur et leur traitement. Rev Prat 8:3835–3844
670. Rénier JC (1973) Les algodystrophies (notions générales). Arch Med Ouest 5:95–106
671. Rénier JC, Bernat M, Moreau R, Morer T (1979) Dynamic isotopic studies in algodystrophy. (Transient osteoporosis) (Abstr. 435) IX European Congress of Rheumatology, Wiesbaden
672. Rénier JC, Bregeon CH, Boasson M, Billabert C (1973) Algodystrophie du membre inférieur. Etude de 65 observations. Arch Med Ouest 5:107–118
673. Rénier JC, Cheguillaume J (1966) Une observation associant des paraostéoarthropathies et un rhumatisme neurotrophique chez une malade opérée d'un glioblastome cérébral. Rev Rhum Mal Osteoartic 33:478–481
674. Rénier JC, Moreau R, Bernat M, Basle M, Jallet P, Minier JF (1979) Apport des explorations isotopiques dynamiques dans l'étude des algodystrophies. Rev Rhum Mal Osteoartic 46:235–241
675. Rénier JC, Oury M, Bregeon C, Tuchais E (1969) Les algodystrophies de la chimiothérapie antituberculeuse. Etude de 24 observations. Rev Rhum Mal Osteoartic 36:605–607
676. Rénier JC, Tonon J, Wellinger C, Simard C, Mazabraud A (1968) Deux observations d'algodystrophie de la hanche avec biopsie synoviale. Rev Rhum Mal Osteoartic 35:258–262
677. Reynolds WA, Karo JJ (1972) Radiologic diagnosis of metabolic bone disease. Orthop Clin North Am 3:521–543
678. Richardson AT (1954) Shoulder-hand syndrom following herpes zoster. Am Phys Med 2:132–134
679. Rickles JA (1977) Ambulatory use of sympathetic nerve blocks: present day clinical indications. Angiology 28:394–402
680. Rieder W (1936) Die akute Knochenatrophie. Dtsch Z Chir 248:269–331
681. Rieder W (1944) Das Sudecksche Syndrom. Zentralbl Chir 71:906–908
682. Riera MT (1964) Contribution à l'étude clinique des algoneurodystrophies des membres inférieurs. MD dissertation, University of Tours
683. Riffat G (1972) Algodystrophie réflexe du pied. Cah Med Lyon 48:1625–1627
684. Riffat G, Berard E, Jacquot F (1973) Algodystrophie réflexe du pied. Rhumatologie (Aix les Bains) 25:61–65
685. Riffat G, Odelin M (1977) Les algodystrophies des membres inférieurs et leur traitement. Lyon Med 237:37–41
686. Rigaud M (1968) Les algodystrophies réflexes (membre supérieur et membre inférieur): traitement médical et kinésithérapique. Cahiers Kinesither 7:383–392
687. Rivelon G (1977) L'algoneurodystrophie de la hanche. MD dissertation, University of Nancy

688. Robecchi A (1955) Le syndrome spalla-mano. Reumatismo 7:153–179
689. Roczniok B, Bresler M, Dwornicki J, Rogala E (1976) Etiology of algodystrophies (in Polish). Pol Tyg Lek 31:1851–1852
690. Rodeck G, Mussgnug G (1955) Über Schweißsekretionsstörungen beim Sudeckschen Syndrom. Arch Klin Chir 280:96–104
691. Rohner A (1958) Contribution à l'étude histopathologique de la dystrophie de Sudeck. Ann Anat Pathol (Paris) 3:477–511
692. Rolandi-Ricci V, Peris G, Gatto E (1957) Contributo alla conoscenza della syndrome spalla-mano associata ad infarto del miocardio. Arch E Maragliano Patol Clin 13:693–701
693. Rose F (1908) Névrite sensitive et trophique à la suite d'un zona. Lésion trophique des os de la main à type de rhumatisme chronique. Rev Neurol (Paris) 16:90–91
694. Rose TF (1953) Sudeck's post-traumatic osteodystrophy of limbs. Med J Aust 1:185–188
695. Rosen PS, Graham W (1957) The shoulder-hand syndrome: historical review with observations on seventy-three patients. Can Mass J 77:86–91
696. Rosen RA (1970) Transitory demineralization of the femoral head. Radiology 94:509–512
697. Rosenthall L, Kaye M (1975) Technetium 99m pyrophosphate kinetics and imaging metabolic bone disease. J Nucl Med 16:33–39
698. Roucayrol JC, Fonroget J, Ghozlan R, Lejeune A (1976) Explorations isotopiques au cours des algoneurodystrophies des membres inférieurs chez l'adulte. In: Rencontre de médecine nucléaire du Val-de-Marne, CHU Henri-Mondor
699. Rougemont de, M (1933) Ostéoporose post-traumatique du pied guérie par sympathectomie périfémorale. Lyon Chir 30:465–467
700. Rouquier A (1941) Les contractures sympathiques réflexes post-traumatiques des membres. Presse Med 49:999–1001
701. Rousseau C (1962) Considérations médico-légales sur les algo-dystrophies réflexes. Cahiers Reeduc Readapt Fonct 2:359–363
702. Rubens-Duval A, Duparc J, Kaplan G, Lubetzki D, Heuleu JN (1973) Les séquelles des syndromes algodystrophiques post-traumatiques. Rhumatologie (Aix les Bains) 25:41–42
703. Rubin LM (1968) Acute post-traumatic bone atrophy (Sudeck's atrophy). J Am Podiatry Assoc 58:266–267
704. Ruffié R, Fournié A, Ayrolles C (1970) La hanche neurotrophique isolée et primitive. Rev CHU Toulouse 12:33–36
705. Russeck HI (1958) Shoulder-hand syndrome following myocardial infarction. Med Clin North Am 42:1554–1566
706. Russeck HI, Russeck AS, Doerner AA, Zohman BI (1953) Cortisone in treatment of shoulder-hand syndrome following acute myocardial infarction. Arch Intern Med 91:487–493
707. Rutishauser E (1947) Ostéopathies post-traumatiques. Brux Med 27:516–521
708. Rutishauser E, Vernet A, Mazabraud A (1956) Etude histopathologique de l'ostéoporose posttraumatique. Acta Chir Belg [Suppl] 1:123–148
709. Sabetta F, Giachi LM (1970) Le osteoartropatie neurogene (aspetti radiografici). Chir Organi Mov 59:29–56
710. Salomon A (1963) Le pied décalcifié douloureux. Entretiens de Bichat Medecine (Paris) 327–330
711. Samuel J (1970) Principes généraux du traitement masso-kinésithérapique des syndromes algoneurodystrophiques. J Kinesitherapie 180:9–12
712. Sany J, Fraissine B, Serre H, Collet H, Suquet P (1976) Scintigraphie osseuse au cours des algodystrophies reflexes des membres. In: Rencontres de médecine nucléaire du Val de Marne, CHU Henri-Mondor
713. Sany J, Serre H (1976) Les algodystrophies réflexes des membres. Aspects cliniques et therapeutiques. Sem Hop Paris 52:503–506
714. Sarkozi A, Bartosiewicz G (1979) Pathogenesis of Sudeck's syndrom and a new possibility for its treatment (in Hungarian). Magy Traumatol Orthop 22:95–103
715. Saudan Y, Chavannes F, Schelling JL (1971) Algoneurodystrophies du traitement aux barbituriques. Un cas particulier de pseudo-rhumatisme médicamenteux. Praxis 60:1330–1333
716. Savin R (1974) La responsabilité de la rééducation fontionelle dans le déclenchement des algodystrophies réflexes posttraumatiques des membres. Mémoire CES Rhumatologie, University of Paris
717. Scarfi G, Sassi N (1974) L'algoporosi transitoria dell'anca. Arch Putti Chir Organi Mov 61:627–635
718. Schabitz J, Teichmann W, Rikirsch P (1971) Zur Frage der Koinzidenz von Herzinfarkt und Schulter Hand Symptomatik. Dtsch Gesundheitswes 26:1726–1728
719. Scheibe G (1956) Über die Kontralateralen Sudeck nach Frakturen. Arch Klin Chir 284:57–61
720. Scheibe G (1957) Der kontrolaterale Sudeck nach Frakturen. Zschr Aerztl Fortbild (Jena) 51:378–381
721. Scheibe G (1957) Die Kapillarschädigung bei der Sudeckschen Krankheit. Arch Klin Chir 283:693–707
722. Scheibe G (1966) Behandlung des Sudeck-Syndroms mit Reparil. Landarzt 42:439–443
723. Scheibe G (1969) Oszillographische Untersuchungen bei Sudeck-Syndrom. Chirurg 40:227–232
724. Scheibe G, Karitzky B (1954) Das funktionelle Hautkapillarbild bei der Sudeckschen Krankheit. Chirurg 25:202–206
725. Scheinberg MA, Aristides RS, Svartman C (1978)

Transient regional osteoporosis of the hip treated with Calcitonin. J Rheumatol 5 (2):236–238
726. Schiano A (1974) Les algodystrophies. Données actuelles: acquisitions thérapeutiques récentes. A propos de 103 cas. MD dissertation, University of Marseille
727. Schiano A, Eisinger J, Acquaviva PC (1976) Les algodystrophies. Laboratoire Armour-Montagu, Paris
728. Schilling F (1973) Reflexdystrophien und dystrophische Pseudoarthritiden der unteren Extremitäten. Z Rheumaforsch 32:375–385
729. Schlomka G, Optz H (1955) Zur Pathogenese des Sudeckschen Syndroms. Chirurg 26:55–57
730. Schmitt HW (1977) Erfahrungen mit Piracetam bei therapieresistenten Schulter-Arm-Syndrom. Fortschr Dtsch Med 95:2578–2580
731. Schönbach G (1956) Ätiologische Betrachtungen zur Sudeckschen Dystrophie auf Grund klinischer und experimenteller Untersuchungen. Arch Klin Chir 284:53–55
732. Schönbach G, Volkmann D (1969) Zur Behandlung der posttraumatischen Schwellungszustände und des Sudeck-Syndroms. Chirurg 40:232–235
733. Schrodi L (1980) Traitement de l'algodystrophie par l'acupuncture. Personnal communication
734. Schrötter G (1953) Das Sudecksche Syndrom als berufsbedingte Erkrankung. Z Inn Med 8: 69–72
735. Secretan H (1903) Oedème dur traumatique. Rev Med Suisse Romande 23:240–245
736. Segre GV (1927) L'atrofia ossea di Sudeck. Ann Ital Chir 6:555–575
737. Semb H (1966) Experimental disuse osteoporosis. Oxygen saturation and oxygentension in intermedullary blood from immobilized rabbit tibial bones. Acta Soc Med Ups 71:96–107
738. Semm K (1954) Sudeck und Tuberkulose im Lichte der Unfallbegutachtung. Arch Klin Chir 279:173–177
739. Serratrice G (1967) Les algodystrophies dans leur cadre général. Cahiers Reeduc Readapt Fonct 2:337–341
740. Serratrice G, Lapousse JC, Gastaut JL, Baret J (1971) Algodystrophie au cours de deux cas de syndrome de Guillain-Barré, dont un récidivant. Marseille Med 108:603–604
741. Serratrice G, Schiano A (1977) Manifestations ostéo-articulaires chez les parkinsoniens. Rhumatologie (Paris) 29:349–351
742. Serre H (1961) Algodystrophie réflexe du membre supérieur, premier signe d'un syndrome de Brown-Séquard par métastase médullaire. Montpellier Med 104:42
743. Serre H, Claustre J, Simon L (1977) L'algodystrophie réflexe du pied. In: Le pied inflammatoire. Maloine, Paris
744. Serre H, Simon L (1959) Le syndrome épaule-main du zona cervicobrachial. Montpellier Med 56:232–237
745. Serre H, Simon L (1961) Syndrome épaule-main d'origine coronarienne. Sem Med Prof Med Soc 37:464–466
746. Serre H, Simon L, Barjon MC (1962) L'action thérapeutique de la Griséofulvine en rhumatologie. Rev. Rhum Mal Osteoartic 29:9–19
747. Serre H, Simon L, Barjon C, Claustre J (1968) Algodystrophie extensive du pied au rachis. Rev Rhum Mal Osteoartic 35:120–124
748. Serre H, Simon L, Caillens JP (1962) Périarthrite scapulo-humérale et syndrome épaule-main au cours de la tuberculose pulmonaire. Rev Rhum Mal Osteoartic 29:165–172
749. Serre H, Simon L, Claustre J (1967) Algodystrophie réflexe du pied (A propos de 45 observations). Rev Rhum Mal Osteoartic 34:722–732
750. Serre H, Simon L, Claustre J (1968) Algodystrophie réflexe du pied. Ann Med Phys 11:3–5
751. Serre H, Simon L, Claustre J (1969) Aspects radiographiques des algodystrophies réflexes du pied. J Radiol Electrol Med Nucl 50:547–548
752. Serre H, Simon L, Claustre J (1973) La réadaptation du pied algodystrophique. Rhumatologie (Aix les Bains) 23:81–84
753. Serre H, Simon L, Claustre J, Blotman F (1974) Le rôle de l'algodystrophie réflexe dans l'évolution des ostéopathies raréfiantes vertébrales (Incidences thérapeutiques). Rev Rhum Mal Osteoartic 41:319–324
754. Serre H, Simon L, Claustre J, Sany J (1973) Formes cliniques des algodystrophies sympathiques des membres inférieurs. Rhumatologie (Aix les Bains) 23:43–54
755. Serre H, Simon L, Sany J, Morlock G (1976) Phénobarbital et algodystrophies. Rev Mediterr Sci Med Fr 1:735–743
756. Serre H, Sucquet P, Sany P, Simon L (1973) Hyperfixation au strontium 85 au cours des syndromes algodystrophiques 8:358–362
757. Sèze S de, Auquier L, Françon J (1955) Une nouvelle observation de pasteurellose osteo-articulaire. Contribution à l'étude de névrites ascendantes et des algodystrophies dites réflexes du membre supérieur. Rev Rhum Mal Osteoartic 22:690–692
758. Sèze S de, Rénier JC, Caro H (1960) Les algodystrophies du genou. Rev Rhum Mal Osteoartic 27:9–19
759. Sèze S de, Ryckewaert A (1951) Algodystrophies sympathiques du membre supérieur. In: Maladies des os et des articulation. Flammarion, Paris
760. Sèze S de, Ryckewaert A, Welfling J, Caroit M, Hubault A (1964) Epaule pseudo-paralysée, épaule douloureuse, épaule bloquée. Presse Med 72:1795–1799
761. Sibilly A (1957) Contribution à l'étude de l'ostéo-

porose posttraumatique. MD dissertation, University of Strasbourg
762. Sicard JA (1921) Parkinsonisme et rhumatisme chronique. Rev Neurol (Paris) 37:682–683
763. Sieber E, Meissner F (1954) Stoffwechsel- und pathologisch-anatomische Untersuchungen der Muskulatur beim Sudeckschen Syndrom. Arch Klin Chir 278:123–133
764. Siegel BA, Donavan RL, Alderson RO, Hack GR (1976) Skeletal uptake of 99m Tc diphosphonates in relation to local bone blood flow. Radiology 120:121–123
765. Simon A (1975) Algodystrophie rachidienne. Personnal communication
766. Simon A (1977) Le syndrôme de Kümmell-Verneuil. Personnal communication
767. Simpson BS (1937) Unusual case of post-traumatic decalcification of bones of foot. J Bone Joint Surg 19:223–227
768. Simson G (1974) Propranolol for causalgia and Sudeck's atrophy. JAMA 227:327
769. Singer FR, Keutmann MT, Neer RM, Potts JT, Krane SM (1972) Pharmacological effects of salmon calcitonin in man. In: Talmager V, Munson PL. Calcium Parathyroid hormon and the calcitonin. Excerpta Medica Amsterdam
770. Sitaj S, Kleinova R, Trnarsky K (1957) Les algodystrophies réflexes au cours des hyperthyroïdies traitées par l'Alkiron. Bratisl Lek Listy 37:659–667
771. Solal C (1965) Périarthrite scapulo-humérale et algodystrophie réflexe du membre supérieur au cours de l'hyperthyroïdie. Rhumatologie (Aix les Bains) 17:329–331
772. Soulié P, Tricot R, Degeorge SM (1950) Le syndrome épaule-main et les affections coronariennes. Sem Hop Paris 26:4141–4151
773. Steinberg LB (1964) Sudeck's disease. A case report. J Am Podiatry Assoc 54:34–35
774. Steinbrocker O (1947) Painful homolateral disability of shoulder and hand with swelling and atrophy of hand. Ann Rheum Dis 6:80–84
775. Steinbrocker O (1947) The shoulder-hand syndrome: associated painful homolateral disability of shoulder and hand with swelling and atrophy of hand. Am J Med 3:402–407
776. Steinbrocker O (1968) The shoulder-hand syndrome: present perspective. Arch Phys Med Rehabil 49:388–395
777. Steinbrocker O, Argyros TG (1958) The shoulder-hand syndrome: present status as a diagnostic and therapeutic entity. Med Clin North Am 42:1533–1553
778. Steinbrocker O, Neustadt D, Bosch S (1955) Painful shoulder syndromes. Their diagnosis and treatment. Med Clin North Am 39:563–564
779. Steinbrocker O, Neustadt D, Lapin L (1953) Shoulder-hand syndrome. Sympathetic block compared with corticotropin and cortisone therapy. JAMA 153:788–792
780. Steinbrocker O, Spitzer N, Friedman HH (1948) Shoulder-hand syndrome in reflex dystrophy of the upper extremity. Ann Intern Med 29:22–52
781. Stenger E, Guse U (1950) Sudecksches Syndrom und Bindegewebmassage. Aerztl Wochenschr 5:573–577
782. Stern WG (1936) Acute transverse bone atrophy. J Bone Joint Surg 18:656–666
783. Stoia I, Stoia H (1961) Reflexalgodystrophien der Gliedmassen vom klinischen und therapeutischen Standpunkt. Z Rheumaforsch 20:283–289
784. Stolle H (1955) Die Bedeutung des Sympathicus bei der Sudeckschen Dystrophie. Monatsschr Unfallheilkd Versicher Versorg Verkehrsmed 58:65–83
785. Stoyanon PC (1963) Hinderungsfaktoren für das Auftreten des sogenannten Schulter-Hand-Syndroms nach einem Infarkt des Myokards. Med Klin 58:1799–1800
786. Strashun A, Chaues Z (1979) Migratory osteolysis. J Nucl Med 20:129–132
787. Strauss J (1974) Les algodystrophies de la hanche. Presse Therm Clim 11:75–78
788. Streda A, Hajkova Z (1976) Transient demineralization of hip-bone (in Czech). Cesk Radiol 30:30–31
789. Sturm G (1965) Das Schulter-Arm-Syndrom. Arch Orthop Unfall-Chir 58:98–101
790. Suchomel J, Beran J (1973) Transient osteoporosis of the hip joint (in Czech) Fysiatr Reumatol Vestn 51:140–143
791. Sudeck P (1899–1900) Zur Altersatrophie (einschl. Coxa vara senium) und Inaktivitätsatrophie der Knochen. Fortschr Geb Roentgenstr 3:201–205
792. Sudeck P (1900) Über die akute entzündliche Knochenatrophie. Arch Klin Chir 62:147–156
793. Sudeck P (1901–1902) Über die akute (reflektorische) Knochenatrophie nach Entzündungen und Verletzungen an den Extremitäten und ihre klinischen Erscheinungen. Fortschr Geb Roentgenstr 5:277–293
794. Sudeck P (1931) Die trophische Extremitätenstörung durch periphere (infectiöse und traumatische) Reize. Dtsch Z Chir 234:596–612
795. Sudeck P (1938) Die kollateralen Entzündungreaktionen an den Glied-massen (sog. akute Knochenatrophie). Arch Klin Chir 191:710–753
796. Sudeck P (1942) Die sogenannte akute Knochenatrophie als Entzündungsvorgang. Chirurg 14:449–458
797. Sudeck P (1943) Kollaterale Heilentzündung-dystrophie. Atrophie der Gliedmassen. Fortschr Geb Roentgenstr 68:1–15
798. Sussman N (1952) The use of cortisone in the management of the shoulder-hand syndrom. A case report. Arch Med Phys 33:289–290

799. Swan DM (1954) Shoulder-hand syndrome following hemiplegia. Neurology 4:480–482
800. Swan DM, Mac Gowan JM (1951) Shoulder-hand syndrome following myocardial infarction: treatment by Procaine block of stellate ganglion. JAMA 146:774–777
801. Swezey RL (1970) Transient osteoporosis of the hip, foot and knee. Arthritis Rheum 13:858–868
802. Takats G de (1937) Reflex dystrophy of extremities. Arch Surg 34:939–956
803. Takats G de (1965) Sympathic reflex dystrophy. Med Clin North Am 49:117–129
804. Takats G de, Miller DS (1943) Post-traumatic dystrophy of the extremities; chronic vasodilator mechanism. Arch Surg 46:469–479
805. Tavernier J (1936) Ostéoporose douloureuse post-traumatique grave guérie après deux infiltrations à la novocaïne du sympathique lombaire. Lyon Chir 33:450–452
806. Temesvari M, Temesvari P, Vischer T, Fallet GH (1976) L'algodystrophie décalcifiante isolée de la hanche. Schweiz Med Wochenschr 106:699–703
807. Terlizzi N, Scagliusi P, D'Amore M, Carrozzo M (1974) Sindrome algoneurodistrofica dell'arto superiore in tre soggetti di giovane eta. Reumatismo 26:129–131
808. Terrasse J, Rampon S, Gras H, Janny P, Plagne J, Bertrix E (1959) Algodystrophie réflexe des membres. Rev Rhum Mal Osteoartic 26:168–196
809. Thomas A, Amyot R (1929) Zona du membre supérieur. Oedème. Lésions ostéo-articulaires. Troubles trophiques. Troubles sympathiques. Rev Neurol (Paris) 2:65–70
810. Thomas P (1957) La maladie de Kümmell-Verneuil existe-t-elle? MD dissertation. University of Bordeaux
811. Thompson M (1961) Shoulder-hand syndrome. Proc Roy Soc Med 54:679–681
812. Thorban W (1962) Klinische und experimentelle Untersuchungen zur Ätiologie und Pathogenese der posttraumatischen Sudeckschen Gliedmassendystrophie. Acta Neuroveg 25:1–62
813. Thorban W (1966) Zusammenhang zwischen Sudeck-syndrom und Pleuritis. Landarzt 42:838–839
814. Thurel J (1939) Les ostéo-arthropathies d'origine cérébrale. Rev Rhum Mal Osteoartic 6:95–106
815. Tilden RL, Jackson J, Enneking WF, Deland FH, Mc Vey JT (1979) 99m Tc polyphosphate histological localization in human femur by autoradiography. J Nucl Med 14:576–578
816. Titze A (1956) Das Sudecksche Syndrom. Wien Med Wochenschr 106:647–649
817. Tixier, Froment R, Arnulf G (1936) Contracture physiopathique post-traumatique des fléchisseurs de l'avant-bras guérie par anesthésie à la novocaïne du ganglion stellaire. Lyon Chir 33:350–352
818. Torrente ML (1970) La hanche neurotrophique isolée et primitive. MD dissertation, University of Toulouse
819. Tracy GD (1972) Prolonged disability after compensable injury. Med J Aust 2:1305–1307
820. Trueta J (1956) Etude physiopathologique et expérimentale du mécanisme vasculaire de l'ostéoporose. Acta Chir Belg [Suppl] 1:165–172
821. Tschirdewahn B (1978) Rheumatische Krankheiten nach Herzinfarkt. Med Klin 73:431–434
822. Tuchais E, Bregeon C, Oury M (1969) Les syndromes algodystrophiques de la chimiothérapie anti-tuberculeuse. A propos de 25 observations. Rev Tuberc Pneumol 33:781–792
823. Tuefferd JP (1933) Contribution à l'étude des ostéoporoses post-traumatiques. MD dissertation, University of Strasbourg
824. Uebermuth H (1956) Untersuchungen über die alkalische Serumphosphatase bei Sudeck-Syndrom. Arch Klin Chir 284:39–42
825. Vaernet K (1952) Two cases of shoulder-hand syndrome in meningioma affecting the premotor region. Acta Psychiatr Neurol Scand 27:201–209
826. Vague J, Codaccioni JL (1957) Manifestations rhumatismales évoluant en marge de l'hyperthyroïdie. A propos de 5 observations de périarthrite scapulo-humérale. Ann Endocrinol (Paris) 18:737–744
827. Valenzuela F, Aris H, Jacobelli S (1977) Transient osteoporosis of the hip. J Rheumatol 4:59–64
828. Valverde C (1976) Hypocalcémie aigüe à la Calcitonine de porc et de saumon. MD dissertation, University of Toulouse
829. Van Bogaert A, Tombeur A (1940) Arthropathie scapulaire et angine de poitrine. Cardiologia 4:121–164
830. Van De Korst JK, Colenbrander H, Cats A (1966) Phenobarbital and the shoulder hand syndrom. Ann Rheum Dis 25:553–555
831. Van Doornick R, Geeter L de (1956) Considérations cliniques et étude statistique sur l'ostéoporose post-traumatique chez l'adulte jeune. Acta Chir Belg [Suppl] 1:441–455
832. Vayssairat M, Fiessinger JN, Housset E (1980) Action de la thyrocalcitonine sur le phénomène de Raynaud. Ann Med Nancy 19:205–206
833. Verhaeghe A (1967) Le pied décalcifié. Cahiers Reeduc Readapt Fonct 2:343–349
834. Verhaeghe A, Lebeurre R (1961) Pied décalcifié douloureux idiopathique. A propos d'un cas bilatéral. Lille Med 6:409–412
835. Verneuil, Forestier (1892) Fracture de la colonne vertébrale par cause musculaire, longtemps méconnue et révélée par l'apparition de douleurs névralgiques en ceinture et d'une gibbosité tardive. Bull Acad Nat Med Paris 28:496–506
836. Vetter G (1973) Observations psychologiques dans les dystrophies réflexes. Rhumatologie (Aix les Bains) 25:25–26
837. Vialleton C (1922) L'ostéoporose localisée à dis-

tance dans les lésions traumatiques et inflammatoires des os. MD dissertation, University of Montpellier
838. Vieten H (1956) Möglichkeiten der Strahlentherapie bei Sudeckschem Syndrom. Arch Klin Chir 284:69–74
839. Vignon E, Chapuy M, Courpron P, Colcombet P, Meunier P (1973) Effets chimiques et biologiques de la calcitonine synthétique de saumon dans les algodystrophies des membres. Lyon Med 237:291–296
840. Villiaumey J, Rotterdam M, Avouac B, Lamotte J (1979) Polymyalgia rheumatica et algodystrophie réflexe des membres. (Abstr. 823) IX European Congress of Rheumatology Wiesbaden
841. Vinceneux P, Stevens-Dudragne D, Peckels B, Caplan G (1979) Algodystrophie décalcifiante de la hanche au cours de la grossesse (à propos de 3 cas). Sem Hop Paris 55:1701–1704
842. Vincent G, Cousin J, Oudar H (1962) Un cas de rhumatisme neurotrophique de la hanche. J Sc Med Lille 80:88–92
843. Vincent G, Rogier M, Tellier L, Devienne JM, Stock D (1974) Les syndromes algodystrophiques. J Sc Med Lille 92:207–214
844. Virtana P, Mähönen H (1960) Thickness of the cortical layer as an estimate of mineral content of human finger bones. Br J Radiol 33:60–62
845. Vitiugov IA, Kotenko VU (1977) Sudeck syndrome. A general medical problem (in Russian). Ortop Travmatol Protez 11:86–93
846. Vogl A (1968) Sudecksches Syndrom und Dupuytrensche Kontraktur. Zentralbl Chir 93:498–505
847. Vollmer E (1979) Etude de la minéralisation osseuse par densitométrie directe chez l'hyperthyroïdien. MD dissertation, University of Strasbourg
848. Voloir P (1970) Les algodystrophies post-traumatiques. Bull Mem Soc Chir Paris 60:293–299
849. Vose GP (1969) Estimation of changes in bone calcium content by radiographic densitometry. Radiology 93:841–844
850. Vulpian AEF (1886) Maladies du système nerveux. Doin, Paris
851. Wagner W (1960) Das Sudeck Syndrom. Mandrich, Wien
852. Wagner W (1966) Zur Therapie des Morbus Sudeck. Ther Ggw 105:557–564
853. Welfling J (1963) Périarthrite de l'épaule et affections cardio-vasculaires. Coeur Med Intern 2:431–436
854. Welfling J (1970) Périarthrite scapulo-humérale. In: EMC Appareil locomoteur 14350 A 10. Editions Techniques, Paris
855. Weil MP, Gérard-Marchant PJ (1954) Du danger des immobilisations plâtrées prolongées intempestives. Rev Rhum Mal Osteoartic 21:684–685
856. Weissenbach R (1964) Problèmes diagnostiques du syndrome épaule-main. Vie Med 45:847–856
857. Weissenbach R (1964) Traitement du syndrome épaule-main. Vie Med 45:1021–1026
858. Weissenbach R, Perles L, Françon F (1950) Syndrome épaule main de Steinbrocker avec atteinte du coude. Rev Rhum Mal Osteoartic 17:568–569
859. Wertheimer P, Guillemin P (1941–1942) Ostéoporose douloureuse post-traumatique. Lyon Chir 37:34–36
860. White JC (1974) Neurosurgical treatment of pain in neuralgias of non-malignant etiology. In: Treatment of chronic pain. Davis, Philadelphia
861. Wilde A (1915) Akute Knochenatrophie nach Unfall. Med Klin 11:569
862. Willenegger H, Bircher J (1971) Die Sudecksche Dystrophie des Fusses. Z Unfallmed Berufskr 64:109–112
863. Williams WR (1977) Reflex sympathetic dystrophy. Rheumatol Rehabil 16:119–124
864. Winter S (1954) Sympathetic reflex dystrophies in coronary heart disease. NY State J Med 54:2330–2332
865. Wondrak E (1975) Unser heutiger Standpunkt zur Sudeckschen Dystrophie. Beitr Orthop Traumatol 22:187–190
866. Wright V (1979) Le syndrome épaule-main. Eular Bulletin 8:51–52
867. Wulf A de (1953) Atrophie osseuse de Sudeck et tuberculose. Acta Orthop Belg 19:112–117
868. Wulf A de (1957) Ostéoporoses posttraumatiques. Acta Chir Belg [Suppl] 1:488–489
869. Wulf A de (1957) Remarques sur l'aspect radiologique de l'ostéoporose. Acta Chir Belg [Suppl] 1:216–217
870. Young JH, Pearson AT (1952) The shoulder-hand syndrome. Med J Aus 1:776–780
871. Zarafonetis CJD, Kalas JP (1960) Serotonin degradation by ceruloplasmin and its inhibition by isoniazid and iproniazid. Am J Med Sci 239:203–206
872. Zavodskaya IS (1970) Rôle du système sympathique et des catécholamines dans le développement des processus dystrophiques neurogènes. Actual Pharmacol (Paris) 23:163–174
873. Zedlitz C von (1966) Verkürzung der Behandlungsdauer und Arbeitsunfähigkeit bei Sudeckscher Dystrophie durch Geschlechtshormone. Muench Med Wochenschr 108:209–212
874. Zehnter H (1954) Behandlung der posttraumatischen Knochendystrophie. Dtsch Med Wochenschr 79:1788–1798
875. Ziegler G, Ballester G, Paecht A, Commandre F, Euller L (1979) Béta-bloquants et algodystrophies sympathiques posttraumatiques (à propos de 47 cas). Rhumatologie (Aix les Bains) 31:83–87
876. Ziegler R, Delling G (1972) Effect of Calcitonin on the regeneration of a circumscribed bone defect. Acta Endocrinol (Copenh) 69:497–706

Subject Index

GPSR Compliance
The European Union's (EU) General Product Safety Regulation (GPSR) is a set of rules that requires consumer products to be safe and our obligations to ensure this.

If you have any concerns about our products, you can contact us on

ProductSafety@springernature.com

In case Publisher is established outside the EU, the EU authorized representative is:

Springer Nature Customer Service Center GmbH
Europaplatz 3
69115 Heidelberg, Germany

www.ingramcontent.com/pod-product-compliance
Lightning Source LLC
Chambersburg PA
CBHW061212240926
51846CB00006B/1204
* 9 7 8 3 6 4 2 6 7 9 9 1 9 *